Current Clinical Pathology

Antonio Giordano, MD, PhD

Series Editor

Director, Sbarro Institute for Cancer Research
and Molecular Medicine and Center for Biotechnology
Temple University
Philadelphia, PA, USA

For further volumes:
http://www.springer.com/series/7632

Cristina Basso • Marialuisa Valente
Gaetano Thiene
Editors

Cardiac Tumor Pathology

Humana Press

Editors
Cristina Basso
Pathological Anatomy
Department of Cardiac
Thoracic and Vascular Sciences
Padova, Italy

Marialuisa Valente
Pathological Anatomy
Department of Cardiac
Thoracic and Vascular Sciences
Padova, Italy

Gaetano Thiene
Pathological Anatomy
Department of Cardiac
Thoracic and Vascular Sciences
Padova, Italy

ISBN 978-1-4939-5925-9 ISBN 978-1-62703-143-1 (eBook)
DOI 10.1007/978-1-62703-143-1
Springer New York Heidelberg Dordrecht London

Softcover re-print of the Hardcover 1st edition 2013

Printed on acid-free paper

Humana Press is a brand of Springer
Springer is part of Springer Science+Business Media (www.springer.com)

To the memory of Ivan Mahaim, a visionary in the diagnosis and treatment of cardiac tumors

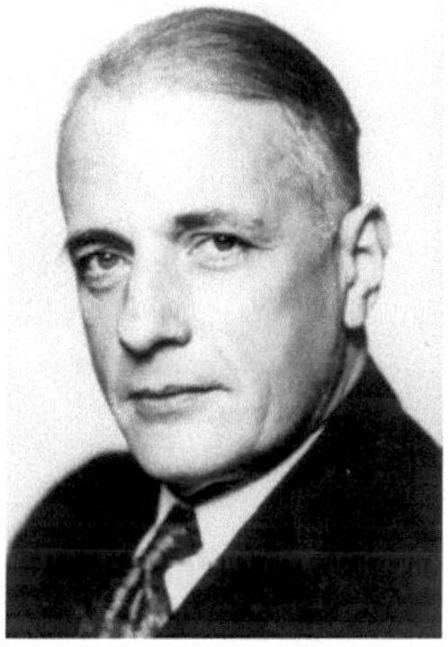

Preface

Cardiac tumors were once considered a nosographic entity of scanty interest because of their rarity, the intrinsic diagnostic difficulty and the therapeutic impossibility. They were mostly fatal or incidental findings at postmortem. Nowadays they have become a topical subject because of the great advances in clinical imaging (echocardiography, magnetic resonance, and computed tomography) and surgical treatment and are a spectacular example of innovation in technology for in vivo diagnosis and therapy.

The present monograph goes over these advances with clinicopathologic correlations. About 90% of primary cardiac tumors are benign and the simple surgical removal is curative forever. Another proof as cardio-pulmonary bypass with cardiac arrest and open-heart surgery was a revolutionary step forward in cardiovascular medicine.

The book covers history, epidemiology, demographics, clinical diagnosis, imaging, surgery, pathology, and basic sciences aspects of both benign and malignant cardiac neoplasms, either primary or secondary. Chemotherapy and radiotherapy of malignant neoplasms is as well as cardiotoxicity are also addressed.

The book is directed to all the researchers and physicians involved in the field of cardiac oncology, from cardiologists to cardiac surgeons, from radiologists to pathologists. In this regard, it must be said that cardiac surgery opened the era of surgical pathology also in the field of cardiac diseases.

As far as cardiac tumors, although tissue characterization with imaging is tempting, histology and immunohistochemistry remain irreplaceable life-saving steps for diagnosis. The presence of an expert cardiovascular pathologist is fundamental in the clinical team dealing with cardiac tumors. This is the reason why pathologists should be interested in reading and consulting the book which however, at difference from previous authoritative books and atlas, include robust clinical and imaging information, with several chapters written by clinicians and surgeons, which represent its peculiarity.

Padua, Italy

Cristina Basso M.D., Ph.D.
Marialuisa Valente M.D.
Gaetano Thiene M.D.

Acknowledgments

The Editors are supported in their research by the Registry of Cardio-cerebro-vascular Pathology, Veneto Region, Venice, Italy.

They also acknowledge Mrs. Chiara Carturan and Mr. Marco Pizzigolotto for their editorial and graphical assistance in preparing this book.

Contents

Contributors

Luigi P. Badano, M.D. Cardiology, Department of Cardiac, Thoracic and Vascular Sciences, Azienda Ospedaliera-University of Padua Medical School, Padua, Italy

Giovanni Bartoloni, M.D. Histopathology Department, "GB Ingrassia" Catania University, Garibaldi-Catania, Catania, Italy

Cristina Basso, M.D., Ph.D. Pathological Anatomy, Department of Cardiac, Thoracic and Vascular Sciences, Azienda Ospedaliera-University of Padua Medical School, Padua, Italy

Tomaso Bottio, M.D., Ph.D. Cardiac Surgery, Department of Cardiac, Thoracic and Vascular Sciences, Azienda Ospedaliera-University of Padua Medical School, Padua, Italy

Rossana Bussani, M.D. Department of Pathologic Anatomy, University of Trieste Medical School, Trieste, Italy

Antonino De Paoli, M.D. Department of Radiation Oncology, Centro di Riferimento Oncologico (CRO), National Cancer Institute, Aviano (PN), Italy

Giuseppe Faggian, M.D. Cardiac Surgery, University of Verona Medical School, Verona, Italy

Gino Gerosa, M.D. Cardiac Surgery, Department of Cardiac, Thoracic and Vascular Sciences, Azienda Ospedaliera-University of Padua Medical School, Padua, Italy

Sabino Iliceto, M.D. Cardiology, Department of Cardiac, Thoracic and Vascular Sciences, University of Padua Medical School, Padua, Italy

Ornella Leone, M.D. Department of Pathology, S. Orsola-Malpighi Hospital, Bologna, Italy

Chiara Lestuzzi, M.D. Department of Cardiology, Centro di Riferimento Oncologico (CRO), National Cancer Institute, Aviano (PN), Italy

Massimo Lombardi, M.D. Cardiovascular MR Unit, Fondazione C.N.R./ Regione Toscana "G. Monasterio", Pisa, Italy

Alessandro Mazzucco, M.D. Cardiac Surgery, University of Verona Medical School, Verona, Italy

Ornella Milanesi, M.D. Pediatric Cardiology, Department of Pediatrics, Azienda Ospedaliera-University of Padua Medical School, Padua, Italy

Gianmaria Miolo, M.D. Department of Medical Oncology, Centro di Riferimento Oncologico (CRO), National Cancer Institute, Aviano (PN), Italy

Denisa Muraru, M.D. Cardiology, Department of Cardiac, Thoracic and Vascular Sciences, University of Padua Medical School, Padua, Italy

Augusto Orlandi, M.D. Department of Biomedicine and Prevention, Institute of Anatomic Pathology, Tor Vergata University, Rome, Italy

Massimo A. Padalino, M.D., Ph.D. Pediatric Cardiac Surgery, Department of Cardiac, Thoracic and Vascular Surgery, Azienda Ospedaliera-University of Padua Medical School, Padua, Italy

Francesco Pizzuto, M.D. Department of Internal Medicine, Section of Cardiology, Tor Vergata University, Rome, Italy

Angela Pucci, M.D. Histopathology Department, Azienda Ospedaliera-Pisa University Hospital, Pisa, Italy

Stefania Rizzo, M.D. Pathological Anatomy, Department of Cardiac, Thoracic and Vascular Sciences, Azienda Ospedaliera-University of Padua Medical School, Padua, Italy

Francesco Santini, M.D. Cardiac Surgery, University of Verona Medical School, Verona, Italy

Furio Silvestri, M.D. Department of Pathologic Anatomy, University of Trieste Medical School, Cattinara Hospital, Trieste, Italy

Gianfranco Sinagra, M.D. Cardiovascular Department, University of Trieste Medical School, Cattinara Hospital, Trieste, Italy

Luigi Giusto Spagnoli, M.D. Department of Biomedicine and Prevention, Institute of Anatomic Pathology, Tor Vergata University, Rome, Italy

Giovanni Stellin, M.D. Pediatric Cardiac Surgery, Department of Cardiac, Thoracic and Vascular Sciences, Azienda Ospedaliera-University of Padua Medical School, Padua, Italy

Mariassunta Telesca, M.D. Cardiac Surgery, University of Verona Medical School, Verona, Italy

Gaetano Thiene, M.D. Pathological Anatomy, Department of Cardiac, Thoracic and Vascular Sciences, Azienda Ospedaliera-University of Padua Medical School, Padua, Italy

Marialuisa Valente, M.D. Pathological Anatomy, Department of Cardiac, Thoracic and Vascular Sciences, Azienda Ospedaliera-University of Padua Medical School, Padua, Italy

Paolo Voci, M.D. Department of Internal Medicine, Section of Cardiology, Tor Vergata University, Rome, Italy

Cardiac Tumors: From Autoptic Observations to Surgical Pathology in the Era of Advanced Cardiac Imaging

1

Gaetano Thiene, Marialuisa Valente, and Cristina Basso

In the popular mind, the term "tumor" recalls the concept of "cancer," i.e., a highly aggressive biological process eventually leading to body consumption due to malignant infiltration and metastasis.

This is not the case at the heart level, since malignant primary cardiac tumors are rare (about 10% of all primary cardiac tumors). Malignancy is hemodynamic rather than biological, due to obstruction of the blood circulation because of intracavitary growth and embolism of neoplastic fragments with potentially devasting ischemic damage to several organs.

Before the advent of cardiac imaging and of open heart surgery, cardiac neoplasms were not diagnosed in vivo and were mostly fatal due to complications along their natural history and, as such, diagnosed by the pathologist only at postmortem.

Noteworthy, the first description of cardiac tumors was made by Matteo Realdo Colombo in 1559 in his book *De Re Anatomica* [1]. While performing the autopsy of the body of Cardinal Gambaro from Brescia, since he was the archiater in Rome at that time, he discovered a left ventricular mass described as follows in Latin "*In Cardinali Gambara Brixiano tumorem praedurum, et ad ovi magnitudinem in sinistro cordis ventricolo Romae vidi, ubi illum in affinium gratiam dissecarem*" ("*in Rome I saw a solid tumour, large like an egg, in the left ventricle of Cardinal Gambaro of whom I was committed by the Pope to make autopsy*") (Fig. 1.1). Most likely it was a post-infarction endocavitary apical mural thrombus rather than a true neoplasm.

In the famous article entitled *Tumors of the heart: review of the subject and report of one hundred and fifty cases*, dated 1951 [2], Richard Prichard wrote "*…the most common cardiac tumour (cardiac myxoma) has never been diagnosed antemortem…*". Noteworthy, in the Mayo Clinic experience published in 1980, 23% of surgically resected cardiac myxomas were referred to surgery on the basis of auscultatory signs and symptoms suggestive of rheumatic mitral valve stenosis [3].

The first book on cardiac tumors was published by Ivan Mahaim in 1945 (Fig. 1.2) with the title *Les tumeurs et les polypes du coeur: etude anatomo-clinique* [4].

At the Institute of Pathological Anatomy of the peaceful Lausanne, spared by the second world war due to the neutral position of Switzerland, the young cardiac pathologist Mahaim wrote an extraordinary book, that was a collection of personal observations at postmortem as well as of

G. Thiene, M.D. (✉) • M. Valente, M.D.
• C. Basso, M.D., Ph.D.
Pathological Anatomy, Department of Cardiac, Thoracic and Vascular Sciences,
Azienda Ospedaliera-University of Padua
Medical School, via A. Gabelli, 61, Padua 35121, Italy
e-mail: gaetano.thiene@unipd.it

C. Basso et al. (eds.), *Cardiac Tumor Pathology*, Current Clinical Pathology,
DOI 10.1007/978-1-62703-143-1_1, © Springer Science+Business Media New York 2013

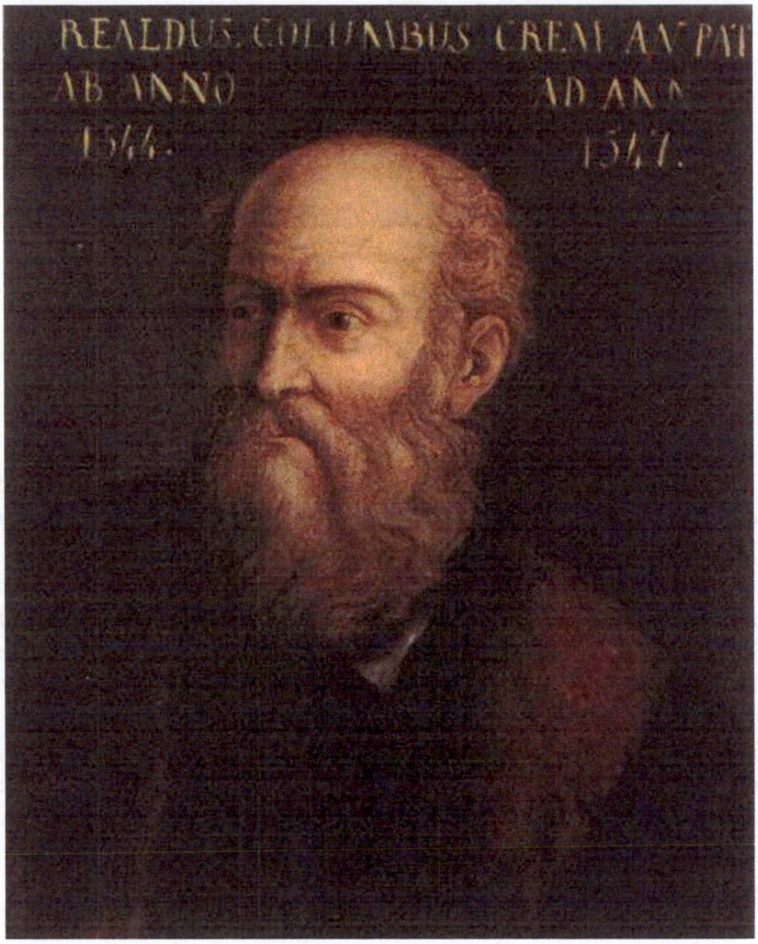

Fig. 1.1 Portrait of Realdo Colombo, Faculty of Medicine Hall, -University of Padua. Reprinted with permission of the Italian Society of Cardiology

literature review, and represented a milestone publication on the topic of cardiac tumors for several generations of pathologists and physicians involved in the field. From him we learned that cardiac myxoma (called in French "*le polype*" due to its resemblance to a pedunculated gastro-enteric polyp), can have a clinical presentation with syncope or dyspnea due to atrio-ventricular valve orifice occlusion (functional mitral stenosis), with peripheral artery occlusion due to embolic phenomena, or can be totally asymptomatic being an incidental finding ("*les polypes silencieux*"). Although these were all autopsy cases, Mahaim was optimist on the perspectives of Medicine. While treating atrial myxoma ("*Le polype du coeur*"), the most frequent cardiac tumor (nearly two-thirds of primary heart neoplasms), he said "*…surgical resection of atrial polyp encounters apparently unsurmountable difficulties. However, we should not give up because of this feeling. In any field of science, with technological progress, the impossible is just a moment during the evolution of our powers. As Mummery said about alpinism, the inaccessible peak becomes an easy route for ladies…*" [4].

On the contrary, in 1951 Prichard manifested a pessimistic attitude by saying "*…of the surgical treatment of these tumours we never heard*" [2]. Surprisingly, in the same year 1951 Goldberg et al. [5] for the first time successfully made a

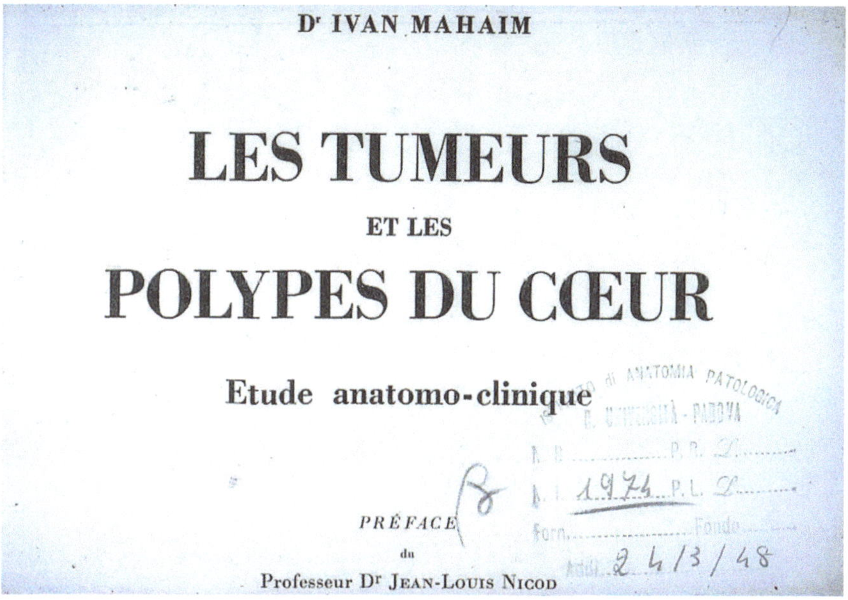
Dr IVAN MAHAIM

LES TUMEURS

ET LES

POLYPES DU CŒUR

Etude anatomo-clinique

PRÉFACE

du

Professeur Dr JEAN-LOUIS NICOD

Fig. 1.2 Title page of the book by Ivan Mahaim on cardiac tumors, published in 1945. Reprinted with permission of the Italian Society of Cardiology

clinical diagnosis of left atrial myxoma using angiography and in 1954 Crafoord resected a myxoma using extracorporeal circulation [6].

Thus, the era of "surgical pathology" started with clinical diagnosis mostly based upon angiography (Fig. 1.3) and the pathologist on call to establish in vivo the nature and histotype of the neoplasm, as in any other field of oncology.

However, the historical watershed in the diagnosis and treatment came in the 1980s, with the advent of non-invasive imaging, i.e., echocardiography (Fig. 1.4) which, together with computed tomography and cardiac magnetic resonance (MRI), substantially improved diagnosis and subsequent treatment. It is possible to easily visualize cardiac tumors at the first onset of symptoms or even incidentally, during routine diagnostic procedures, and send the patient promptly to the surgeon for resection with a nearly 100% success in the benign forms. Before the 1980s cardiac myxomas were a postmortem finding, thereafter they became almost exclusively a clinical and surgical observation.

The role of the pathologists is now to establish the nature of the resected mass (non-neoplastic, benign, or malignant neoplasms) and, last but not least, to make the differential diagnosis with secondary neoplasms. The advent of immunohistochemistry to characterize the antigenic markers, by using monoclonal and polyclonal antibodies, leads to major advances in the diagnosis of primary and secondary cardiac tumors as in other fields of oncology, but particularly of malignant primary sarcomas, where the tumor cell of origin can be the endothelial cell, fibroblast, cardiomyocyte, smooth muscle cell, adipocyte, etc. [7].

We report some anecdotal cases collected along the last 35 years at our center in Padua, which are emblematic of the historical evolution in the field of cardiac oncology.

In 1976 a 61-year-old man died during angiographic examination performed due

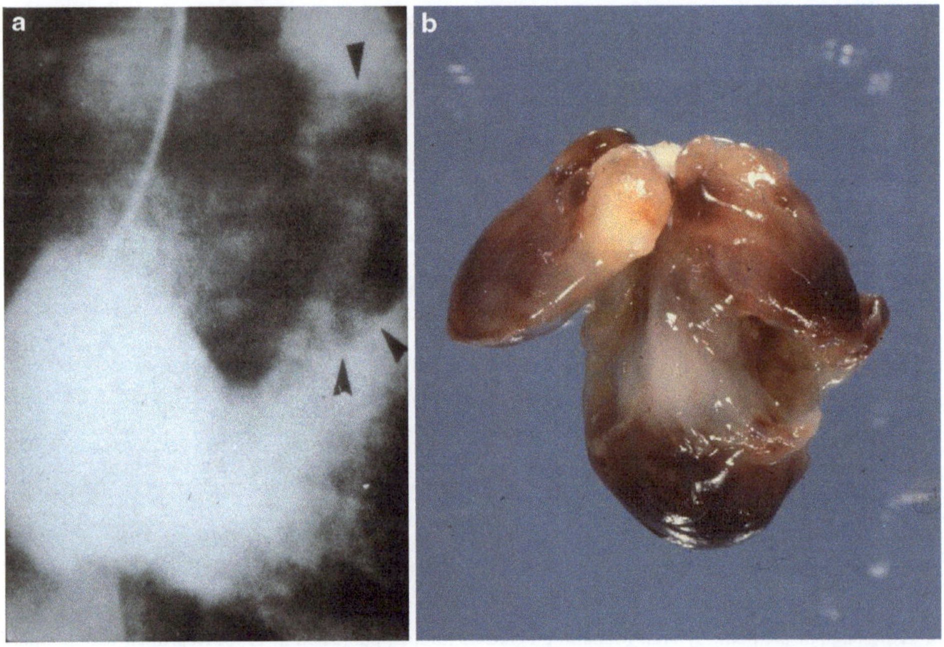

Fig. 1.3 Angiographic diagnosis of right ventricular myxoma in a 21-year-old male (from Bortolotti et al. [20] modified). Reprinted with permission of the Italian Society of Cardiology. (**a**) Angiographic image showing a contrast medium defect at the level of the right outflow tract. (**b**) At surgery, a bi-lobated myxoma was found

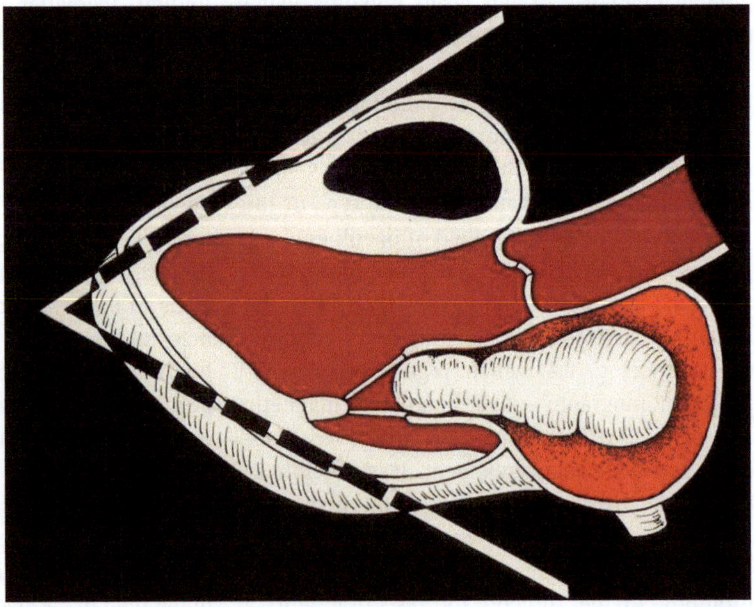

Fig. 1.4 Diagram illustrating a left atrial myxoma as viewed in the long-axis *parasternal* view by two-dimensional echocardiography. Reprinted with permission of the Italian Society of Cardiology

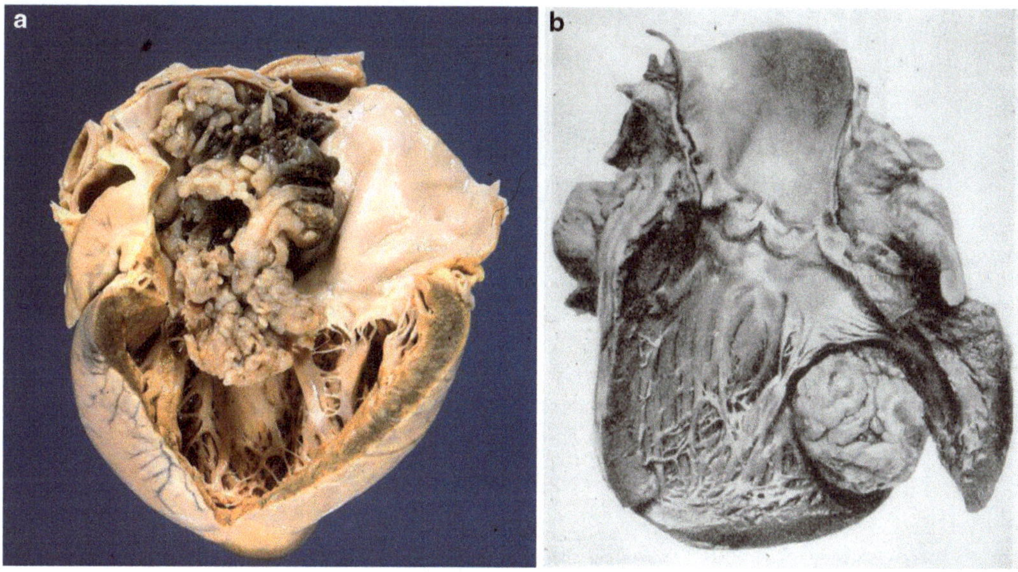

Fig. 1.5 A 61-year-old man who died due to acute pulmonary edema in 1976. (**a**) A giant left atrial, cluster-shaped myxoma was found occupying the left atrio-ventricular valve orifice. (**b**) A similar drawing is available in the book by Mahaim (observation by Ferrari E. *Sui tumori poliposi dell'endocardio atriale*. Arch Sc Mediche 1941;72:75). Reprinted with permission of the Italian Society of Cardiology

to acute pulmonary edema and peripheral embolisms. The need to wait for angiography before referring the patient to surgery resulted to be fatal. A giant villous left atrial myxoma occupied the mitral atrio-ventricular orifice, herniating and protruding into the left ventricle (Fig.1.5).

In 1979 a 45-year-old man suffered a sudden left leg ischemia. An embolus was retrieved by Fogarty, and histology showed the a thrombotic composition. Two days later the patient had an embolic "storm," including the cerebral arteries and died. At autopsy a smooth left atrial myxoma, covered by a stratified thrombus as the probable source of multiple embolisms, was found (Fig. 1.6). Since then, we learned that the true nature of the embolic source cannot be derived with certainty from the histological examination of emboli fragments alone. An echocardiographic examination should have been performed to look at the heart and save the life of the patient by emergency operation to resect the embolic source.

In 1978, a 15-year-old boy had a diagnosis of myocarditis due to chest pain with cardiac enzymes release and ST segment elevation on 12 lead ECG. Discharged at home 20 days later, he suffered an embolic stroke while playing soccer and died suddenly. Autopsy examination revealed a bi-atrial myxoma (Fig. 1.7a, b) with myxomatous embolisms of the cerebral and right coronary artery, the latter being the cause of the previously misdiagnosed inferior myocardial infarction (Fig. 1.7c). Again, echocardiography examination should have identified the cardiac mass, with prompt indication to surgical resection thus preventing the second fatal embolic episode.

In 1979, a 43-year-old man, brother of a distinguished surgeon at the University of Padua, complained of malaise and leg arthralgias. Although the brother reassured him by saying that he was only stressed, the patient asked a chiromancer who, by massaging his legs, told that his problems came from far away, i.e., from the heart. Few days later, he suffered bi-lateral leg

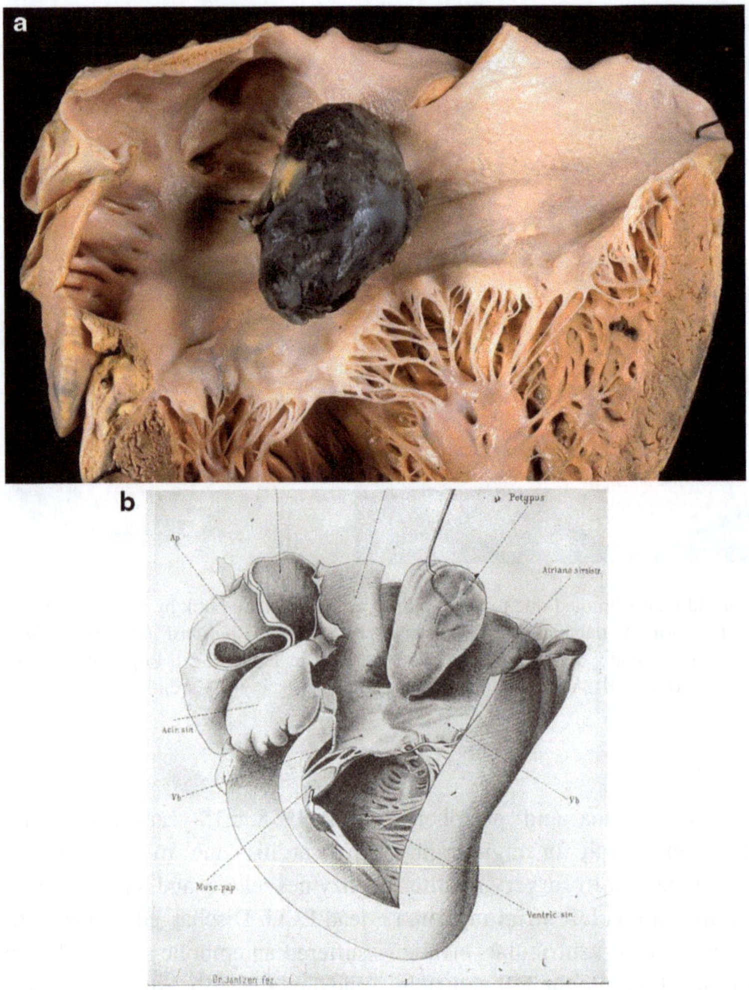

Fig. 1.6 A 45-year-old man who died in 1979 after several episodes of peripheral embolism. (**a**) A left atrial myxoma was found at autopsy ("polyp") with the endocardial surface covered by thrombus. Histological examination of peripheral embolisms retrieved during life was negative for myxoma (only thrombus). (**b**) Drawing of a left atrial myxoma in the book by Mahaim, herein described as a "pedunculated polyp" accounting for functional mitral stenosis. Note the similarity between the two cases. Reprinted with permission of the Italian Society of Cardiology

ischemia and the infra-renal abdominal aorta appeared occluded at angiography. At emergency vascular surgery, a big white–gray embolus, of gelatinous consistency in keeping with myxomatous material at histology, was retrieved from the aortic carrefour. At angiography, a left atrial mass was found and cardiac surgery was immediately performed with resection of a huge villous myxoma from the left atrial cavity (Fig. 1.8).

Some anecdotal cases belong also to the so-called echocardiographic era.

A 6-year-old boy suffered a stroke with hemiplegia and echocardiographic examination detected a left atrial mass. The surgically resected mass revealed to be at histology a vil-

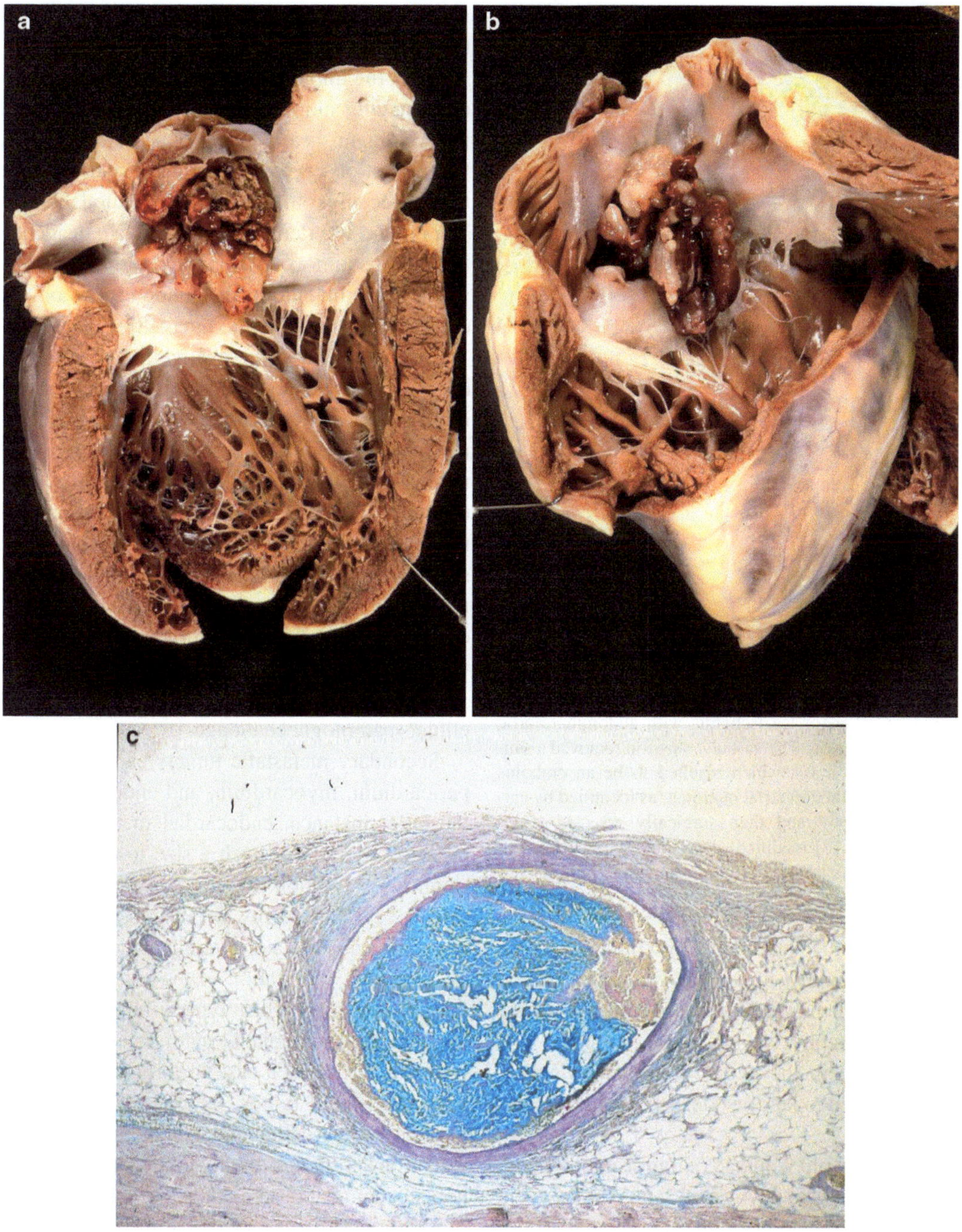

Fig. 1.7 A 15-year-old boy who died due to cerebral embolism after a "myocarditis-like" presentation (from Valente and Montaguti [24] modified). Reprinted with permission of the Italian Society of Cardiology. (**a**) Villous left atrial myxoma; (**b**) villous right atrial myxoma, covered by thrombi; and (**c**) right coronary artery occluded by myxomatous embolism (Alcian PAS ×15)

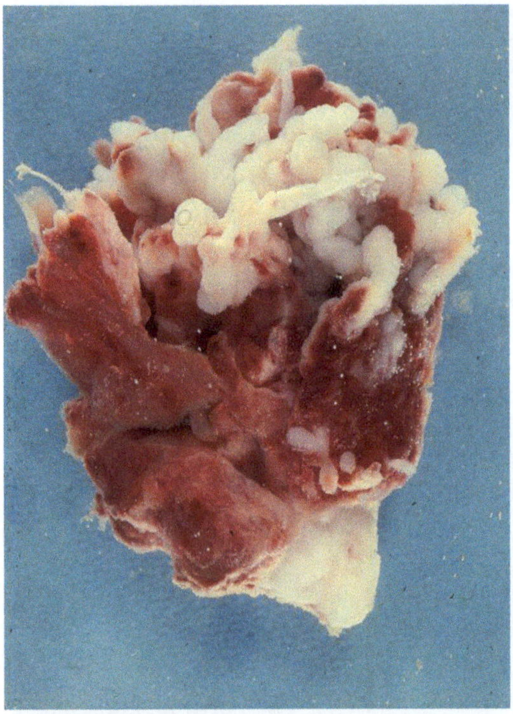

Fig. 1.8 A 43-year-old man with villous left atrial myxoma accounting for leg ischemia with abdominal aortic carrefour occlusion. The vascular surgeon removed a sausage-like huge mass, which resulted to be an embolus detached from the left atrial myxoma, as identified by cardiac angiography and then surgically resected (from Ballotta et al. [18] modified). Reprinted with permission of the Italian Society of Cardiology

lous, gelatinous, and friable myxoma (Fig. 1.9). During the follow-up, the boy well recovered without neurological sequelae. Since then, echocardiography is always performed in any patient, even in the pediatric age, with neurological or syncopal episodes, to exclude a cardiac source.

A 47- year-old woman coming from the South of Italy to Padua as devotee of Saint Antony, went to the Church in Padua with malaise and arthralgias; while kneeling to Saint Antony, she had loss of consciousness and fainted. Promptly transferred to the Intensive Care Unit in Padua, echocardiography disclosed a left atrial mass wedging into the mitral valve orifice (Fig. 1.10). She had emergency operation and survived without any complication: a joint venture between the Patavian Medical School and the thaumaturgical power of the Saint!

After the implementation of non-invasive cardiac imaging and with the exponential increase of in vivo diagnosis and "surgical pathology" cases, we did not observe anymore autopsy deaths due to cardiac myxomas along the natural history. The rare postmortem observations were incidental findings of tumors of small size or of myxoma with calcific involution, a condition for whom we coined the term "lithomyxoma" [8] (Fig. 1.11).

On the contrary, the availability of echocardiography performed as a routine/screening test in several conditions due to its non-invasiveness, led to the frequent casual identification of many small benign endocavitary tumors, particularly fibroelastomas (or fibroelastic papillomas). When localized in the left chambers, surgical resection is always indicated, for primary prevention of embolic phenomena. On the contrary, right-sided papillomas can be followed up.

Malignant cardiac tumors represent a different clinico-pathologic challenge.

Secondary metastatic tumors can involve the pericardium, myocardium, and endocardium. In the latter instance, endocardial metastases may be also observed of such a size to create endocavitary obstruction like primary cardiac tumors (Fig. 1.12). Noteworthy, the diagnosis of secondary cardiac mass is no so rarely achieved only by histological examination of the resected cardiac mass that reveals a histotype different from that of primary malignant cardiac tumors. For instance, we recall a case of a right atrial endocavitary villous tumor, labeled as myxoma at naked eye observation and then diagnosed as testis corion carcinoma after histological and immunohistochemical investigation; as well as the case of a right atrial mass located at the orifice of the inferior caval vein, subsequently diagnosed as clear cell renal carcinoma (Fig. 1.13). In both instances, a total body imaging (echo, CT) has been then performed with discovery of the primary malignant tumors and orchiectomy and nephrectomy were carried out, respectively, with adjuvant chemotherapy.

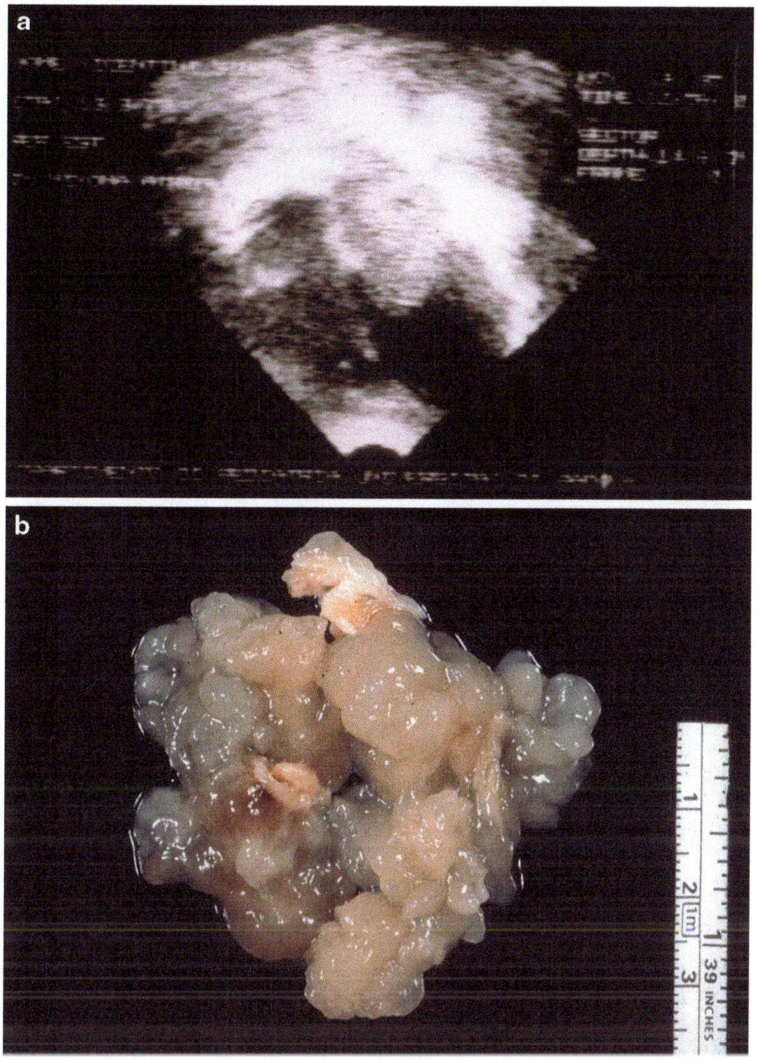

Fig. 1.9 Left atrial myxoma in a 6-year-old child with cerebral stroke and hemiplegia. Two-dimensional echocardiography revealed a left atrial mass (**a**). At surgical pathology examination, a friable, villous left atrial myxoma was diagnosed (**b**). Reprinted with permission of the Italian Society of Cardiology

Primary malignant cardiac tumors are mostly infiltrating masses with inherent difficulties in achieving a complete surgical resection and as such with a poor prognosis. An exception is represented by the rare primary malignant cardiac tumors with an endocavitary growth and a clinical presentation mimicking myxoma due to obstructive symptoms and signs. The patient can even present with cardiogenic shock, when the intracardiac mass occupies the atrio-ventricular orifices or the pulmonary artery, mimicking pulmonary embolism. Histological examination of the resected "embolus" is mandatory, to assess the benign or malignant nature of the process and characterize the histotype [7].

In the last two decades, there have been many steps forward in the clinical diagnosis and treatment of cardiac tumors:

1. *Endomyocardial biopsy*. Tissue sampling to assess the neoplastic nature of the mass during

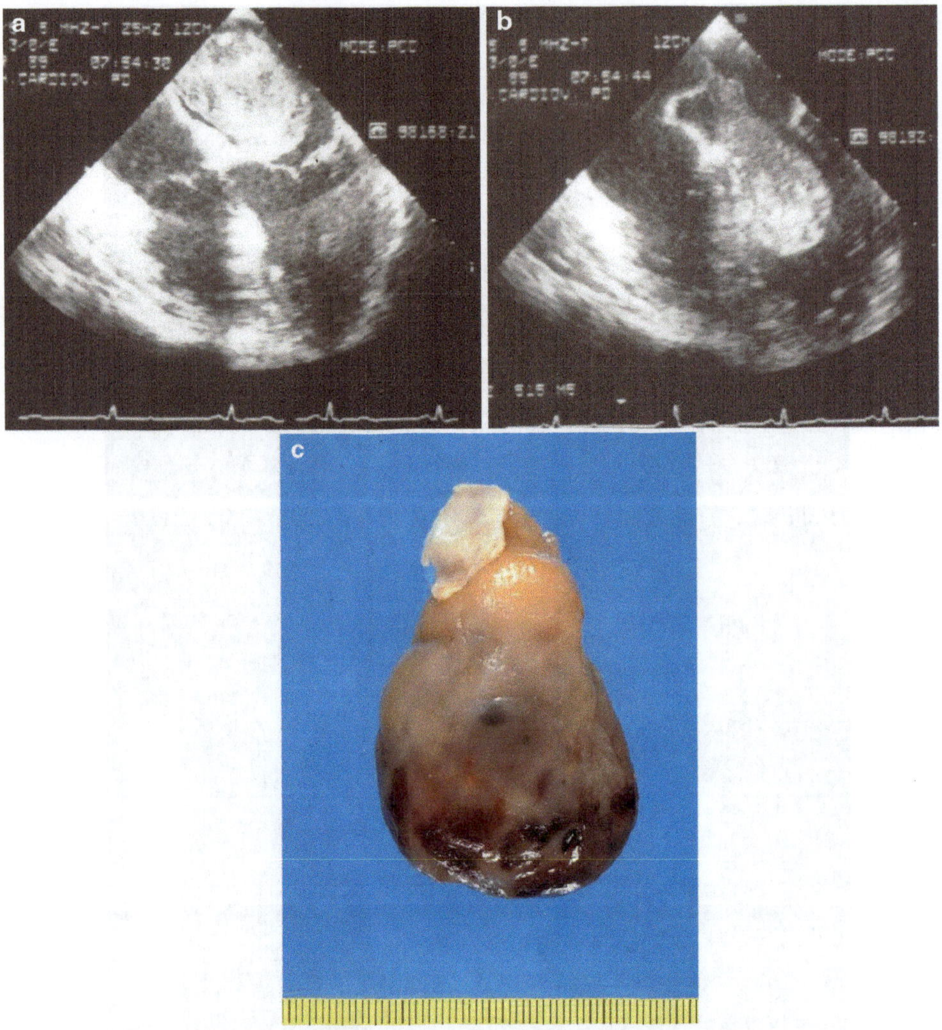

Fig. 1.10 A 47-year-old woman with syncopal episodes. The prompt echocardiographic examination (**a**, **b**) detected a polypous left atrial mass, impinging during diastole into the mitral valve orifice. The successfully resected mass revealed to be a smooth myxoma ("polyp") (**c**). Reprinted with permission of the Italian Society of Cardiology

life can be achieved through either surgical thoracotomy or endomyocardial biopsy. With the latter technique, tissue samples may be taken with the bioptome introduced antegrade in the right cardiac chambers either through femoral or jugular veins or, more rarely, retrograde in the left chambers through femoral arteries [9]. The procedure is under echocardiographic guidance and avoids thoracotomy for diagnosis, allowing therapeutic planning, including cardiac transplantation, in cases of malignant neoplasm without extra-cardiac metastasis. Moreover, endomyocardial biopsy can be useful in the setting of tumors which are unresectable or require histological characterization before chemotherapy is started, such as lymphomas. An adequate number and size of samples (4–5 pieces, 1–2 mm each) is

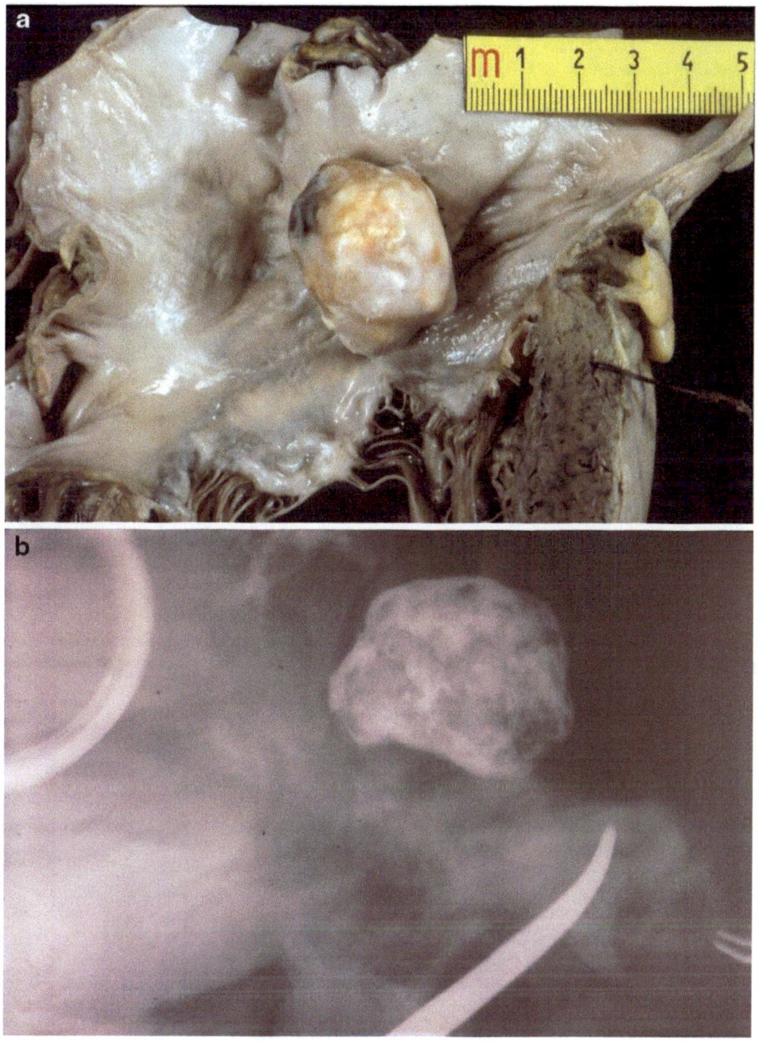

Fig. 1.11 Incidental autopsy finding of left atrial myxoma with calcific involution (lithomyxoma) in a 72-year-old woman who died due to ischemic heart disease (from Basso et al. [8] modified). Reprinted with permission of the Italian Society of Cardiology. (a) gross view; (b) ex vivo X-Ray

usually enough for a thorough histological investigation, including immuno-histochemistry, to achieve a precise diagnosis (Fig. 1.14).

2. *Prenatal echocardiographic diagnosis*. Nowadays, prenatal echography is a routine examination during pregnancy and the request for fetal echocardiography is increasing. Many congenital heart diseases are diagnosed before birth, including cardiac tumors [10]. They consist mostly of teratomas, fibromas, rhabdomyomas either intramural or endocavitary, and more frequent indications include arrhythmias, hydrops, retarded intrauterine growth, and familiarity of tuberous sclerosis. Prenatal diagnosis is essential to plan the surgical intervention soon after delivery.
3. *Cardiac transplantation*. Organ replacement with orthotopic cardiac transplantation is an

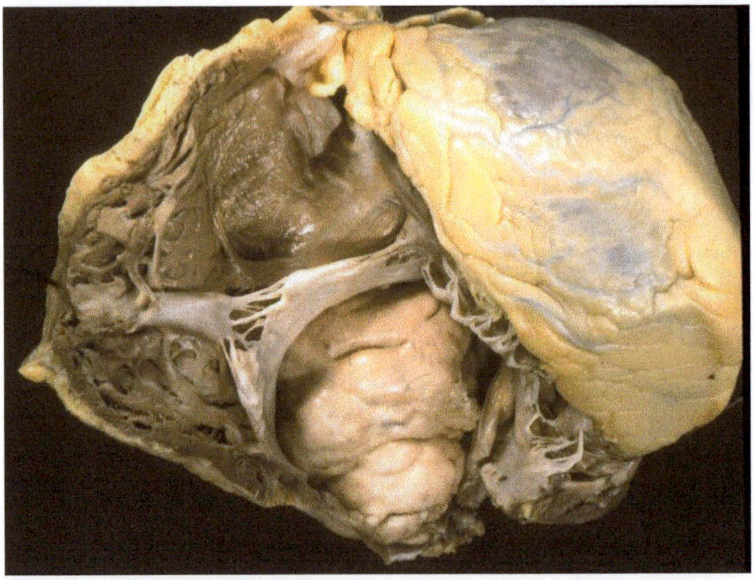

Fig. 1.12 Huge endocavitary right atrial mass, herniating into the tricuspid valve orifice in a 77-year-old man with a history of cirrhosis. At histology, a metastasis of hepatocarcinoma was identified. Reprinted with permission of the Italian Society of Cardiology

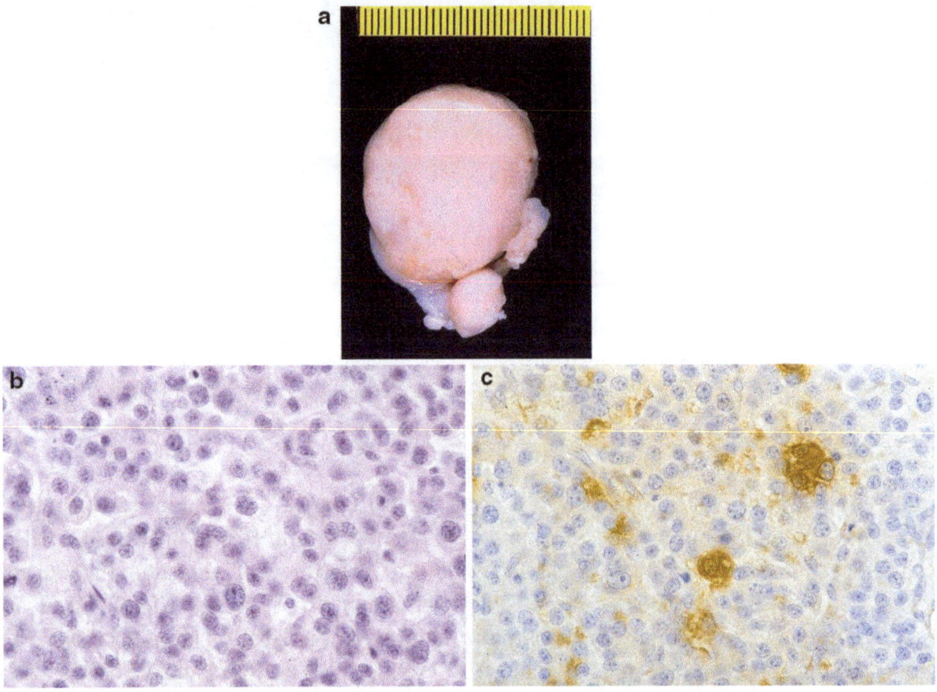

Fig. 1.13 Right atrial mass with pre-operative diagnosis of cardiac myxoma in a 42-year-old woman. Reprinted with permission of the Italian Society of Cardiology. (**a**) Gross view of the surgically resected mass with a smooth surface. (**b**) At histology, clear cells with round nuclei and vacuolated cytoplasm, aggregated in cordon-like structures are visible (hematoxylin–eosin). (**c**) At immunohistochemistry, a few cells are positive for vimentin. A final diagnosis of cardiac metastasis of clear cell renal carcinoma was done

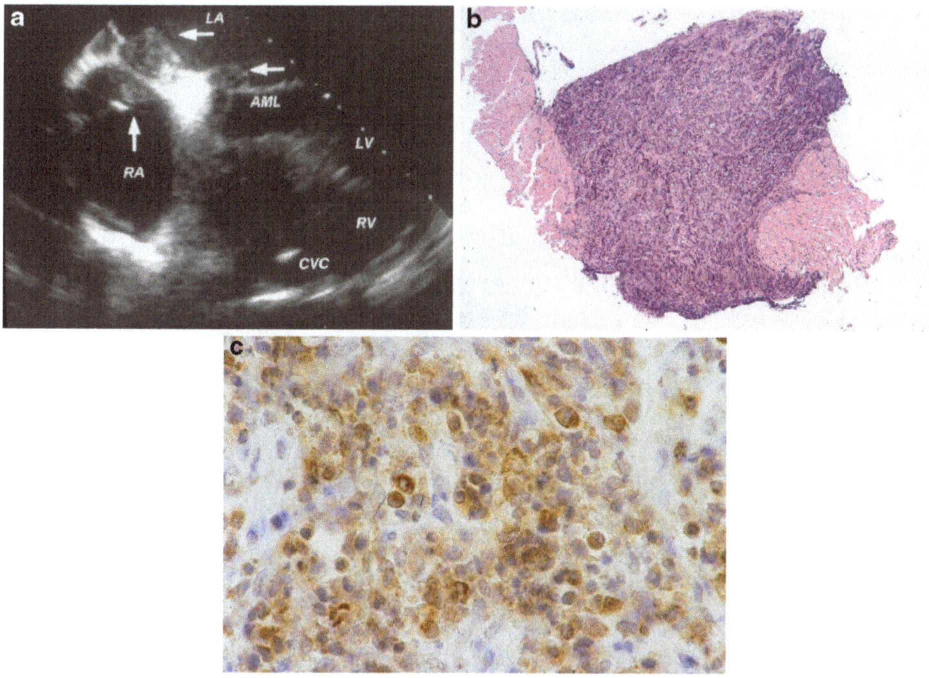

Fig. 1.14 Histologic diagnosis of cardiac metastasis by T-cell lymphoma through endomyocardial biopsy in a 36-year-old woman (from Testolin et al. [40] modified). Reprinted with permission of the Italian Society of Cardiology. (**a**) Trans-esophageal echocardiography, four-chamber view: a mass on both side of the interatrial septum is visible (arrows). (**b**) Right ventricular endomyocardial biopsy shows a lympho-proliferative lesion infiltrating the myocardium. (**c**) At immunohistochemistry, the cells are positive for T lymphocytes (CD3) (AML anterior mitral leaflet, CVC central venous catheter, RA right atrium, RV right ventricle, LA left atrium, LV left ventricle)

extreme therapeutic option which is indicated in the setting of non-resectable benign cardiac tumors, or in cases of infiltrating primary malignant neoplasms without extra-cardiac metastasis. The ideal situation is typically represented by cardiac fibroma, which is usually located within the interventricular septum (Fig. 1.15) or the left ventricular free wall [10]; total heart removal with ex vivo repair on the bench, followed by auto-transplant, can be also carried out. A different situation is represented by infiltrating primary malignant cardiac tumors, where cardiac transplantation is considered only in the absence of metastases. However, the cardiac surgeon has always to take into consideration the low number of donors and the high number of patients in the waiting list with a potentially better long-term prognosis.

4. *Cardiac magnetic resonance imaging* (MRI) *and computed tomography* (CT). MRI is the best available non-invasive procedure for cardiac tumor diagnosis in terms of site, morphology, dimensions, extension, topographic relations, and infiltration of surrounding structures. It may also help for tissue characterization (adipose tissue, necrosis, hemorrhage, vascularization, calcification), although the specificity is still low [11]. A "probabilistic" histopathological diagnosis is more reliable and the term "mass" should be employed, leaving the final answer to histology. In case of lipoma, with hyper-intensity signal in T1 imaging, the precise histotype may be established by MRI, with a very high diagnostic probability. Use of contrast medium may be of help to detect highly vascularized tumors, like

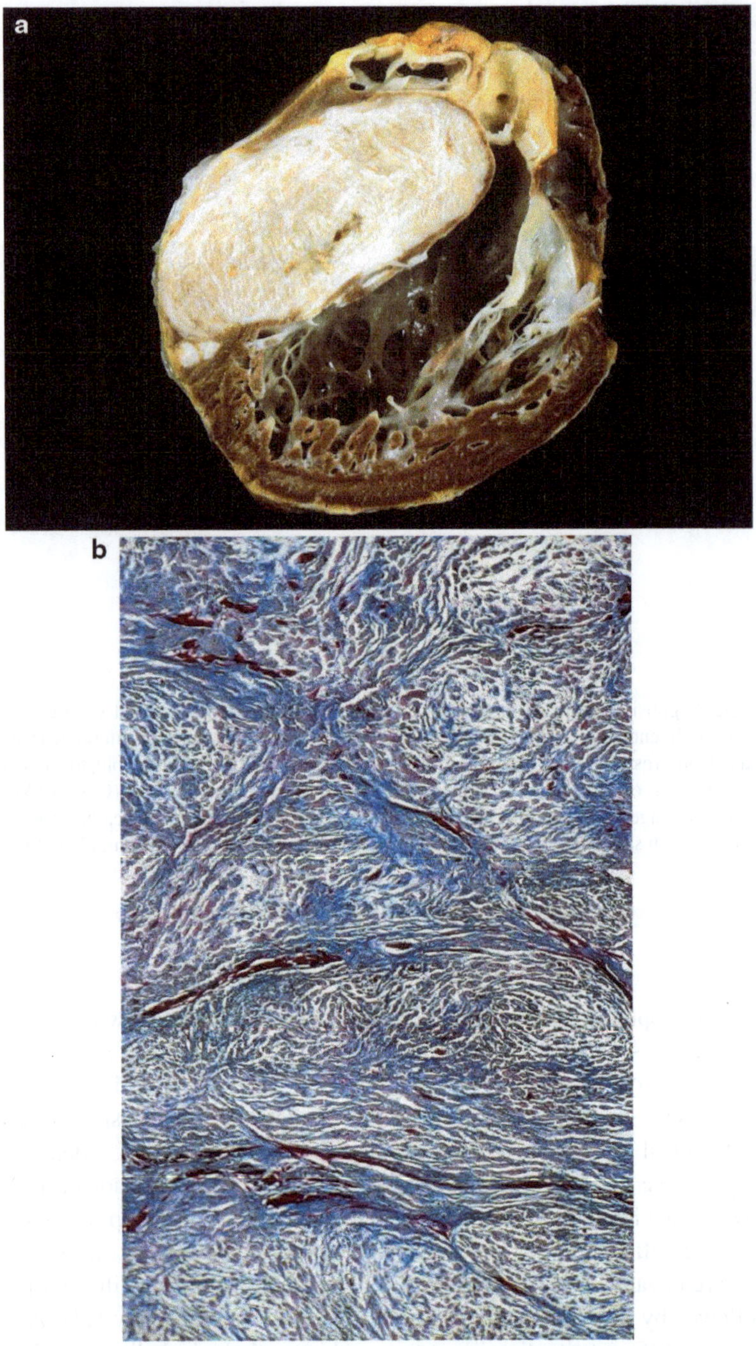

Fig. 1.15 A 40-year-old woman, with echocardiographic diagnosis of asymmetric hypertrophic cardiomyopathy, underwent cardiac transplantation due to refractory congestive heart failure (from Valente et al. [10]). Reprinted with permission of the Italian Society of Cardiology. (**a**) Long axis section of the native heart showing a huge oval shape whitish mass occupying the interventricular septum and accounting for subaortic bulging/obstruction. (**b**) At histology, a cardiac fibroma was diagnosed (Heidenhain trichrome)

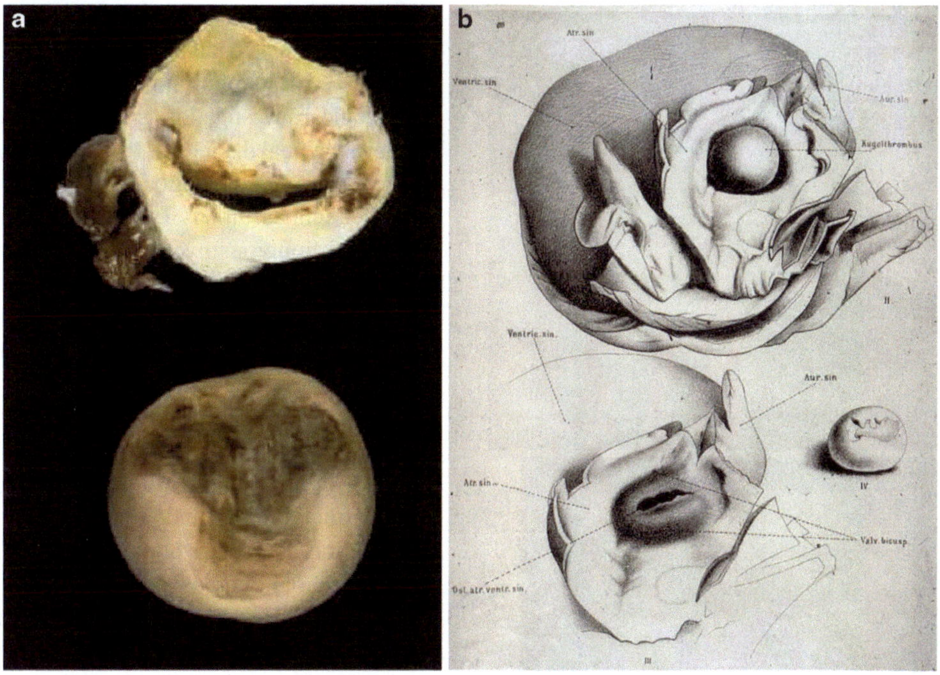

Fig. 1.16 (**a**) Rheumatic mitral valve stenosis with left atrial ball-thrombus, mimicking a myxoma (a 72- year-old woman with history of peripheral embolism who underwent mitral valve replacement). (**b**) Similar drawing in the original book by Mahaim. Reprinted with permission of the Italian Society of Cardiology

myxomas, angiomas, and angiosarcomas. In case of fibroma, delayed contrast enhancement shows homogeneous uptake of gadolinium, indicating fibrous tissue.

Multi-slice CT has the advantage of a better spatial resolution in case of possible lung, pleural, and mediastinal involvement. Moreover, calcification is easily detected within the mass and may point to fibroma, in case of mural mass, myxoma in case of an intracavitary atrial mass in the elderly, or teratoma in case of pericardial mass in infancy. MRI and CT can also differentiate serous from hemorrhagic pericardial effusion.

However, multi-slice CT does not allow to fully investigate involvement of cardiac valves, and presents the limitation of high dosage radiation, so as to preclude its employment in the follow-up of young subjects. Fast heart rates and arrhythmias may jeopardize the quality of imaging of both MRI and multi-slice CT.

Obviously, two-dimensional echocardiography remains the first diagnostic approach for detection of cardiac masses, whereas MRI and CT may be complementary tools, with their own advantages and limitations. Due to their non-invasiveness and lack of radiation, two-dimensional echo and MRI are also the gold standard for follow-up studies.

Non-neoplastic Cardiac Masses

Only histological examination may establish whether a cardiac mass is neoplastic in nature, either benign or malignant. When seen by clinical imaging, the use of term "mass" is advisable, since it may have several explanations other than cardiac tumors.

1. *Thrombi.* An isolated mass inside an atrial appendage is almost exclusively a thrombus. In the left atrium, free floating masses like "ball thrombus" should point to a mitral valve pathology, usually rheumatic in origin (Fig. 1.16). However, differential diagnosis with left atrial

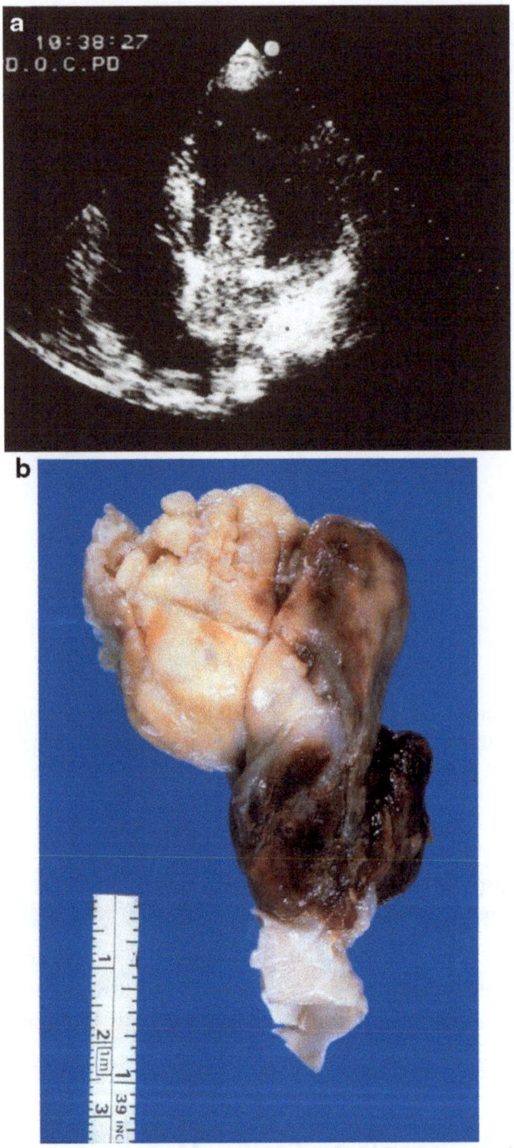

Fig. 1.17 A 61-year-old man with pulmonary edema. Reprinted with permission of the Italian Society of Cardiology. (**a**) Two-dimensional echocardiography, four-chamber view shows a mass occupying the mitral valve orifice. (**b**) At surgery, a myxoma with strangulation corresponding to the sphincter contraction of the mitral valve anulus is found

myxoma is always needed (Fig. 1.17). Small mural thrombi may be observed at the apex of the left ventricle, even in the setting of a preserved contractility, and misinterpreted clinically as left ventricular myxomas (Fig. 1.18). Non-bacterial thrombotic endocarditis may mimic valve papillary fibroelastoma. Valvular and non-valvular endocardial thrombosis may be observed in antiphospholipid syndrome [12]. Histological investigation is always needed to achieve the final diagnosis [13] (Fig. 1.19).

2. *Cardiomyopathies*. Endocardial fibroplastic Loeffler endocarditis is a restrictive (obliterative) cardiomyopathy, usually associated with eosinophilia, hypersensitivity, or eosinophilic leukemia, consisting of a mural thrombus filling the apical and inflow portions of the ventricles to such an extent to entrap the mitral and/or tricuspid valves apparatus. Cardiac imaging may mis-diagnose an apical form of hypertrophic cardiomyopathy or an endocardial tumor. Endomyocardial biopsy with tissue characterization may be of help for differential diagnosis (Fig. 1.20).
3. *Infections*. Infective vegetations of cardiac valves may mimic papillary fibroelastoma, and sometimes at the mitral level they may be so huge as to simulate embolizing atrial myxoma. Free floating masses may not necessarily be thrombotic, but even septic (fungal in immunosuppressed patients) (Fig. 1.21). Pericardial or myocardial cysts may be hydatid cysts by echinococcosis, to be treated cautiously during the surgery to avoid rupture and spread of infection (Fig. 1.22).
4. *Calcium*. Calcium stones, intramural or intracavitary, may occur and not necessarily are the outcome of dystrophic calcification of previous infections/tumors, as in the case of lithomyxoma. The phenomenon may be so massive to transform the heart into a sort of a stone quarry. Dystrophic calcification of the mitral valve annulus can also account for misdiagnosis of an atrio-ventricular mass by echocardiography. Endocavitary calcific masses have been reported even in the pediatric age as a consequence of calcific involution of thrombi upon central venous catheters.

The single center experience collected at the University of Padua since 1970, when the first surgical intervention for resection of a cardiac myxoma was accomplished [15], is witnessed by the numerous publications on the topic, available in the literature [16–55].

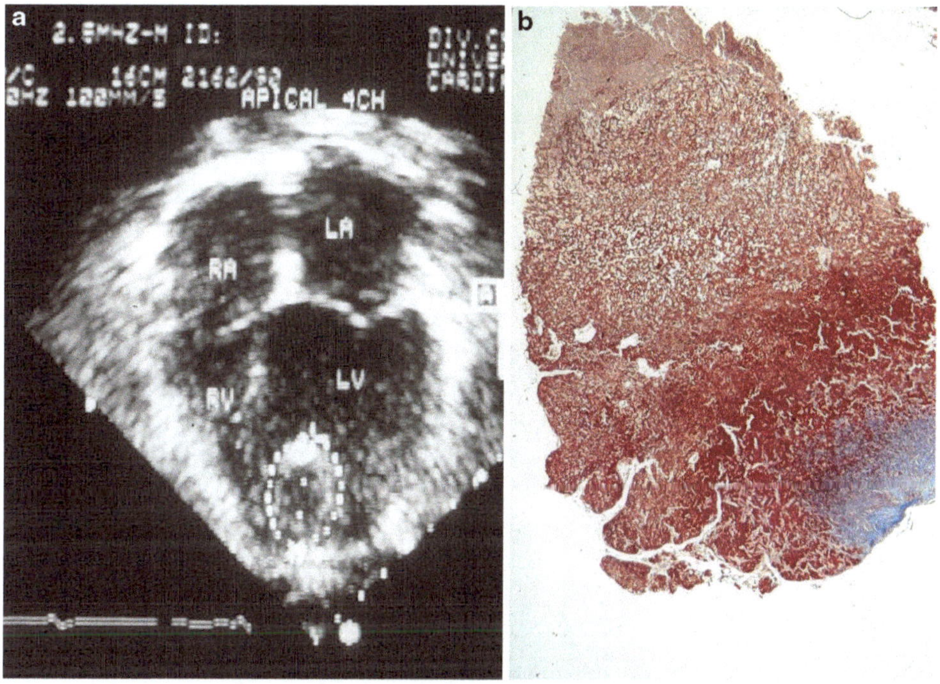

Fig. 1.18 A 33-year-old woman with recurrent left ventricular apex thrombosis, mimicking a endocardial tumor. Reprinted with permission of the Italian Society of Cardiology. (**a**) Two-dimensional echocardiography, four-chamber view (*LA* left atrium, *LV* left ventricle, *RA* right atrium, *RV* right ventricle). (**b**) At histology, the resected mass consists of thrombotic material (Heidenhain trichrome)

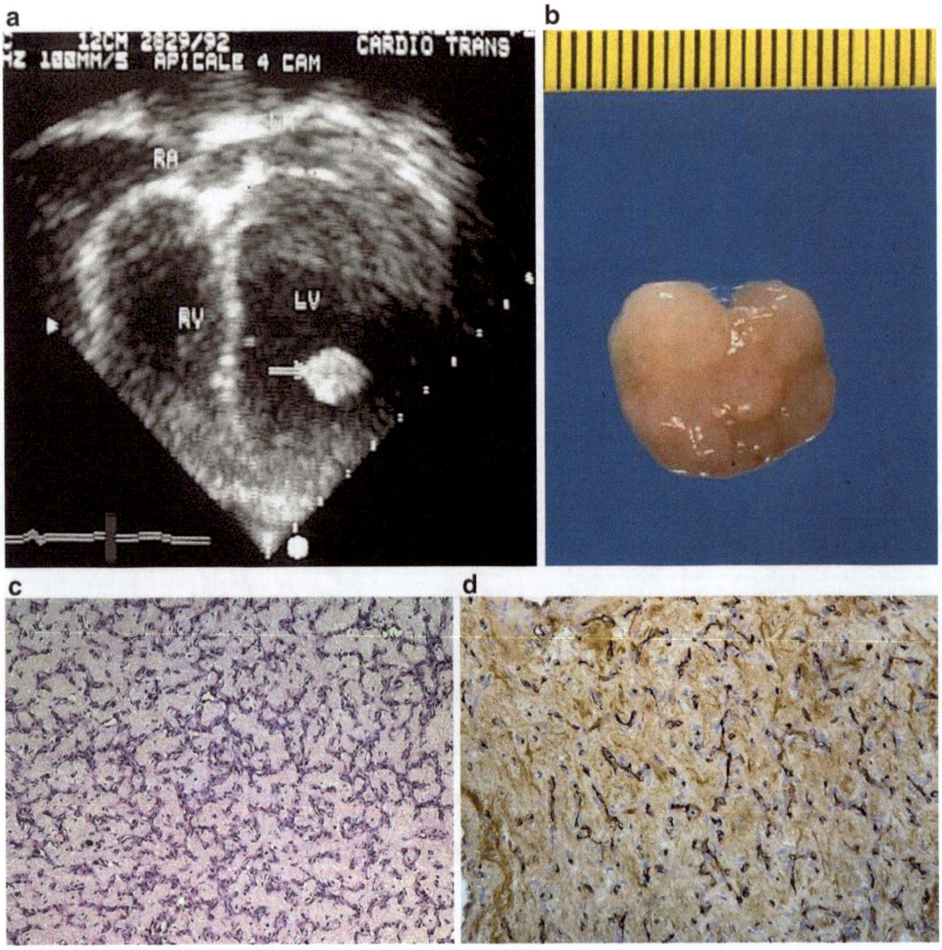

Fig. 1.19 A 20-year-old patient with a small left ventricular apical mass (from Basso et al. [12] modified). Reprinted with permission of the Italian Society of Cardiology. (**a**) Two-dimensional echocardiography, apical four-chamber view shows a round mass at the left ventricular apex (*arrow*) (*LA* left atrium, *LV* left ventricle, *RA* right atrium, *RV* right ventricle). (**b**) Gross view of the surgically resected mass: note the smooth surface and the *pink color*. (**c**, **d**) At histology and immunohistochemistry, the benign proliferation shows a myxoid background with vessel proliferation in keeping with myxomatous angioma (hematoxylin–eosin and CD31)

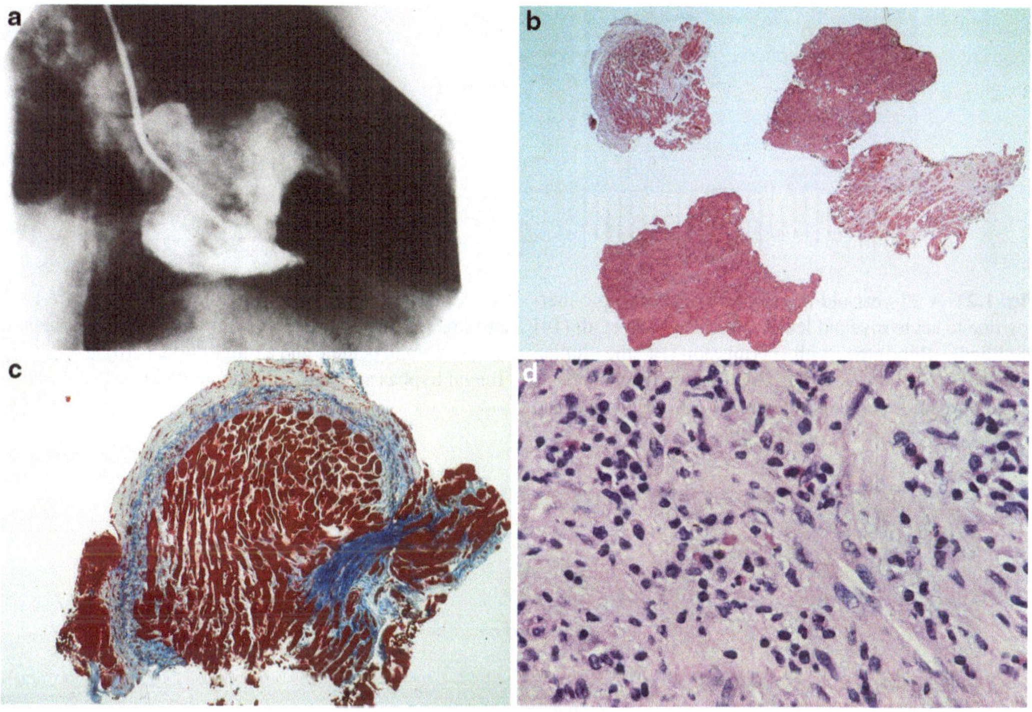

Fig. 1.20 A 61-year-old man affected by Loeffler fibroplastic endocarditis (from Basso et al. [36] modified). Reprinted with permission of the Italian Society of Cardiology. (**a**) Left ventricular angiography showing a contrast medium defect at the apex corresponding to a round oval mass. (**b**) Four samples retrieved by endomyocardial biopsy, two of which consist of thrombotic material (hematoxylin–eosin). (**c**) One of the endomyocardial biopsy samples shows endocardial fibrous thickening (Heidenhain trichrome). (**d**) At higher magnification, eosinophilic infiltrates are visible (hematoxylin–eosin)

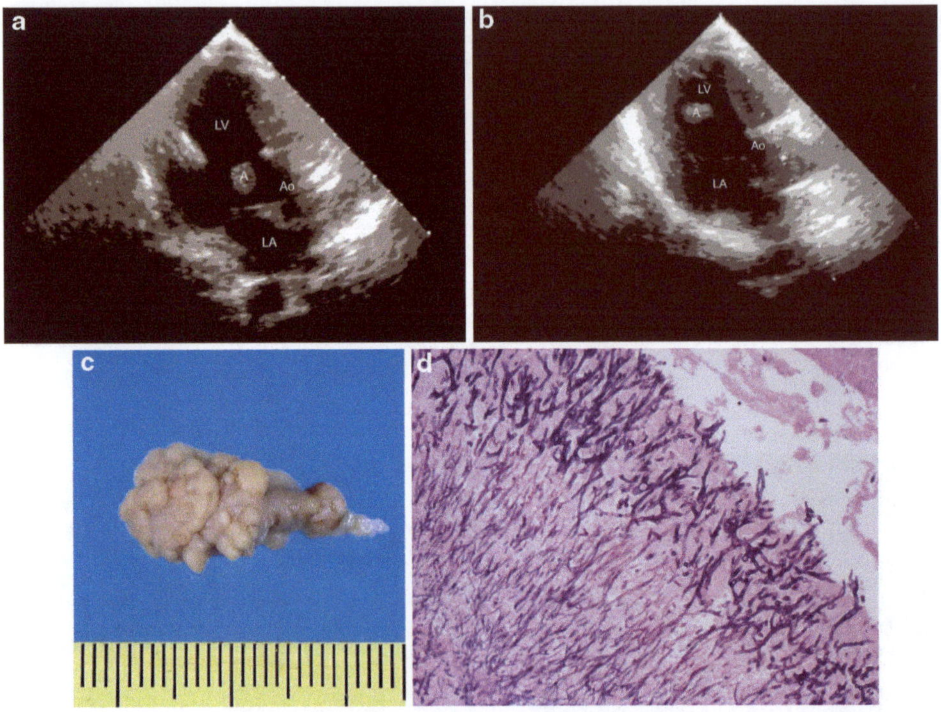

Fig. 1.21 A 23-year-old man under chemotherapic therapy due to acute myeloid leukemia (from Vida et al. [14] modified). Reprinted with permission of the Italian Society of Cardiology. (**a**, **b**) at two-dimensional echocardiography, a free-floating round mass is visible within the left ventricular cavity (*A* aspergilloma, *Ao* aorta, *LA* left atrium, *LV* left ventricle); (**c**) the resected whitish mass shows a small pedicle and a rough surface; (**d**) at histology, fungal hyphas are detected (Alcian PAS)

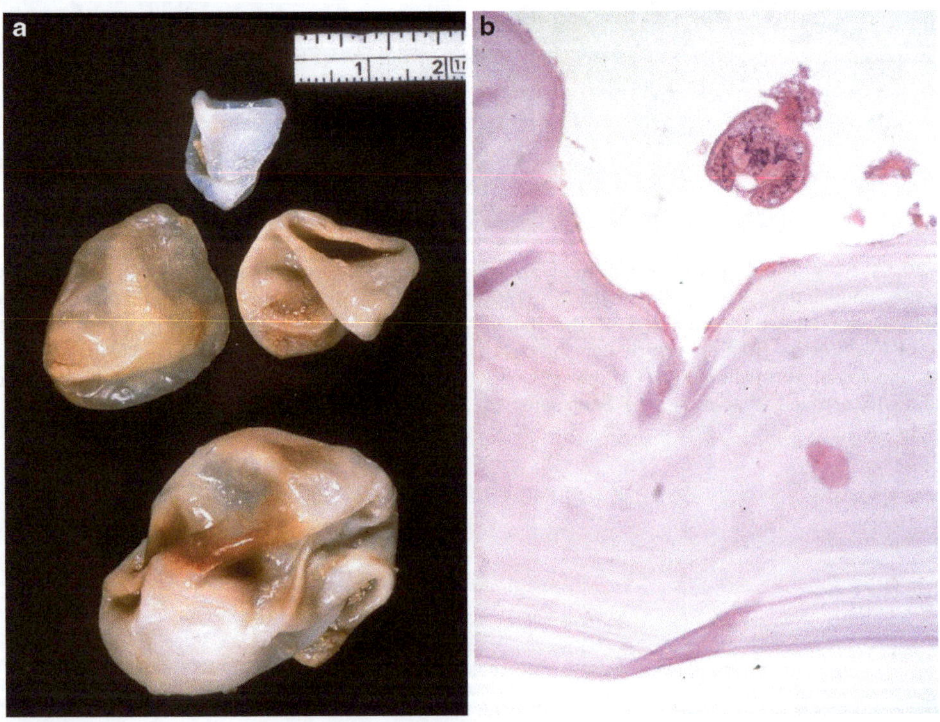

Fig. 1.22 Echinococcus cyst is surgically removed from the paricardial cavity in a 55-year-old man (**a**). At histology, the external membrane and the scolices inside the cyst are appreciable (**b**, hematoxylin–eosin). Reprinted with permission of the Italian Society of Cardiology

References

1. Columbus MR. De Re Anatomica, Libri XV. Venice: N Bevilacque,1559, p 269.
2. Prichard RW. Tumors of the heart: review of the subject and report of 150 cases. Arch Pathol. 1951;51:98–128.
3. Wold LE, Lie JT. Cardiac myxomas: a clinicopathologic profile. Am J Pathol. 1980;101:219–40.
4. Mahaim I. Le tumeurs et les polypes du coeur: etude anatomoclinique. Paris: Masson; 1945.
5. Goldberg HP, Glenn F, Dotter CT, Steinberg I. Myxoma of the left atrium: diagnosis made during life with operative and post-mortem findings. Circulation. 1952;6:762–7.
6. Crafoord C. Panel discussion on late results of mitral commissurotomy. In: Lam CR, editor. International symposium on cardiovascular surgery. Philadelphia, PA: Saunders; 1955. p. 161–78
7. Basso C, Valente M, Poletti A, Casarotto D, Thiene G. Surgical pathology of primary cardiac and pericardial tumors. Eur J Cardiothorac Surg. 1997;12:730–7.
8. Basso C, Valente M, Casarotto D, Thiene G. Cardiac lithomyxoma. Am J Cardiol. 1997;80:1249–51.
9. Poletti A, Cocco P, Valente M, Fasoli G, Chioin R, Thiene G. In vivo diagnosis of cardiac angiosarcoma by endomyocardial biopsy. Cardiovasc Pathol. 1993;2:89–91.
10. Valente M, Cocco P, Thiene G, Casula R, Poletti A, Milanesi O, Fasoli G, Livi U. Cardiac fibroma and heart transplantation. J Thorac Cardiovasc Surg. 1993;106:1208–12.
11. Hoffmann U, Globits S, Schima W, Loewe C, Puig S, Oberhuber G, Frank H. Usefulness of magnetic resonance imaging of cardiac and paracardiac masses. Am J Cardiol. 2003;92:890–5.
12. Basso C, Fasoli G, Casarotto D, Thiene G. Unusual left ventricular mass. Circulation. 1998;98:1036–7.
13. Basso C, Bottio T, Rubino M, Ruffatti A, Pittarello D, Thiene G, Gerosa G. Antiphospholipid sindrome and right atrial mass. J Thorac Cardiovasc Surg. 2005;130:1462–3.
14. Vida V, Biffanti R, Thiene G, Stellin G, Milanesi O, Basso C. Left ventricular mass after treatment with chemotherapic drugs. Circulation. 2004;109:e300–1.
15. Casarotto D. Mixoma dell'atrio sinistro. Chirurgia Triveneta. 1971;11:279–87.
16. Thiene G, Miraglia G, Menghetti L, Nava A, Rossi L. Multiple lesions of the conduction system in a case of cardiac rhabdomyosarcoma with complex arrhythmias. An anatomic and clinical study. Chest. 1976;70:378–81.
17. Casarotto D, Bortolotti U, Russo D, Betti D, Schivazappa L, Thiene G. Surgical removal of a left atrial myxoma during pregnancy. Chest. 1979;75:390–2.
18. Ballotta E, Thiene G, Valente M, Deriu GP. Mixoma dell'atrio sinistro rivelato da un'occlusione acuta del carrefour aortico. G Ital Cardiol. 1979;9:627–30.
19. Stritoni P, Daliento L, Fasoli G, Schivazappa L, Chioin R, Fusaro A, Casarotto D, Bortolotti U, Valente M, Thiene G. Mixoma atriale. Esperienza clinica, diagnostico-strumentale, chirurgica e patologica in 13 casi. G Ital Cardiol. 1979;9:1001–16.
20. Gallucci V, Stritoni P, Fasoli G, Thiene G. Giant blood cyst of tricuspid valve. Successful excision in an infant. Br Heart J. 1976;38:990–2.
21. Bortolotti U, Mazzucco A, Valfrè C, Valente M, Pennelli N, Gallucci V. Right ventricular myxoma: review of the literature and report of two patients. Am Thorac Surg. 1982;33:277–84.
22. Stellin G, Bortolotti U, Valfré C, Mazzucco A, Thiene G, Cavarzerani A, Gallucci V. Mural papilloma of the left ventricle and floppy mitral valve: report of an unusual association. Texas Heart Inst J. 1983;10:89–92.
23. Valente M. Structural profile of cardiac myxoma. Appl Pathol. 1983;1:251–63.
24. Valente M, Montaguti A. Il mixoma cardiaco nell'adolescenza. Studio anatomo-patologico in tre pazienti. Pathologica. 1984;76:323–32.
25. Livi U, Bortolotti U, Milano A, Valente M, Prandi A, Frugoni C, De Mozzi P, Valfré C, Mazzucco A, Gallucci V. Cardiac myxomas: results of 14 years experience. Thorac Cardiovasc Surg. 1984;32:143–7.
26. Thiene G, Valente M. I tumori primitivi del cuore e del pericardio nell'esperienza dell'Istituto di Anatomia Patologica dell'Università di Padova (1972–1984). In: Pansini R, editors. Progressi Clinici: Medicina. Padova: Piccin Ed., 1985;2/2–3: p. 169–207.
27. Bortolotti U, Mazzucco A, Rubino M, Maraglino G, Sturaro M, Milano A, Stellin G, Thiene G, Gallucci V. I mixomi dell'atrio destro. Tecnica operatoria, risultati e follow-up a distanza. Chir Torac. 1989;42:371–2.
28. Mazzucco A, Bortolotti U, Thiene G, Dan M, Stritoni P, Scutari M, Stellin G. Left ventricular papillary fibroelastoma with coronary embolization. Eur J Cardio-Thorac Surg. 1989;3:471–3.
29. De Dominicis E, Frigiola A, Thiene G, Menicanti L, Bozzola L, Finocchi G. Subaortic stenosis by solitary rhabdomyoma. Successful excision in an infant following 2D echocardiogram and Doppler diagnosis. Chest. 1989;95:470–2.
30. Bortolotti U, Maraglino G, Rubino M, Santini F, Mazzucco A, Milano A, Fasoli G, Livi U, Thiene G, Gallucci V. Surgical excision of intracardiac myxomas: a 20-year follow-up. Ann Thorac Surg. 1990;49:449–53.
31. Bortolotti U, Faggian G, Mazzucco A, Milano A, Thiene G, Fasoli G, Gallucci V. Right atrial myxoma originating from the inferior vena cava. Ann Thorac Surg. 1990;49:1000–2.
32. Cocco P, Valente M, Thiene G. I tumori primitivi del cuore nell'era cardiochirurgica: dall'autopsia al trapianto cardiaco. Riv Anat Pat Oncol. 1991;49–50:135–72.
33. Mazzucco A, Faggian G, Bortolotti U, Bonato R, Pittarello D, Centonze G, Thiene G. Embolizing

papillary fibroelastoma of the mitral valve. Texas Heart Inst J. 1991;18:62–6.
34. Valente M, Basso C, Thiene G, Bressan M, Stritoni P, Cocco P, Fasoli G. Fibroelastic papilloma: a not-so-benign cardiac tumor. Cardiovasc Pathol. 1992;1:161–6.
35. Basso C, Stefani A, Calabrese F, Fasoli G, Valente M. Primary right atrial fibrosarcoma diagnosed by endocardial biopsy. Am Heart J. 1996;131:399–402.
36. Basso C, Poletti A, Valente M, Thiene G. Diagnosi di tumore cardiaco tramite biopsia endomiocardica. In: Baroldi G, Thiene G, editors. Testo Atlante Biopsia Endomiocardica. Padova: Piccin Ed; 1996. p. 178–96.
37. Basso C, Valente M, Poletti A, Casarotto D, Thiene G. Surgical pathology of primary cardiac and pericardial tumors. Eur J Cardio-thorac Surg. 1997;12:730–8.
38. Scalia D, Basso C, Rizzoli G, Lupia M, Budano S, Thiene G, Venturini A. Should right-sided fibroelastomas be operated upon? J Heart Valve Dis. 1997;6:647–50.
39. Basso C, Barbazza R, Thiene G. Lipomatous hypertrophy of the atrial septum. Circulation. 1998;97:1423.
40. Testolin L, Basso C, Pittarello D, Casarotto D, Valente M. Cardiogenic shock due to metastatic cardiac lymphoma: still a diagnostic and therapeutic challenge. Eur J Cardiothorac Surg. 2001;19:365–8.
41. Bottio T, Basso C, Rizzoli G, Casarotto D, Thiene G. Case report: fibroelastoma of the papillary muscle of the mitral valve: diagnostic implications and review of the literature. J Heart Valve Dis. 2002;11:288–91.
42. Basso C, Valente M, Thiene G. Aspetti anatomo-clinici dei tumori del cuore e del pericardio. In: Crepaldi G, Baritussio A, editors. Trattato di Medicina Interna: Malattie del cuore e dei vasi. Padova: Piccin Editore; 2002. p. 757–68.
43. Padalino MA, Basso C, Thiene G, Stellin G. Images in cardiovascular medicine: Giant right ventricular fibroma in an infant. Circulation. 2002;106:386.
44. Padalino MA, Basso C, Moreolo GS, Thiene G, Stellin G. Left atrial myxoma in a child: case report and review of the literature. Cardiovasc Pathol. 2003;12:233–6.
45. Basso C, Bottio T, Valente M, Bonato R, Casarotto D, Thiene G. Primary cardiac valve tumours. Heart. 2003;89:1259–60.
46. Rizzoli G, Bottio T, Pittarello D, Napodano M, Thiene G, Basso C. Atrial septal mass: transesophageal echocardiographic assessment. J Thorac Cardiovasc Surg. 2004;128:767–9.
47. Bottio T, Pittarello D, Bonato R, Thiene G, Gerosa G, Casarotto D, Basso C. Echocardiographic diagnosis of aortic valve papillary fibroelastoma. Tex Heart Inst J. 2004;31:322–323
48. Vida V, Cerutti A, Thiene G, Stellin S, Milanesi O, Basso C. Calcified mass in the right atrium. Ann Thorac Surg. 2005;79:717.
49. Padalino M, Basso C, Milanesi O, Vida VL, Svaluto Moreolo G, Thiene G, Stellin G. Surgically treated primary cardiac tumors in early infancy and childhood. J Thorac Cardiovasc Surg. 2005;129:1358–63.
50. Mazzola A, Spano JP, Valente M, Gregorini R, Villani C, Di Eusanio M, Ciocca M, Minuti U, Giancola R, Basso C, Thiene G. Leiomyosarcoma of the left atrium mimicking a left atrial myxoma. J Thorac Cardiovasc Surg. 2006;131:224–6.
51. Thiene G, Valente M, Lombardi M, Basso C. Tumours of the heart. In: Camm JA, Luscher TF, Serruys PV, editors. ESC textbook of cardiovascular medicine. Oxford: Oxford University Press; 2009.
52. Rickelt S, Rizzo S, Doerflinger Y, Zentgraf H, Basso C, Gerosa G, Thiene G, Moll R, Franke WW. A novel kind of tumor type-characteristic junction: plakophilin-2 as a major protein of adherens junctions in cardiac myxomata. Mod Pathol. 2010;23:1429–37.
53. Padalino MA, Vida VL, Bhattarai A, Reffo E, Milanesi O, Thiene G, Stellin G, Basso C. Giant intramural left ventricular rhabdomyoma in a newborn. Circulation. 2011;124:2275–7.
54. Perazzolo M, Thiene G, De Lazzari M, Calabrese F, Lacognata C, Rizzo S, Cacciavillani L, Tona F, Corbetti F, Iliceto S, Basso C. Concealed metastatic lung carcinoma presenting as acute coronary syndrome with progressive conduction abnormalities. Circulation. 2012;125:e499–502.
55. Padalino MA, Vida VL, Boccuzzo G, Tonello M, Sarris GE, Berggren H, Comas JV, Di Carlo D, Di Donato RM, Ebels T, Hraska V, Jacobs JP, Gaynor JW, Metras D, Pretre R, Pozzi M, Rubay J, Sairanen H, Schreiber C, Maruszewski B, Basso C, Stellin G. Surgery for primary cardiac tumors in children: early and late results in a multicenter European congenital heart surgeons association study. Circulation. 2012;126:22–30.

Cardiac Tumors: Classification and Epidemiology

2

Gaetano Thiene, Cristina Basso, Stefania Rizzo, Gino Gerosa, Giovanni Stellin, and Marialuisa Valente

Introduction

The precise prevalence of primary cardiac tumors in the general population is still unknown and is based on old postmortem studies.

In a study of 12,485 autopsies carried out in the time interval 1972–1991, Lam et al. reported a rate of 0.056% for primary (56 cases per 100,000 autopsies), and of 1.23% for secondary tumors (123 cases per 10,000 autopsies) [1]. However, epidemiological data are strongly influenced by when and where the data have been collected and do not necessarily reflect the real incidence in the population.

For instance, at the Mayo Clinic the autopsy prevalence of primary cardiac tumors was 0.05% in the time interval 1915–1930; when, with the advent of cardiac surgery, it became a referral center for diagnostic and therapeutic purposes, the autopsy prevalence had a threefold increase up to 0.17%, in the time interval 1954–1970 [2].

As far as secondary cardiac tumors, an investigation performed at our University in the time interval 1967–1976 revealed that among 7,460 autopsies the cause of death was malignancies in 1,181 cases (15.33%) [3], in 74 of which cardiac metastases occurred. This accounted for 1% of all autopsies and 6% of those with malignancies.

Anyway, it is generally agreed that autopsy prevalence of primary cardiac tumors is 1 out of 2,000 and that of secondary cardiac tumors is 1 out of 100 autopsies, with a secondary/primary cardiac tumors ratio of 20:1.

Classification of Cardiac Tumors

Although a classification of tumors can be based upon cellular organization (proliferative reaction, hamartoma, cyst, and true neoplasm, either benign or malignant) or tumor histotype (mesenchymal, epithelial, mesothelial), it is easier to follow the classic distinction between benign and malignant, differentiating cardiac and pericardial tumors [4].

The World Health Organization recently convened a group of pathologists to put forward a new classification of primary cardiac tumors (Table 2.1).

Although some neoplasms or tumor-like lesions have been ignored (cysts of pericardium,

G. Thiene, M.D. (✉) • C. Basso, M.D., Ph.D.
S. Rizzo, M.D. • M. Valente, M.D.
Pathological Anatomy, Department of Cardiac, Thoracic and Vascular Sciences, Azienda Ospedaliera-University of Padua Medical School, via A. Gabelli, 61, Padua 35121, Italy
e-mail: gaetano.thiene@unipd.it

G. Gerosa, M.D.
Cardiac Surgery, Department of Cardiac, Thoracic and Vascular Sciences, Azienda Ospedaliera-University of Padua Medical School, via N. Giustiniani, 2, Padua 35128, Italy

G. Stellin, M.D.
Pediatric Cardiac Surgery, Department of Cardiac, Thoracic and Vascular Sciences, Azienda Ospedaliera-University of Padua Medical School, via N. Giustiniani, 2, Padua 35128, Italy

C. Basso et al. (eds.), *Cardiac Tumor Pathology*, Current Clinical Pathology,
DOI 10.1007/978-1-62703-143-1_2, © Springer Science+Business Media New York 2013

Table 2.1 Histological classification of tumors of the heart, World Health Organization (from Travis et al. [4])

Benign tumors and tumor-like lesions	
Rhabdomyoma	8,900/0
Histiocytoid cardiomyopathy (Purkinje cell tumor)	
Hamartoma of mature cardiac myocytes	
Adult cellular rhabdomyoma	8,904/0
Cardiac myxoma	8,840/0
Papillary fibroelastoma	
Hemangioma	9,120/0
Cardiac fibroma	8,810/0
Inflammatory myofibroblastic tumor	8,825/1
Lipoma	8,850/0
Cystic tumor of the atrioventricular node	
Malignant tumors	
Angiosarcoma	9,120/3
Epithelioid hemangioendothelioma	9,133/3
Malignant pleomorphic fibrous histiocytoma (MFH)/undifferentiated pleomorphic sarcoma	8,830/3
Fibrosarcoma and myxoid fibrosarcoma	8,840/3
Rhabdomyosarcoma	8,900/3
Leiomyosarcoma	8,890/3
Synovial sarcoma	9,040/3
Liposarcoma	8,854/3
Cardiac lymphoma	
Metastatic tumors	
Pericardial tumors	
Solitary fibrous tumor	8,815/1
Malignant mesothelioma	9,050/3
Germ cell tumors	
Metastatic pericardial tumors	

blood cysts), this classification has the merit of unifying the terminology. Since cardiac tumors have been variously named, we will add the synonym for each histotype. According to this last classification, cardiac tumors are grouped into three categories, i.e., benign tumors and tumor-like lesions; malignant tumors; and pericardial tumors.

According to the morphology code of the International Classification of Diseases for Oncology (ICD-0) [5] and the Systematized Nomenclature of Medicine (http://snomed.org) the biological behavior is coded /0 for benign tumors, /3 for malignant tumors, and /1 for "borderline" or uncertain behavior.

Malignant Cardiac Tumors, Grading and Staging

Given their low frequency, there is no grading system for malignant cardiac tumors and we have to refer to the criteria used for soft tissue neoplasms [6]. The main parameters in non-cardiac soft tissue tumors are the mitotic index and the extent of tumor necrosis [7, 8].

Three grades of malignancy are usually recognized: G1, low grade; G2, intermediate grade; G3, high grade.

The FNCLCC (Fédération Nationale des Centre de Lutte Contre le Cancer) system is based on a score obtained by evaluating three features: tumor differentiation, mitotic rate, and amount of tumor necrosis. A score is attributed independently to each of the three parameters and the final histological grade is the sum of the three attributed scores (Table 2.2) [8].

As a general rule, grading should be used only for untreated primary soft tissue sarcomas and should be performed on representative material (for instance, tissue obtained through endomyocardial biopsy cannot be used for grading purposes).

Concerning the epidemiology and prevalence of various tumor histotypes, the data are also not uniform in the literature. Being a rare disease, the published numbers of primary cardiac tumors frequently reflect a referral bias. This is for instance the case of the data reported by the series of the Armed Force Institute of Pathology (AFIP) in Washington [9], which remains the most quoted histopathology publication on cardiac tumors, based upon 386 cases of primary cardiac tumors. The rates of 35% for primary sarcomas and of only 29% for myxomas, clearly reflect the referral bias of data derived from pathology tertiary centers, where only the most difficult cases are sent for expert opinion.

The difficulty in obtaining real epidemiological data on primary cardiac tumors is emphasized by the nonreliability of both autopsy and surgical pathology series, since in the former there is the selection bias of dead patients during hospitalization and in the latter that of indication to surgery

Table 2.2 Parameters of the grading system for sarcomas of the Féderation Nationale des Centres de Lutte contre le Cancer (FNCLCC)

Tumor differentiation	
Score 1	Sarcomas closely resembling normal adult mesenchymal tissue (e.g., low-grade leiomyosarcoma)
Score 2	Sarcomas for which histological typing is certain (e.g., myxoid fibrosarcoma)
Score 3	Undifferentiated sarcoma, angiosarcoma
Mitotic count	
Score 1	0–9 mitoses per 10 HPF[a]
Score 2	10–19 mitoses per 10 HPF[a]
Score 3	≥20 mitoses per 10 HPF[a]
Tumor necrosis	
Score 0	No necrosis
Score 1	<50% tumor necrosis
Score 2	≥50% tumor necrosis
Histological grade	
Grade 1 (G1)	Total score 2, 3
Grade 2 (G2)	Total score 4, 5
Grade 3 (G3)	Total score 6, 7, 8

Modified from Trojani et al. [8]
[a]A high-power field (HPF) measures 0.1734 mm^2

(see for instance rhabdomyoma) or tumor resectability (see for instance primary malignant cardiac tumors with infiltration and metastases).

We herein refer to the clinicopathologic experience of the University of Padua, Italy in the time interval 1970–2010.

Epidemiology of Primary Cardiac Tumors 1970–2010 at the University of Padua

In the time interval 1970–2010, 267 primary cardiac and pericardial tumors have been studied, including 239 bioptic (89.5%) and 28 autoptic (10.5%) (Fig. 2.1). This is mostly a biopsy-based experience, thus emphasizing that nowadays cardiac tumors are uncommonly fatal, with the exception of the rare primary malignant forms.

Among the consecutive 239 bioptic primary cardiac tumors (135 female, age ranging 1 day–85 years, mean 48 ± 22 years, median 53), only 26 (10.5%) were malignant and 213 (89.5%) benign (Fig. 2.2).

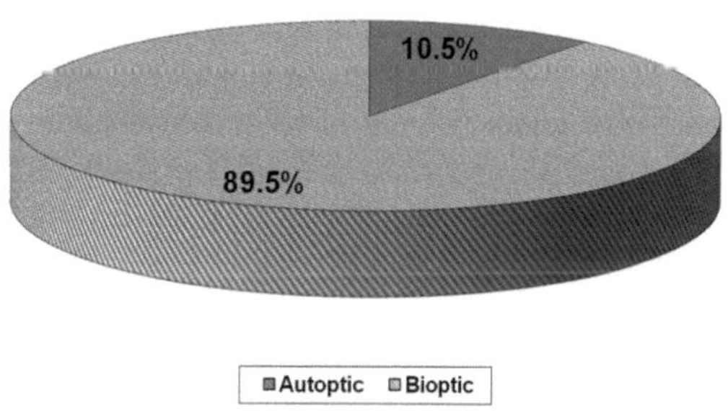

Fig. 2.1 Primary cardiac and pericardial tumors, University of Padua Medical School (1970–2010): 267 cases, 239 (89.5%) bioptic and 28 (10.5%) autoptic

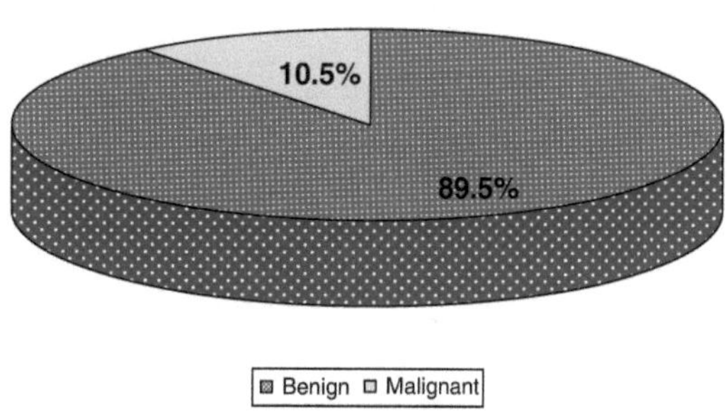

Fig. 2.2 Primary bioptic cardiac and pericardial tumors, University of Padua Medical School (1970–2010): 239 cases, 213 (89.5%) benign and 26 (10.5%) malignant

In eight cases (3.5%) the diagnosis was achieved through preoperative biopsy: endomyocardial in four cases (right atrium angiosarcoma in three and fibrosarcoma in one, respectively) and thoracotomic in four cases (two right ventricular fibromas, one left ventricular hemangioma, and one left atrial malignant schwannoma). Cardiac transplantation was performed in three cases (1.25%, all with cardiac fibroma).

Primary Malignant Bioptic Cardiac Tumors

The population consists of 26 patients, 15 male and 11 female, age ranging 21–80 years, mean 50±13. They died within 6 months from clinical onset, with the exception of three cases, i.e., a 21-year-old woman with left atrial leiomyosarcoma, who was still alive 96 months after surgical resection and adjuvant chemotherapy [10]; and two cases operated of right atrial angiosarcoma who were alive at a follow-up of 12 and 18 months, respectively. The most prevalent histotype was leiomyosarcoma and angiosarcoma (19% each) and undifferentiated sarcoma (15.5%). The various tumor histotypes are illustrated in Fig. 2.3.

Tumor location was the left atrium in eight (three undifferentiated sarcomas, two leiomyosarcomas, one fibrosarcoma, one malignant fibrous histiocytoma, and one malignant schwannoma); the right atrium in eight (five angiosarcomas, one B cell lymphoma, one fibrosarcoma, and one malignant fibrous histiocytoma), the right ventricle in two (one leiomyosarcoma, one malignant fibrous histiocytoma), the pulmonary artery in two (leiomyosarcoma), and the pericardium in four (malignant mesothelioma in three and undifferentiated sarcoma in one); finally, in two lymphomas cardiac involvement was diffuse without any chamber predilection.

Primary Benign Bioptic Cardiac Tumors

A consecutive series of 213 bioptic benign cardiac tumors have been studied in the same years, mean 48.1±22.5, median 53 years. Figure 2.4 illustrates the various histotypes.

Cardiac myxoma is the most frequent primary cardiac tumor. A consecutive series of 141 surgi-

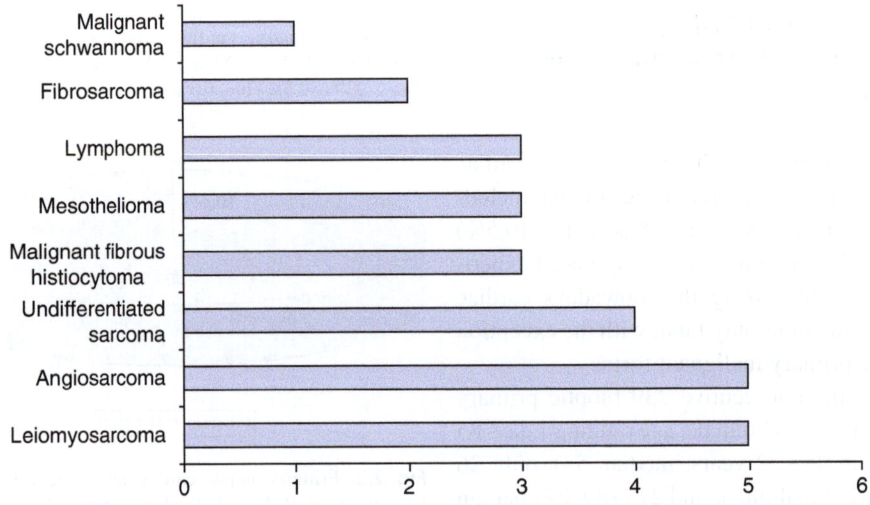

Fig. 2.3 Primary bioptic malignant cardiac and pericardial tumors, University of Padua Medical School (1970–2010): 26 cases. Prevalence of various tumor histotypes

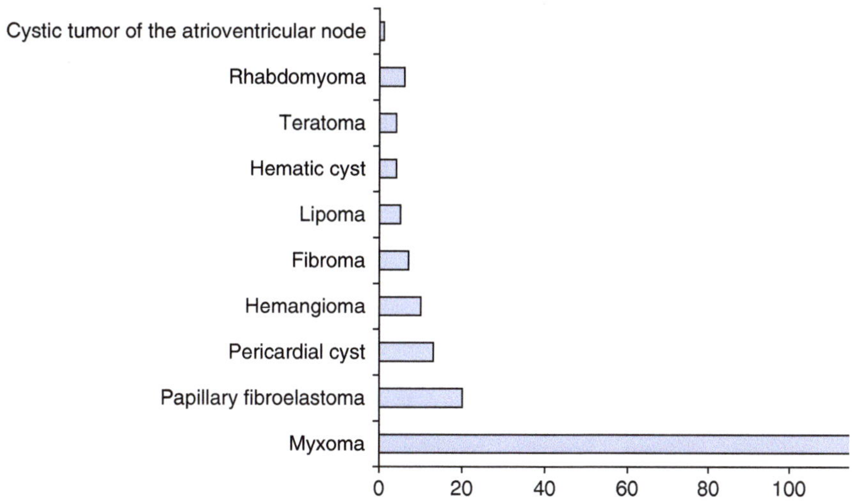

Fig. 2.4 Primary bioptic benign cardiac and pericardial tumors, University of Padua Medical School (1970–2010): 213 cases. Prevalence of various tumor histotypes

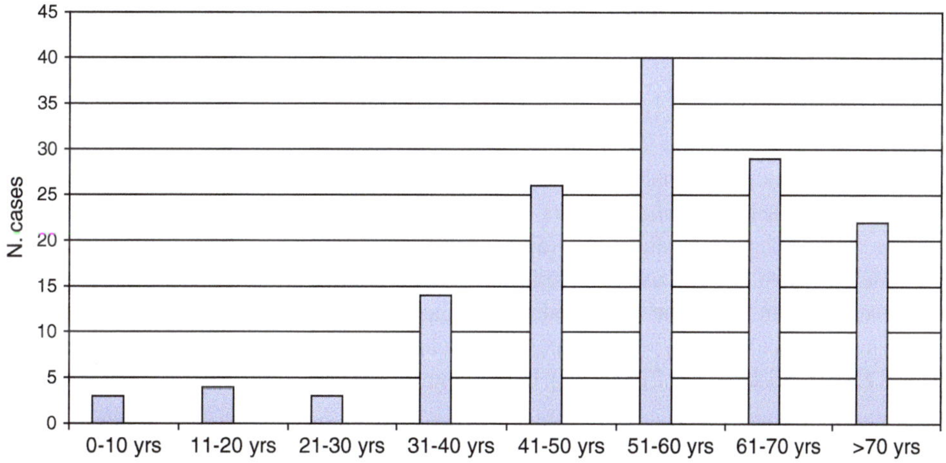

Fig. 2.5 Cardiac myxoma, University of Padua Medical School (1970–2010): 141 bioptic cases. Distribution according to age intervals

cally resected myxomas has been collected, representing 59% of all primary bioptic cardiac tumors and 66% of benign bioptic cardiac tumors. The majority were female (88, 62.5%), the age range was 2–85 years (mean 54 ± 16, median 56).

Figure 2.5 reports the distribution of cardiac myxomas per age, showing a peak of incidence in people 50–60 years of age; only six cases (4%) have been surgically resected in the pediatric age (<18 years).

Location of cardiac myxoma was mostly the left atrium (116 cases, 82.5%), followed by the right atrium (22 cases, 15.5%), and exceptionally the ventricles (the right ventricle in two cases and the left ventricle in one case, 2%) (Fig. 2.6). In our experience, a valvular location was never observed. The weight ranged from 2 to 125 g (mean 38 ± 24) and the surface was smooth in 65% and villous in 35% of cases.

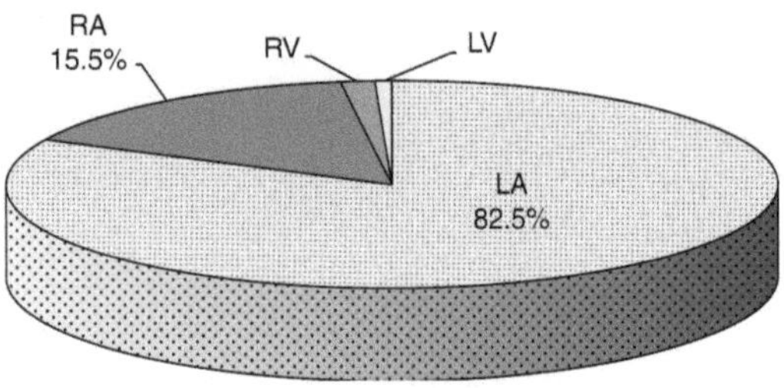

Fig. 2.6 Cardiac myxoma, University of Padua Medical School (1970–2010): 141 bioptic cases. Distribution according to tumor location (LA left atrium; LV left ventricle; RA right atrium; RV right ventricle)

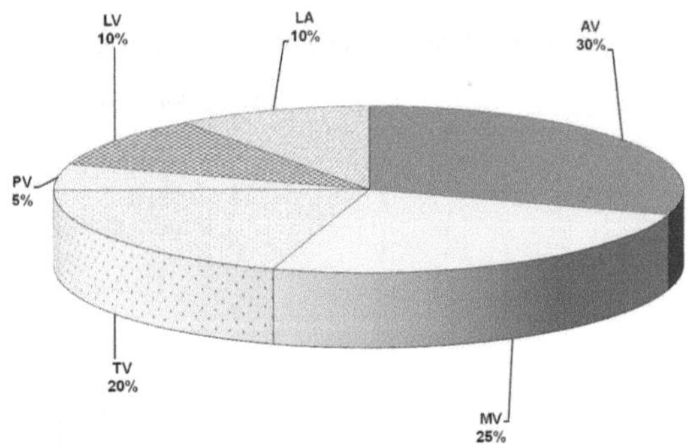

Fig. 2.8 Papillary fibroelastoma, University of Padua Medical School (1970–2010): 20 bioptic cases. Distribution according to tumor location (*AV* aortic valve, *LA* left atrium, *LV* left ventricle, *MV* mitral valve, *PV* pulmonary valve, *TV* tricuspid valve)

As far as clinical presentation is concerned, signs and symptoms of hemodynamic obstruction were present in 60% of cases, constitutional symptoms in 30%, embolic phenomena in 16%, while one-fourth of patients were asymptomatic and myxoma was an incidental finding during echocardiographic examination (Fig. 2.7).

Papillary fibroelastoma (or endocardial papilloma) represents the second most frequent primary cardiac tumor after myxoma. Twenty cases have been surgically resected in 19 patients (8.5% of all primary bioptic cardiac tumors and 9.5% of benign bioptic cardiac tumors), 11 female, age ranging 24–78 years, mean 57 ± 17, median 52.5 years. The location was the valvular endocardium in 16 (aortic valve in 6, mitral valve in 5, tricuspid valve in 4, and pulmonary valve in 1) and the mural endocardium in 4 (left ventricular cavity and/or papillary muscles in 2 and left atrial cavity in 2) (Fig. 2.8). In 10 patients, the diagnosis was incidental during routine echocardiograpy (seven) or during cardiac surgery (three), while in the remaining nine patients it was achieved due to signs and symptoms of myocardial ischemia (six cases), heart failure (two cases) or arrhythmias (one case).

Hemangioma. Ten patients were studied, 4 males, age ranging from 2 days to 73 years, mean 30 ± 30 years, median 19 years. Cardiac hemangioma was intramural in 2 (left ventricular free wall and atrial septum, one each), intracavitary in 7 (right atrium in 2, right ventricle in 2, left atrium in 1, left ventricle in 1, mitral valve in 1), and pericardial in 1. The diagnosis was achieved during echocardiographic examination (nine cases) or intraoperatively (one case).

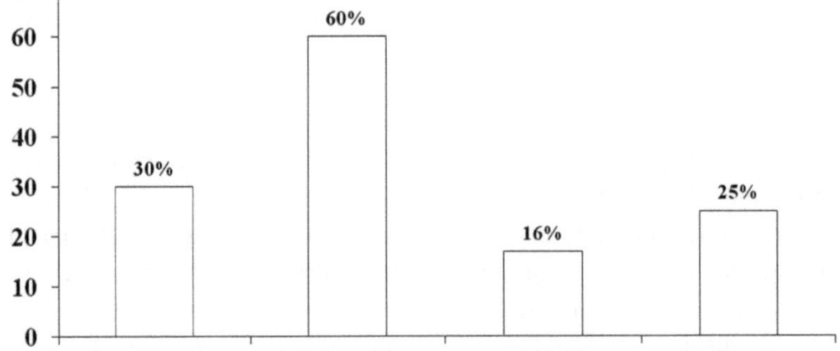

Fig. 2.7 Cardiac myxoma, University of Padua Medical School (1970–2010): 141 bioptic cases. Clinical presentation

Fibroma. Seven patients, four female, age ranging 1 month–40 years (mean 6 ± 14 years, median 6 months) were studied. The fibroma was located in the interventricular septum in three, right ventricular free wall in two, and left ventricular free wall in two. In three cases, surgical resection was not feasible and cardiac transplantation was performed.

Hematic cyst. Four cases were collected, all in infants (two male and one female, age ranging 4–11 months) but one (a 70-year-old woman). Two of them occurred in the setting of a congenital heart disease (hypoplastic right heart and tetralogy of Fallot, respectively). They were located at the level of the tricuspid valve in two, of the right atrium in one, and of inferior vena cava orifice in one.

Teratoma. Four patients, one male and three female, age ranging 1 month–35 years (median 1 month) were operated, all but one presenting with congestive heart failure since birth and with radiographic and echocardiographic evidence of pericardial mass.

Rhabdomyoma. Six patients, three female and three male, age ranging 7 days–4 months (mean 46 ± 47 days, median 22 days), had a surgically resected rhabdomyoma. In all, cardiac rhabdomyoma had an intracavitary growth with obstructive symptoms, at the level of the left ventricular outflow tract in four and of the right ventricular outflow tract in two.

Lipoma. Five surgically resected cases have been studied, including a 75 year old woman with lipomatous hypertrophy of the interatrial septum. The remaining four cases are true lipomas, with either an intracavitary growth (on the mitral valve-male 24 year old—and in the right atrium—male 61year old and female 85 year old) or pericardial (male 64 year old).

Cystic tumor of the atrioventricular node (or Tawarioma). One surgically resected case has been examined in a full heart specimen coming from cardiectomy for heart transplantation (male 39 year old, dilated cardiomyopathy).

Pericardial cyst. Thirteen cases, 10 male and three female, age ranging 22–68 years, mean 48.5 ± 13, median 52 years have been collected. These tumors represent the third most common primary cardiac and pericardial tumor in our bioptic experience, after myxoma and papilloma.

Primary Cardiac Tumors in the Pediatric Age (<18 years)

The pediatric experience (<18 years) consists of 29 cases (12% of all primary bioptic cardiac tumors), 13 female and 16 male, age ranging 1 day–18 years, mean 43 months, median 4 months.

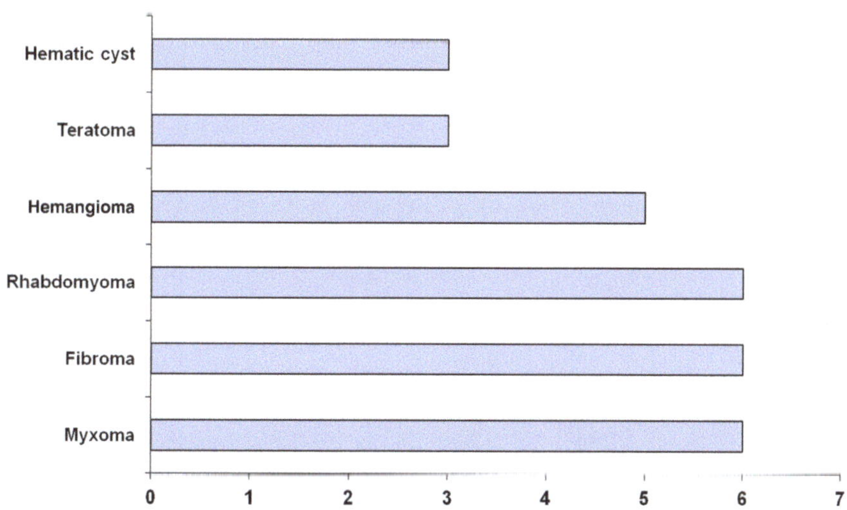

Fig. 2.9 Primary cardiac tumors in the pediatric age, University of Padua Medical School (1970–2010): 29 bioptic cases (12%). Prevalence of various tumor histotypes

They are all benign primary cardiac tumors, consisting of 6 myxomas (21%), 6 fibromas (21%), 6 rhabdomyomas (21%), 5 hemangiomas (17%), 3 pericardial teratomas (10%), and 3 hematic cysts (10%) (Fig. 2.9).

References

1. Lam KY, Dickens P, Chan AC. Tumors of the heart. A 20-year experience with a review of 12,485 consecutive autopsies. Arch Pathol Lab Med. 1993;117:1027–31.
2. Wold LE, Lie JT. Cardiac myxomas: a clinicopathologic profile. Am J Pathol. 1980;101:219–40.
3. Terribile V, Fassina A. Le neoplasie secondarie del cuore. In: Il problema delle metastasi. Atti del XIV Congresso Nazionale della Società Italiana di Patologia (Catania, 3–6 novembre 1977). Roma: Società Editrice Universo, 1978. p. 426–31
4. Travis WD, Brambilla E, Muller-Hermelink H, Harris CC. Pathology and genetics of tumours of the lung, pleura, thymus and heart. Lyon: IARC Press; 2004.
5. Fritz A, Jack A, Parkin DM, Percy C, Shanmugarathan S, Sobin L, Whelan S. International classification of diseases for oncology. 3rd ed. Geneva: World Health Organization; 2000.
6. Fletcher CDM, Unni KK, Mertens F. World Health Organization classification of tumours. Pathology and genetics of tumours of soft tissue and bone. Lyon: IARC Press; 2002.
7. van Unnik JA, Coindre JM, Contesso C, Albus-Lutter CE, Schiodt T, Sylvester R, Thomas D, Bramwell V, Mouridsen HT. Grading of soft tissue sarcomas: experience of the EORTC soft tissue and bone sarcoma group. Eur J Cancer. 1993;29:2089–93.
8. Trojani M, Contesso G, Coindre JM, Rodesse J, Bui NB, de Mascarel A, Goussot JF, David M, Bonichon F, Lagarde C. Soft-tissue sarcomas of adults: study of pathological prognostic variables and definition of a histopathological grading system. Int J Cancer. 1984;33:37–42.
9. Burke AP, Virmani R. Tumours of the heart and great vessels. 3rd ed. Washington, DC: Armed Forces Institute of Pathology; 1996.
10. Mazzola A, Spano JP, Valente M, Gregoriani R, Villani C, Di Eusanio M, Ciocca M, Minuti U, Giancola R, Basso C, Thiene G. Leiomyosarcoma of the left atrium mimicking a left atrial myxoma. J Thorac Cardiovasc Surg. 2006;131:224–6.

3 Cardiac Myxoma

Giovanni Bartoloni and Angela Pucci

Introduction

Primary cardiac tumors are rare and cardiac myxomas represent the most common neoplasms among these [1–4]. The mean age at diagnosis is 50 years, but occasionally they can be seen in younger patients, and they are mainly found in females, localized to *foramen ovale* in the left atrium and in up to 5% of cases overriding it and apparently looking as a biatrial tumor [5–8]. Cardiac myxomas are usually single tumors [4, 6], but rarely they can be multiple and familial as part of Carney complex [9–13]. They have uncertain histogenesis and show a wide range of clinical presentations that may mimic a variety of neoplastic and nonneoplastic conditions [14, 15]. Cardiac myxomas may cause recurrent strokes, peripheral or pulmonary embolism, and constitutional symptoms (i.e., fever, weight loss, high sedimentation rate, anemia, and/or leucocytosis), syncope, or even sudden death [16]. These tumor characteristics, together with possible tumor relapse following incomplete surgical resection, have contributed to the controversial issue of *malignant myxomas or metastatic potential of cardiac myxomas* [17–19]. Several histological, cytogenetic, and molecular studies have been investigating their pathological and biological characteristics, including mechanisms of growth and embolic potential, and increasing evidences are confirming the benign biology of cardiac myxoma. Modern histological criteria and diagnostic tools (i.e., immunohistochemistry and molecular biology) are helpful for differential diagnosis from *myxoid sarcomas* that may share similar gross features but have malignant behavior and often poor prognosis [17, 20].

G. Bartoloni, M.D. (✉)
Histopathology Department, "GB Ingrassia" Catania University, via Santa Sofia, 87, Catania 95123, Italy
e-mail: gbartolo@unict.it

A. Pucci, M.D.
Histopathology Department, Azienda Ospedaliera-Pisa University Hospital, via Roma, Pisa 56126, Italy
e-mail: angelapucci@libero.it

Epidemiology

Primary tumors of the heart are rare, their reported incidence ranging between 0.0017 and 0.03% in autopsy series, and 50% of them are represented by myxoma [2, 6, 14]. This percentage value might be underestimated, because in surgical series they represent up to 78% of primary heart tumors [1, 4]. They show a female preponderance, with *F*/*M* ratio of 1.8/1, a mean age at diagnosis of 50 years, most patients being in 30–60 age range [5, 17]. Nevertheless they are reported also in pediatric age, and as a part of a genetic disease (i.e., Carney complex) they are diagnosed in young patients without sex predilection [13, 21, 22].

C. Basso et al. (eds.), *Cardiac Tumor Pathology*, Current Clinical Pathology,
DOI 10.1007/978-1-62703-143-1_3, © Springer Science+Business Media New York 2013

Clinical Aspects

The clinical features are determined by their location, size, and mobility, and there is no any pathognomonic sign or symptom [2, 14, 15]. The most common presenting symptom is systemic embolism (30–50% of cases) requiring histology for etiological diagnosis, followed by congestive heart failure because of mitral valve obstruction with possible supraventricular arrhythmias [15]. Atrial myxomas may cause obstruction of (pulmonary or systemic) venous drainage or of atrio-ventricular valves with valve stenosis, syncope, and even sudden death after abrupt mitral valve obstruction [16, 23].

Nonspecific constitutional symptoms and signs may occur in up to 90% of cases. They include myalgia, muscle weakness, arthralgia, fever, weight loss, fatigue, and skin manifestations, and may be associated with elevated serum levels of inflammatory cytokines (in particular IL-6) [24, 25]. Such signs and symptoms do occur in a variety of other infectious (endocarditis or rheumatic fever), or immunologic (rheumatoid arthritis, vasculitis, connective tissue) diseases but also in other neoplastic conditions (often associated with malignant tumors).

Unusual clinical presentations have been described in a few cases of cardiac myxomas, including infected cardiac myxomas that are very fragile and may lead to a catastrophic disorder with systemic bacteremia, mycotic embolism, and disseminated intravascular coagulation [26] or anecdotical cases with pulsatile tinnitus, back pain, and hair loss [27].

In a minority of cases, cardiac myxomas are asymptomatic representing an incidental finding at autopsy or in vivo, this latter event being quite frequent nowadays because of the widespread use of echocardiography in routinely diagnostic investigations [14].

Multiple cardiac myxomas are rare [6, 14]. They may be localized to the ventricles, show a high recurrence rate and be part of Carney complex, a familial disorder with autosomical dominant transmission including NAME (naevi, atrial myxoma, myxoid neurofibromata, and ephelides) [28] or LAMB (lentigines, atrial myxoma, mucocutaneous myxoma, and blue naevi) [10] syndrome and associated with the germline mutation PRKAR1A [29, 30]. Carney complex has been firstly described in 1985 by Carney, it represents about 10% of total cardiac myxoma cases and is usually diagnosed in younger patients with no sex differences [13]. Approximately 30–60% of Carney complex patients will develop cardiac myxomas and cardiac complications are the cause of death in more than half of them [31–33].

The most recent diagnostic criteria of Carney complex include spotty skin pigmentation, cutaneous and cardiac myxomas, breast myxomatosis, paradoxical positive response of urinary glucocorticosteroids to dexamethasone administration during liddle's test, acromegaly, blue nevus and epithelioid blue nevus, osteochondromyxoma and/or thyroid carcinoma [12, 29, 34, 35].

Tumor Biology

The growth speed of cardiac myxoma is estimated to be quite low, about 0.15 cm per month or 1.8 cm per year, corresponding to a monthly weight increase of 1.2 g or 14 g per year, but recent echocardiographic data have raised the issue of a possible higher growth rate [36, 37]. On the other hand, growth may be influenced by the possible overlapping of various phenomena such as thrombosis, hemorrhage, or fragmentation causing tumor detachment and embolism.

Metalloproteases (MMP)-2 and MMP-9 overexpression has been found in embolic cardiac myxomas; it might increase the risk of embolism by contributing to excessive degradation of tumor extracellular matrix [38].

Mucins are expressed within myxoma matrix and their presence could favor tumor embolism [39]. In particular, expression of membrane-associated MUC1 has been reported to be higher than that of the secreted mucins, MUC2 and MUC5AC, the latter one having been related to lesser embolism.

Increased IL-6 and/or α1-globulin serum levels can be found in patients with cardiac myxoma, and have been proposed as predictive markers of embolic accidents; they represent activated immunological phenomena influencing tumor remodeling and increasing embolic potential [24, 25]. Moreover, a correlation has been seen between the preoperative tumor size (i.e., maximum diameter) and IL-6 and/or α1-globulin levels ($P < 0.005$) [25].

Recently, plakophilin-2 has been identified as a major protein of adherens junctions in cardiac myxomas [40]. So far, this type of junction has only sporadically been noted in some isolated cells or cell groups in a rhabdomyosarcoma, and general occurrence of plakophilin-2, associated with cadherin-11 in myxoma adherens junctions discloses new clues as to cell–cell adhesion and tumor growth and to new possible therapeutic concepts.

Histopathogenesis

Origin and histopathogenesis of cardiac myxoma are controversial, the two main hypotheses suggesting an origin from multipotent mesenchymal cells or from neural endocardial tissue [1–4, 41–49]. Their preferential site (i.e., *foramen ovale*) is considered to be consistent with an origin from multipotent mesenchymal cells or from embryonic rests [42, 43]. Kodama et al. have shown the expression of gene transcript in myxoma cells compatible with a mesenchymal origin [45]. Other authors have shown differentiation patterns and gene expression compatible with an origin form endocardial neural or embryonic tissue [44, 49]. Moreover, cardiac myxomas show peculiar features as compared to their extracardiac counterpart [20]. They share a similar mucopolysaccharide-rich extracellular matrix, but extracardiac myxomas lack the typical vascular and syncytial-like pattern of cardiac myxomas.

Neoplastic theory. Cardiac myxoma is considered an actual neoplasm. It is histologically distinct from thrombus that may echocardiographically and grossly mimic cardiac myxoma. Many evidences are supporting the neoplastic hypothesis, either by showing a definite pattern of differentiation, on the basis of cytological, ultrastructural, and immunohistochemical features, or demonstrating the biological characteristics by using experimental models such as in vitro cell cultures comparing thrombus and cardiac myxomas [50–52].

Thrombotic theory. Development of cardiac myxomas from thrombus has been hypothesized [53]. Myxomas apparently have a slow growth rate as mural intracardiac thrombus, often are partially covered by thrombotic depositions (similar to Lambl excrescences at gross examination) and share common features with organized thrombus (i.e., mucoid deposits, possible cartilaginous and/or osseous metaplasia) [54]. But cardiac myxomas are characterized by the typical neoplastic *lepidic* cells and by a well-defined vascularization.

Dysembryoplastic theory. Cardiac myxoma has been supposed to represent a hamartoma originating from endocardial embryonic myxoid rests localized to *foramen ovale* [16]. But, differently from other cardiac hamartomas such as rhabdomyomas, they are not present at birth, being usually diagnosed late in life, and do not spontaneously regress [7, 8].

Histopathogenesis of glandular cells in myxoma. Glandular structures may be rarely found within an otherwise typical cardiac myxoma. Morphological and immunohistochemical studies support two histopathogenetic hypotheses, that is a possible origin from embryonic foregut rests [46, 55] or a progressive differentiation from neoplastic multipotent myxoma cells [17]. During the embryonic development, the foregut and the primitive heart tube lie adjacent and in the same area as most cardiac myxomas, i.e., the *foramen ovale*, therefore glandular foregut rests might result to be embedded within myxoma, although embryonic glandular structures have never been described in the interatrial septum so far. Finally, lack of other cell lines and the different localization of myxomas are not consistent with teratoma hypothesis.

Genetics

PRKAR1A gene mutations in chromosome 2, band p16 and in chromosome 17, bands q22–24 are found in cardiac myxomas associated with Carney complex [29, 56], whereas most sporadic, non-familial myxomas do not show mutations [57]. Casey et al. demonstrated that mutations of PRKAR1A gene, codifying the regulatory subunit R1α of protein kinase A c-AMP dependent, acting as a tumor suppressor gene, are responsible of Carney complex [31, 34]. The Carney complex gene 1 was identified 10 years ago as the regulatory subunit 1A of protein kinase A (PRKAR1A) located at 17q22–24 [30, 31]. An inactivating heterozygous germline mutation of PRKAR1A is observed in about two-thirds of Carney complex patients [31–33]. Such mutations cause haploinsufficiency and reduction of protein with predisposition to tumorigenesis.

As to DNA analysis, many sporadic cases of cardiac myxomas have been shown to be diploid [58, 59].

Gross Features

Myxomas are intracardiac tumors and are more frequently found in the left atrium (about 75% of the cases), localized to the interatrial septum and adjacent to *foramen ovale*, although they may be found in any other cardiac chamber, i.e., right atrium (15–29%) or ventricles, whereas they are rare on a cardiac valves [1–4]. In this latter case, for a correct differential diagnosis, it has to be excluded the most frequent valve tumor, i.e., papillary fibroelastoma that may show gross features similar to myxoma, or the rare myxoid fibrosarcoma of the heart [2].

Cardiac myxomas have a highly variable size, in most cases the maximum diameter is

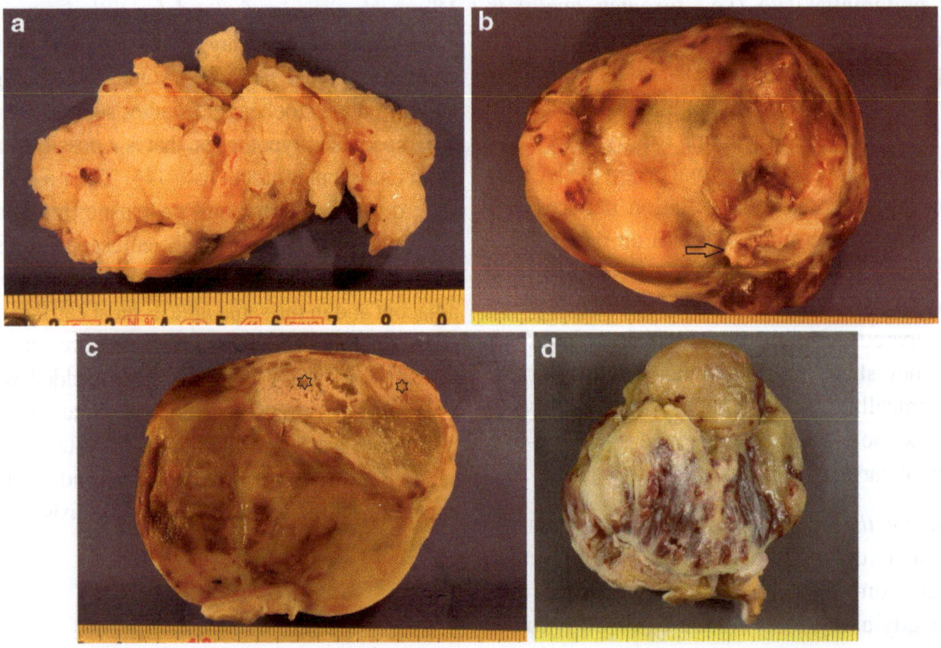

Fig. 3.1 Gross features of cardiac myxomas. (**a**) Myxoma with villous features, showing friable and soft projections on the surface. (**b**) Polypoid, oval myxoma with smooth and lobulated surface. Tumor attachment on the interatrial septum has been resected (*arrow*). (**c**) Cross-section of the same tumor evidencing attachment base, hemorrhagic foci, myxoid aspects, and a well-defined, necrotic area just beneath the tumor surface (*asterisks*). (**d**) Lobulated myxoma external surface; *dark hemorrhagic* foci are intermingled with *pale yellow* myxoid areas

between 6 and 7 cm with a mean weight of 40 g. Myxoma often presents as a smooth, oval and lobulated, or villous, friable and soft or gelatinous-like mass (Fig. 3.1). Flat and sessile myxomas are rare, and might result from embolization of most tumor mass. Rarely, cardiac myxomas show extensive calcifications with stone-like consistency, the so-called *lithomyxoma* [60], which is usually asymptomatic although complete embolization has been reported after pedicle detachment with floatation into the aorta causing patient death [61].

Histology

Common features. Cardiac myxoma is largely made up by amorphous mucopolysaccharide-rich matrix conferring the typically myxoid aspect. Within the myxoid stroma, few fibrillary structures and numerous thin-walled blood vessels are found together with the characteristic myxoma cells, or *lepidic cells* [2, 4, 17] (Fig. 3.2) indicating (see ancient Greek *lepis* term) the scale-like cell shape. *Lepidic* cells are stretched or star-shaped, show round or oval nucleus with often evident nucleolus, may be binucleated and even display syncytial features, but they lack mitotic figures. They can be single, scattered cells or more frequently, they constitute small nests, cord-like or perivascular structures. Perivascular structures are made up of single or multiple *lepidic* cell layer/s surrounding a central lumen with endothelial lining, with alcian-blue amorphous substance deposits between the *lepidic* cell layers. Associated features consist of hemorrhage, extramedullary hematopoiesis, inflammatory infiltrates (made up of granulocytes, lymphocytes, plasma cells, macrophages, and hemosiderin-laden macrophages), hemosiderin deposits,

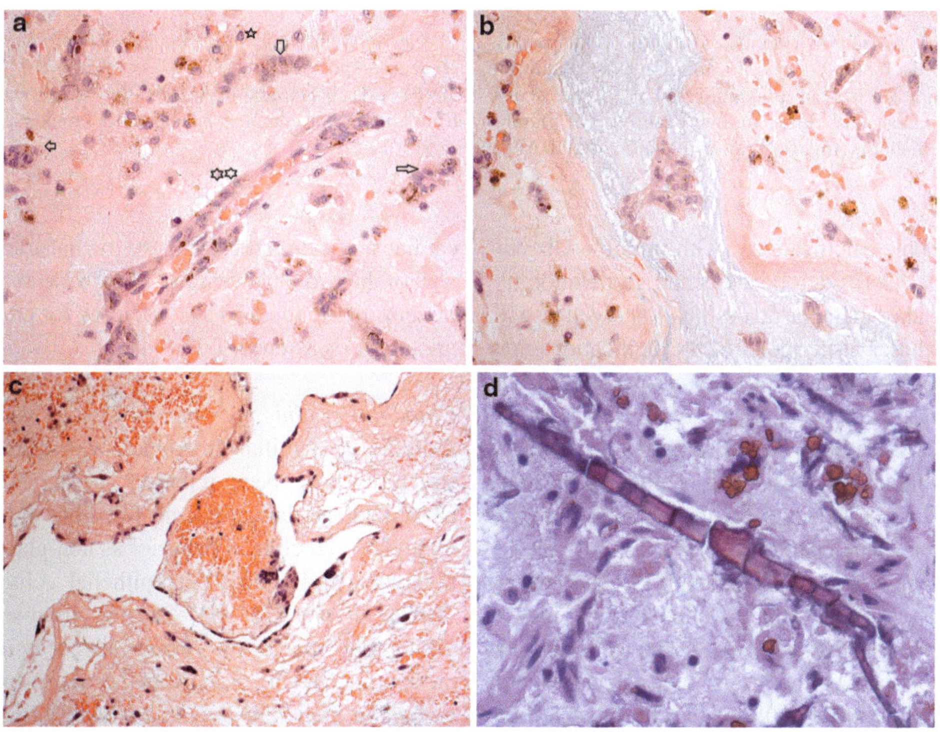

Fig. 3.2 Histologic features of cardiac myxomas. (**a**, **b**) Myxoma (*lepidic*) cells are embedded within myxoid stroma, as scattered single cells (*asterisk*), small solid nests (*arrow*) or in layers around vessels (*double asterisk*). Hemosiderin deposits and hemorrhage are also present. (**c**) Myxoma cells with syncytial-like features. (**d**) Extracellular deposits of hemosiderin with stretched structure (*bamboo-shaped* pattern)

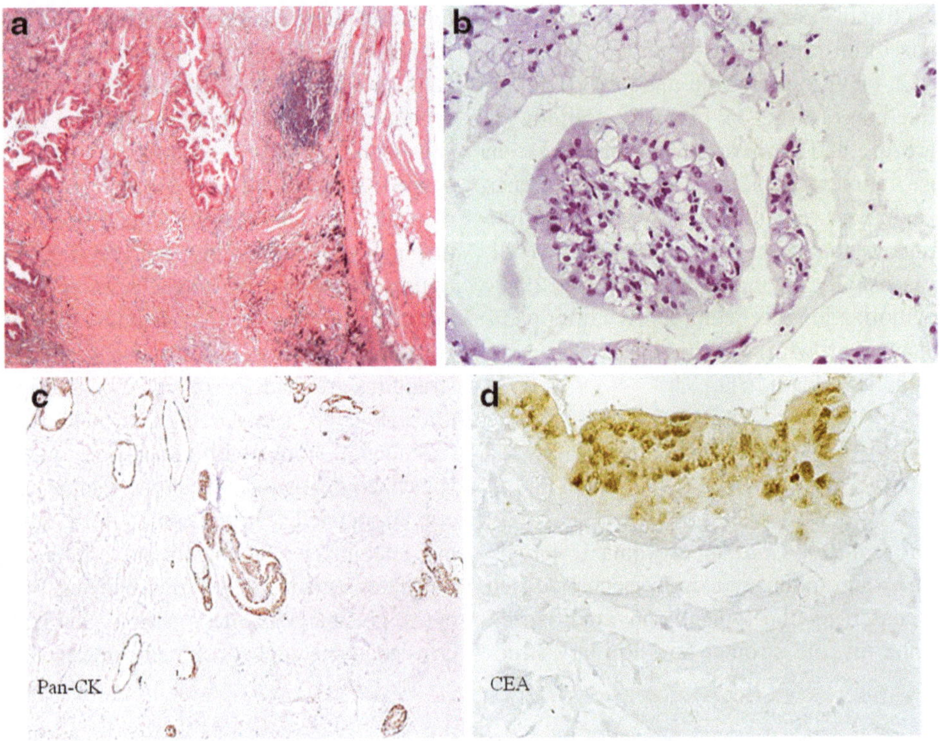

Fig. 3.3 *Glandular* myxomass .Reprinted with permission of the Italian Society of Cardiology. (**a**) Glands are present at the base of a myxoma. (**b**) High power view of glandular epithelium. Immunoreactivity of glandular epithelium for (**c**) pan-cytokeratin (AE1/AE3), (**d**) carcynoembryonic antigen (CEA), (**e**) protein S100, (**f**) neuron-specific enolase (NSE), cytokeratins 7 (**g**) and 20 (**h**) or (**i**) chromogranin A. Hematoxylin and eosin (**a**, **b**) avidin–biotin complex, hematoxylin counterstaining (**c–i**)

dystrophic calcifications (with possible Ghandi-Gamna sclerosiderotic areas and granulation tissue) and/or metaplastic ossification together with limited foci of necrosis [62]. Calcifications may develop also within cell cords or pseudovascular cuffings, with characteristic stripe or ring shapes, both of them showing faded edges. Finally, the extracellular deposits of hemosiderin may develop a stretched structure, i.e., the so-called bamboo-shaped pattern.

The myxoma pedicle is mainly constituted by fibrous tissue with thick-walled vessels, including arterioles with possible medial and/or intimal hyperplasia. At tumor basis, myxoma may microscopically infiltrate the adjacent endocardium and the underlying myocardium. Histologically, the infiltration is characterized by a stromal myxoid intercellular substance, which together with rare *lepidic* cells, makes its way through the cardiac myocytes and also in the medial arteriolar wall of the peduncle vessels. Then, wide excision margins of myxoma basis is required for preventing tumor recurrence.

Glandular cardiac myxoma. At least 28 cases of sporadic or familiar myxomas with glandular structures have been reported so far [50, 55, 63–65]. Glandular cardiac myxoma has the same biological and clinical behavior as non-glandular myxoma [9, 17, 55], but epithelial cells may display atypia [55, 63] causing troublesome differential diagnosis from adenocarcinoma metastasis [64] (Fig. 3.3). As to the rarely reported *malignant* glandular myxomas [66–69], in most cases the malignant behavior appears to be actually dependent upon embolism, local recurrence, or multifocality of tumor associated with incomplete excision [43, 70]. The glands are

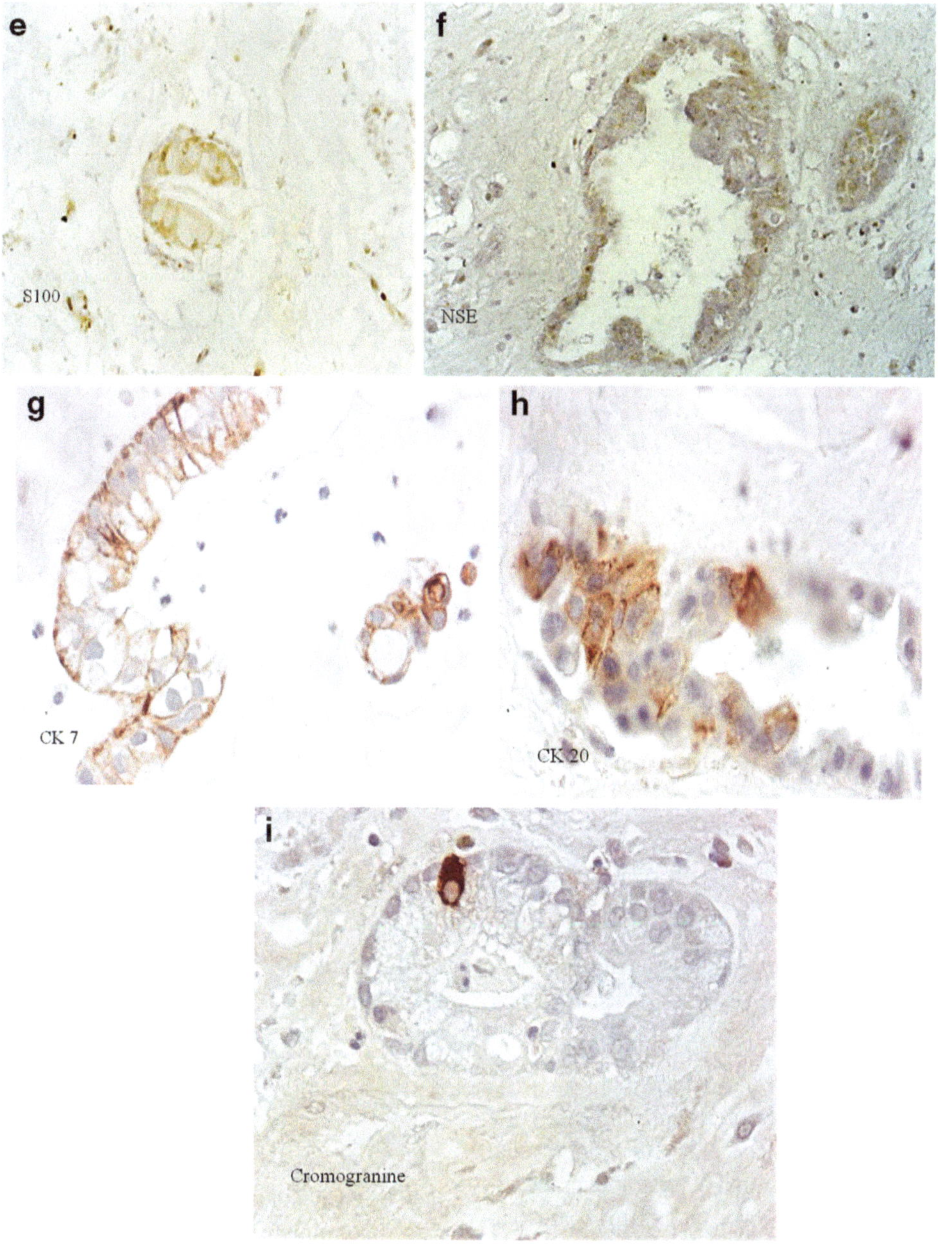

Fig. 3.3 (continued)

mainly localized close to tumor base, either scattered in a loose myxoid stroma or within myxoma cell islands. In the former pattern, single glandular structures or glandular clusters are found in the loose myxoid stroma, adjacent to the classical polygonal cell clusters of cardiac myxomas. The latter pattern is characterized by round or elongated glands usually centrally located in myxoma cell islands. Chronic inflammatory infiltrates may be present, around the glands or as intraepithelial granulocytes similar to active inflammation of the gastrointestinal mucosa. We have observed three cases of glandular myxoma, including a case with mild cellular atypia,

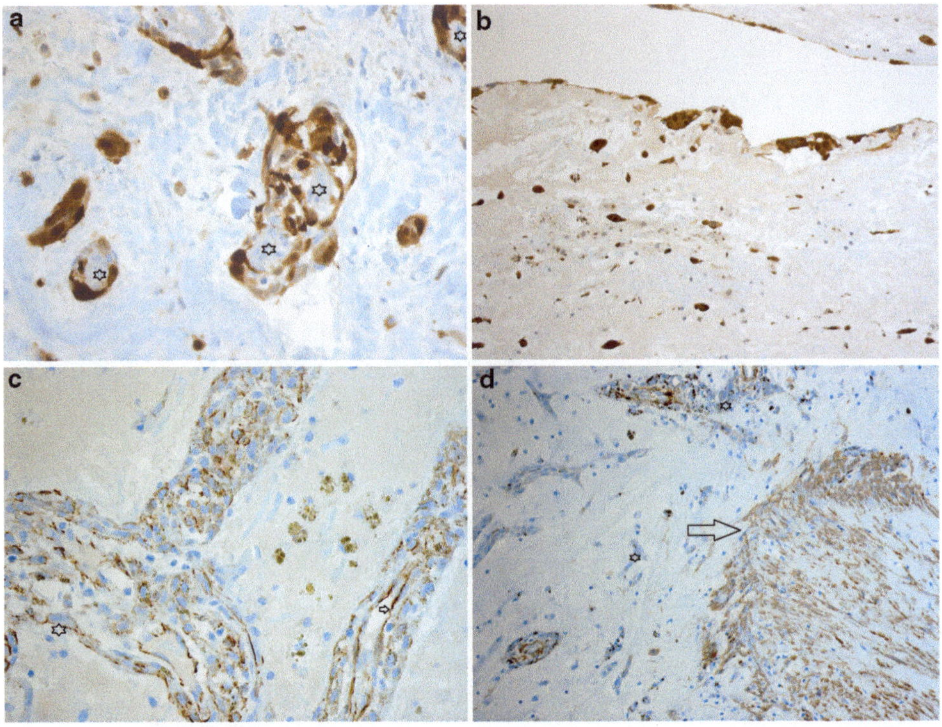

Fig. 3.4 Other immunohistochemical features of cardiac myxomas (**a**) S100-immunoreactivity is shown in *lepidic* myxoma cells whereas the inner endothelial cell layer (*asterisk*) is negative. (**b**) Calretinin-immunoreactivity in syncytial-like myxoma cells. (**c**) CD31 endothelial antigen immunoreactivity is shown in the inner endothelial cells (*arrow*) and in few myxoma cells (*asterisk*). (**d**) alpha-actin immunoreactivity in a group of smooth muscle cells (*arrow*) adjacent to myxoma *lepidic* (*asterisk*) cells

all of them undergoing complete excision without recurrence and free of events at a >5-year follow-up [55].

Other unusual features. Calcifications may be present in cardiac myxomas and rarely they are so extensive to be consistent with *lithomyxoma* which may require throughout histological examinations for diagnosis, the typical myxoma features (*lepidic cells*) being very limited [60, 61]. Recently, thymic rests with neoplastic transformation have been described in two. otherwise typical cardiac myxomas [71].

Immunohistochemistry

Lepidic cells. Neoplastic cells of myxoma have been shown to be immunoreactive for Calretinin, PGP 9.5 (protein gene product), NSE (neuron-specific enolase), protein S100, and synaptophysin, but also for vimentin and endothelin-1 [17, 43, 44, 50, 72] (Fig. 3.4). Epithelial and monocyte/macrophage markers are usually negative. Endothelial markers (FVIII, UEA, CD31, CD34, and UEA-1) are expressed by the endothelium of vessels present within myxoma, including the inner endothelial layer of myxoma cell nests, but immunoreactivity has been variably detected in the *lepidic* cells [43, 73, 74]. Such immunoreactivity pattern highlights the differentiation capabilities of *lepidic cells* and may support the most recent histogenetic hypotheses to origin from multipotent or embryonic stem cells, even if it has to be pointed out that neoplastic cells might express aberrant histotypes which do not always correlate to cell origin.

Glandular cells. Epithelial glandular cells, rarely present in myxomas, show an epithelial immunore-

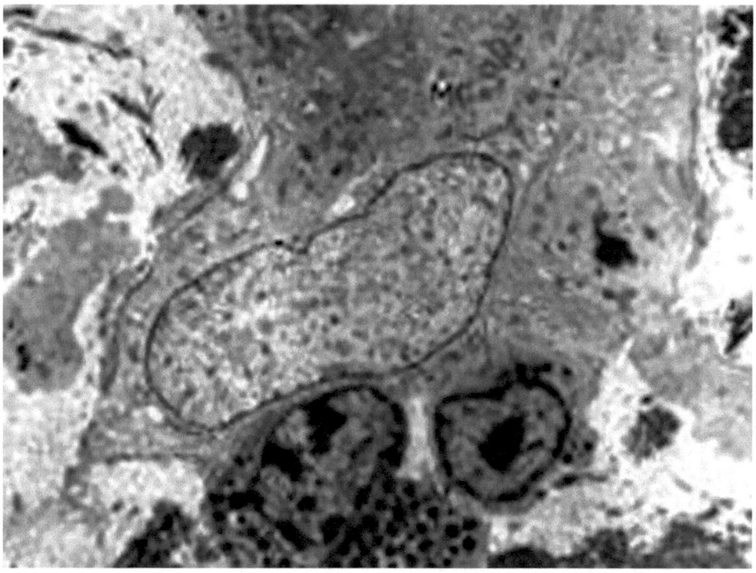

Fig. 3.5 Electron microscopy features of cardiac myxomas, lepidic cell of a cardiac myxoma (MC): rough endoplasmic reticulum, lysosomes, and iron deposits are shown in the cytoplasm. Mast cells (*M*) and collagen bundles are present within osmiophilic stroma (Uranyl acetate and lead citrate counterstaining)

activity pattern, i.e., cytokeratines 7 and 20, EMA, CEA, NSE, S100, and (focally) chromogranin positivity that is similar to the fundic mucous cells of the upper gastrointestinal tract [17, 18, 50, 55, 65] (Fig. 3.3).

Other cell elements. Within tumor, vessels of small and medium size (the latter ones usually close to the base), and smooth muscle cells, localized to the media of blood vessels or in groups of cells interspersed in the myxoid stroma, are variably detected (Fig. 3.4). They display their usual immunohistochemical differentiation pattern, being immunoreactive for endothelial (FVIII, EUA, CD31, and CD34) and muscular (muscle-specific actin and α-smooth muscle actin) markers, respectively [43, 74].

Electron Microscopy

Lepidic cells show a single, round, or elongated nucleus, with or without an evident nucleolus, and unevenly distributed cytoplasmic organelles (Fig. 3.5). They are characterized by a secretory pattern. Secretion activity of the myxoma neoplastic cell is in fact expressed in the synthesis of the neoplastic stroma. The cytoplasm shows abundant smooth and rough endoplasmic reticulum, free ribosomes, polyribosomes, and lysosomes, aside from pinocytotic vesicles [75, 76]. Moreover, mitochondria of variable shape and dimension are found, together with numerous filaments of 85–125 Å diameter, and up to 80 Å periodicity, focally showing myofibril-like arrangement. Iron deposits are frequently present in these cells.

Differential Diagnosis and Peculiar Clinical Aspects

Differential diagnosis of intracardiac myxoid masses requires histology. Myxoid tumors of the heart may correspond to biologically benign myxoma, to myxoid sarcomas, or even to cardiac metastasis [70, 77, 78]. The presence of myxoid stroma is not a pathognomonic feature and diagnosis of myxoma requires the presence of *lepidic* cells and the absence of mitosis. Hemorrhage,

Table 3.1 Cardiac myxoma: gross and histopathological criteria for differential diagnosis of the main intracardiac myxoid and non-myxoid tumors

Tumors	Myxoma	Fibrosarcoma	Angiosarcoma	Undifferenziated pleomorphic sarcoma (ex-malignant fibrous histiocytoma)	Osteosarcoma
Gross features	Occasional infiltration of attachment base	Almost usual infiltration of implant base	Mural infiltration and intracavitary growth	Mural infiltration	Mural infiltration
Histological features					
Cellularity	Isolated cells with inconspicuous cellular borders, mild or no atypia, no mitosis	Spindle cells with mild atypia and variable mitotic figures	Anastomosed vascular channels, endothelial cell pleomorphism, frequent mitoses	Severe atypia with numerous pleomorphic and multinucleated cells	Atypical cells (spindle shaped, epithelioid, rounded, plasmacytoid, etc.)
Architecture	Syncytial aggregates cell cords	Fasciculated pattern, frequent herringbone arrangement	Variable and pleomorphic pattern	Wide storiform arrangement	Mild fasciculated arrangement with osteoid foci
Vascular pattern	Perivascular structures	Plexiform or arborized capillary network	Anastomosed vascular channels	Hemangiopericytoma-like	Preponderant stroma compared to vascular component
Immunoreactivity	Vimentin, variable endothelial or neural markers	Vimentin, variable neural markers	Endothelial markers (CD34, CD31)	Variable (according or not to the different subtypes or cellular differentiation)	Osteonectin, osteocalcin
Other histological features	Inflammatory infiltrate with hemosiderin Calcifications, extramedullary hemopoyesis, metaplastic bone	Several (including myxoid) histological subtypes	Extravascular erythrocytes	Inflammatory infiltrates	Cartilagineous and/or fibrous tissue

hemosiderin deposits, and inflammatory cells are frequently found in myxomas but are not specific. Base infiltration may be microscopically observed in myxomas, whereas in sarcomas and malignant tumors it is often quite extensive and grossly evident [1–4].

Few reports have raised the controversial issue whether malignant variants of cardiac myxomas with metastatic potential do exist [18, 19, 50, 67–70, 79, 80]. In the most recent and updated soft tissue tumor classifications, cardiac myxoma is considered and classified as a benign neoplasm [20]. Lack of both marked atypias and mitosis, slow growth rate, absent recurrence after radical excision (except in familial forms, i.e., Carney complex, that are often multicentric) are in favor of benign biology [1–4, 6]. The *metastatic potential* of cardiac myxomas might rather correspond to clinical consequences of tumor embolism and depend upon morphology of tumor, soft consistency, thrombotic depositions on the tumor surface and hemodynamic forces that may cause detachment of even conspicuous tumor fragments with embolism and even occlusion of peripheral arteries causing ischemic damage of organs or tissues [14, 15, 17, 81]. Moreover, complete resection of cardiac myxoma is curative also in embolic cases, whereas in malignant tumors, proliferative phenomena cause distant metastases without ischemic occurrences, and surgical therapy is not curative and is not appropriate in most cases with metastatic disease.

Cardiac myxoma may also cause mitral valve occlusion with severe clinical consequences such as syncope and sudden death, similar to benign meningiomas of central nervous system that may determine intracranial hypertension and compressive phenomena [14, 15].

As other benign tumors of soft tissues, cardiac myxomas do not show a correspondent malignant counterpart, and *myxosarcoma* is not a recognized entity in the present classifications of soft tissue tumors [20]. In the past, cases of *myxosarcoma* have been reported but today they could rather be classified as myxoid rhabdomyosarcoma, leiomyosarcoma, fibrosarcoma, low-grade fibromyxoid sarcoma, etc. by using the modern diagnostic criteria (Table 3.1) [1, 18, 20, 70, 77, 78]. Then, a relapsing myxoid cardiac tumor has to be differentiated from a myxoid sarcoma after excluding incomplete resection of a myxoma or a multicentric myxoma in the case of Carney complex.

Conclusions

Cardiac myxoma has to be considered a benign neoplasm of still controversial histogenesis, although recent histological and molecular studies have highlighted a few differentiation aspects. Reported cases of *malignant* and *metastatic myxomas* might rather represent misdiagnosed *myxoid sarcomas* or embolic phenomena of biologically benign cardiac myxomas. Finally, modern imaging techniques are fundamental for diagnosis of cardiac masses and histology is mandatory for either the definitive diagnosis of cardiac myxoma or the differential diagnosis from myxoid imitators.

References

1. Basso C, Valente M, Poletti A. Surgical pathology of primary cardiac and pericardial tumors. Eur J Cardiothorac Surg. 1997;12:730–7.
2. Burke AP, Virmani R. Atlas of tumor pathology. Tumors of the heart and great vessels. 3rd series, fascicle 16. Washington, DC: Armed Forces Institute of Pathology; 1996.
3. McAllister Jr HA. Primary tumors of the heart and pericardium. Pathol Annu. 1979;14:335–66.
4. Tazelaar HD, Locke TJ, McGregor CGA. Pathology of surgically excised primary cardiac tumors. Mayo Clin Proc. 1992;67:957–65.
5. Yoon DH, Roberts W. Sex distribution in cardiac myxomas. Am J Cardiol. 2002;90:563–5.
6. Burke A, Jeudy Jr J, Virmani R. Cardiac tumors: an update. Heart. 2008;94:117–23.
7. Becker AE. Primary heart tumors in the pediatric age group: a review of salient pathologic features relevant for clinicians. Pediatr Cardiol. 2000;21:317–23.
8. Isaacs Jr H. Fetal and neonatal cardiac tumors. Pediatr Cardiol. 2004;25:252–73.
9. Carney JA, Gordon H, Carpenter PC, Shenoy BV, Go VL. The complex of myxomas, spotty pigmentation, and endocrine overactivity. Medicine. 1985;64:270–83.

10. Rhodes AR, Silverman RA, Harrist TJ, Perez-Atayde AR. Mucocutaneous lentigines, cardiomucocutaneous myxomas and multiple blue nevi: the "LAMB" syndrome. J Am Acad Dermatol. 1984;10:72–82.
11. Carney JA, Hruska LS, Beauchamp GD, Gordon H. Dominant inheritance of the complex of myxomas, spotty pigmentation, and endocrine overactivity. Mayo Clin Proc. 1986;61:165–72.
12. Stratakis CA, Carney JA, Lin JP, Papanicolaou DA, Karl M, Kastner DL, Pras E, Chrousos GP. Carney complex, a familial multiple neoplasia and lentiginosis syndrome. Analysis of 11 kindreds and linkage to the short arm of chromosome 2. J Clin Invest. 1996;97:699–705.
13. Carney JA. Differences between non-familial and familial cardiac myxoma. Am J Surg Pathol. 1985;9:53–5.
14. Reynen K. Cardiac myxomas. N Engl J Med. 1995;333:1610–7.
15. Pinede L, Duhaut P, Loire R. Clinical presentation of left atrial cardiac myxoma. A series of 112 consecutive cases. Medicine. 2001;80:159–72.
16. Modi K, Venkatesh P, Agnani S, Rowland T, Reddy P. Sudden death in a patient with left atrial myxoma: report of two cases and review of literature. BJMP. 2010;3:311–8.
17. Burke AP, Virmani R. Cardiac myxomas. A clinicopathologic study. Am J Clin Pathol. 1993;100:671–80.
18. Curschellas E, Toia D, Borner M. Cardiac myxomas: immunohistochemical study of benign and malignant variants. Virch Arch A Pathol Anat. 1991;418:485–91.
19. Altundag MB, Ertas G, Ucer AR, Durmus S, Abanuz H, Calikoğlu T, Ozbagi K, Demirkasimoglu A, Kaya B, Bakkal BH, Altundag K. Brain metastasis of cardiac myxoma: case report and review of the literature. J Neurooncol. 2005;75:181–4.
20. Fletcher CDM, Unni KK, Mertens F. WHO Classification of tumors: pathology and genetics of tumours of soft tissue and bone. Lyon: IARC Press; 2002.
21. Padalino MA, Basso C, Milanesi O, Vida VL, Moreolo GS, Thiene G, Stellin G. Surgically treated primary cardiac tumors in early infancy and childhood. J Thorac Cardiovasc Surg. 2005;129:1358–63.
22. Wu KH, Mo XM, Liu YL. Clinical analysis and surgical results of cardiac myxoma in pediatric patients. J Surg Oncol. 2009;99:48–50.
23. Blondeau P. Primary cardiac tumours-French studies of 533 cases. Thorac Cardiovasc Surg. 1990;38:192–5.
24. Jourdan M, Bataille R, Seguin J, Zhang XG, Chaptal PA, Klein B. Constitutive production of interleukin-6 and immunologic features in cardiac myxomas. Arthritis Rheum. 1990;33:398–402.
25. Yokomuro H, Yoshihara K, Watanabe Y, Shiono N, Koyama N, Takanashi Y. The variations in the immunologic features and interleukin-6 levels for the surgical treatment of cardiac myxomas. Surg Today. 2007;37:750–3.
26. Yoshioka D, Takahashi T, Ishizaka T, Higuchin T. Successful surgical resection of infected left atrial myxoma in a case complicated with disseminated intravascular coagulation and multiple cerebral infarctions: case report. J Cardiothorac Surg. 2011;6:68–71.
27. Rajab TK, Shekar P, Falk RH. Myxoma, dyspnoea, tinnitus, scoliosis, and alopecia. Lancet. 2011;377:1378.
28. Koopman RJ, Happle R. Autosomal dominant transmission of the NAME syndrome (nevi, atrial myxoma, mucinosis of the skin, and endocrine overactivity). Hum Genet. 1991;86:300–4.
29. Stergiopoulos SG, Stratakis CA. Human neoplasms associated with Carney complex and germline PRKAR1A mutations: a protein kinase A disease. FEBS Lett. 2003;546:59–64.
30. Kirschner LS, Sandrini F, Monbo J, Jing-Ping L, Carney A, Stratakis CS. Genetic heterogeneity and spectrum of the PRKAR1A gene in patients with the Carney complex. Hum Mol Genet. 2000;9:3037–46.
31. Casey M, Vaughan CJ, He J, Hatcher CJ, Winter JM, Weremowicz S, Montgomery K, Kucherlapati R, Morton CC, Basson CT. Mutations in the protein kinase A R1alpha regulatory subunit cause familial cardiac myxomas and Carney complex. J Clin Invest. 2000;106:R31–8.
32. Bertherat J. Carney complex (CNC). Orphanet J Rare Dis. 2006;1:21.
33. Stratakis CA, Kirschner LS, Carney JA. Clinical and molecular features of the Carney complex: diagnostic criteria and recommendations for patient evaluation. J Clin Endocrinol Metab. 2001;86:4041–6.
34. Casey M, Mah C, Merliss AD, Kirschner LS, Taymans SE, Denio AE, Korf B, Irvine AD, Hughes A, Carney JA, Stratakis CA, Basson CT. Identification of a novel genetic locus for familial cardiac myxomas and Carney complex. Circulation. 1998;98:2560–6.
35. Carney JA, Ferreiro JA. The epithelioid blue nevus. A multicentric familial tumor with important associations, including cardiac myxoma and psammomatous melanotic schwannoma. Am J Surg Pathol. 1996;20:259–72.
36. Malekzadeh S, Roberts WC. Growth rate of left atial myxoma. Am J Cardiol. 1989;64:1075–6.
37. Walpot J, Shivalkar B, Rodrigus I, Pasteuning WH, Hokken R. Atrial myxomas grow faster than we think. Echocardiography. 2010;27:E128–31.
38. Orlandi A, Ciucci A, Ferlosio A, Pellegrino A, Chiariello L, Spagnoli LG. Increased expression and activity of matrix metalloproteinases characterize embolic cardiac myxomas. Am J Pathol. 2005;166:1619–28.
39. Chu PH, Jung SM, Yeh TS, Lin HS, Chu JJ. MUC1, MUC5AC expressions in cardiac myxoma. Virchows Arch. 2005;446:52–5.
40. Rickelt S, Rizzo S, Doerflinger Y, Zentgraf H, Basso C, Gerosa G, Thiene G, Moll R, Franke WW. A novel kind of tumor type-characteristic junction: plakophilin-2 as a major protein of adherens junctions in cardiac myxomata. Mod Pathol. 2010;23:1429–37.
41. Stout AP. Myxoma, the tumor of primitive mesenchyme. Ann Surg. 1948;127:706–19.
42. Krikler DM, Rode J, Davies MJ, Woolf N, Moss E. Atrial myxoma: a tumour in search of its origin. Br Heart J. 1992;67:89–91.

43. Pucci A, Gagliardotto P, Zanini C, Pansini S, di Summa M, Mollo F. Histopathologic and clinical characterization of cardiac myxoma. Am Heart J. 2000;140:134–8.
44. Terracciano LM, Mhawech P, Suess K, D'Armiento M, Lehmann FS, Jundt G, Moch H, Sauter G, Mihatsch MJ. Calretinin as a marker for cardiac myxoma. Diagnostic and histogenetic considerations. Am J Clin Pathol. 2000;114:754–9.
45. Kodama H, Hirotani T, Suzuki Y, Ogawa S, Yamazaki K. Cardiomyogenic differentiation in cardiac myxoma expressing lineage-specific transcription factor. Am J Pathol. 2002;161:381–9.
46. Johansson L. Histogenesis of cardiac myxomas: an immunohistochemical study of 19 cases, including one with glandular structures, and review of the literature. Arch Pathol Lab Med. 1989;113:735–41.
47. Govoni E, Severi B, Cenacchi G, Laschi R, Pileri S, Rivano MT, Alampi G, Branzi A. Ultrastructural and immunohistochemical contribution to the histogenesis of human cardiac myxoma. Ultrastruct Pathol. 1988;12:221–33.
48. Amano J, Kono T, Wada Y, Zhang T, Koide N, Fujimori M, Ito K. Cardiac myxoma: its origin and tumor characteristics. Ann Thorac Cardiovasc Surg. 2003;9:215–21.
49. Orlandi A, Ciucci A, Ferlosio A, Genta R, Spagnoli LG, Gabbiani G. Cardiac myxoma cells exhibit embryonic endocardial stem cell features. J Pathol. 2006;209:231–9.
50. Deshpande A, Venugopal P, Sampath Kumar A. Phenotypic characterization of cellular components of cardiac myxoma: a light microscopy and immunohistochemistry study. Hum Pathol. 1996;27:1056–9.
51. Landon G, Ordonez NG, Guarda LA. Cardiac myxoma: an immunohistochemical study using endothelial, histiocytic and smooth muscle cell markers. Arch Pathol Lab Med. 1986;110:116–20.
52. Tanimura A, Kitazono M, Nagayama K, Tanaka S, Kosuga K. Cardiac myxoma. Morphologic, histochemical and tissue culture studies. Hum Pathol. 1988;19:316.
53. Salyer WR, Salyer DC. The development of cardiac myxomas and papillary endocardial lesions from mural thrombus. Am Heart J. 1975;89:4–17.
54. Waller BF, Grider L, Rohr TM, McLaughlin T, Taliercio CP, Fetters J. Intracardiac thrombi: frequency, location, etiology, and complications: a morphologic review, part I. Clin Cardiol. 1995;18:477–9.
55. Pucci A, Bartoloni G, Tessitore E, Carney JA, Papotti M. Cytokeratin profile and neuroendocrine cells in the glandular component of cardiac myxoma. Virchows Arch. 2003;443:618–24.
56. Kirschner LS, Carney JA, Pack SD, Taymans SE, Giatzakis C, Cho YS, Cho-Chung YS, Stratakis CA. Mutations of the gene encoding the protein kinase A type I-alpha regulatory subunit in patients with the Carney complex. Nat Genet. 2000;26:89–92.
57. Fogt F, Zimmerman RL, Hartmann CJ, Brown CA, Narula N. Genetic alterations of Carney complex are not present in sporadic cardiac myxoma. Int J Mol Med. 2002;9:59–60.
58. Seidman JD, Berman JJ, Hitchcock CL, Becker RL Jr, Mergner W, Moore GW, Virmani R, Yetter RA. DNA analysis od cardiomyxomas. Hum Pathol. 1991;22:494–500.
59. Rocco M, Pizzolitto S, Luciani M, Antoci B. Quantitative analysis of DNA using flow cytometry and immunocytochemical findings in 16 cases of cardiac myxomas. Pathologica. 1991;83:295–300.
60. Basso C, Valente M, Casarotto D, Thiene G. Cardiac lithomyxoma. Am J Cardiol. 1997;80:1249–51.
61. Veroux P, Mignosa C, Veroux M, Bartoloni G, Bonanno MG, Tumminelli MG. Acute occlusion of abdominal aorta: unusual embolization site for a cardiac tumor mass. Tumori. 2002;88:417–9.
62. Trotter SE, Shore DF, Olsen EG. Gamma-Gandy nodules in a cardiac myxoma. Histopathology. 1990;17:270–2.
63. Abenoza P, Sibley RK. Cardiac myxoma with gland-like structure: an immunohistochemical study. Arch Pathol Lab Med. 1986;110:736–9.
64. Lindner V, Edah-Tally S, Chafkè N, Onody T, Eisemann B, Walter P. Cardiac myxoma with glandular component: case report and review of the literature. Pathol Res Pract. 1999;195:267–72.
65. Goldman BI, Frydman C, Harpaz N. Glandular cardiac myxomas: histologic, immunohistochemical and ultrastructural evidence of epithelial differentiation. Cancer. 1987;59:1767–75.
66. de Morais CF, Falzoni R, Ferreira Alves VA. Myocardial infarct due to a unique atrial myxoma with epithelial-like cells and systemic metastases. Arch Pathol Lab Med. 1988;112:185–90.
67. Scarpelli M, Montironi R, Ricciuti R. Cardiac myxoma with glandular elements metastatic to the brain 12 years after the removal of the original tumor. Clin Neuropathol. 1997;16:190–4.
68. Eckhardt BP, Dommann-Scherrer CC, Stuckmann G, Zollifoker CL, Wenz KU. Giant cardiac myxoma with malignant transformed glandular structures. Eur Radiol. 2003;13:2099–102.
69. Uppin SG, Jambhekar N, Puri A, Kumar R, Agarwal M, Sanghvi D. Bone metastasis of glandular cardiac myxoma mimicking a metastatic carcinoma. Skeletal Radiol. 2011;40:107–11.
70. Attum AA, Johnson GS, Masri Z, Girardet R, Lansing AM. Malignant clinical behavior of cardiac myxomas and "myxoid imitators". Ann Thorac Surg. 1987;44:217–22.
71. Miller DV, Tazelaar HD, Handy JR, Young DA, Hernandez JC. Thymoma arising within cardiac myxoma. Am J Surg Pathol. 2005;29:1208–13.
72. Sakamoto H, Sakamaki T, Sumino H, Sawada Y, Sato H, Sato M, Fujita K, Kanda T,Tamura J, Kurabayashi M. Production of endothelin-1 and big endothelin-1 by human cardiac myxoma cells – Implications for the origin of myxomas. Circ J. 2004;68:1230–2.
73. Boxer ME. Cardiac myxoma: an immunoperoxidase study of histogenesis. Histopathology. 1984;8:861–72.

74. McComb RD. Heterogeneous expression of factor VIII/von Willebrand factor by cardiac myxoma cells. Am J Surg Pathol. 1984;8:539–44.
75. Ferrans VJ, Roberts WC. Structural features of cardiac myxomas. Histology, histochemistry, and electron microscopy. Hum Pathol. 1973;4:111–46.
76. Valente M. Structural profile of cardiac myxoma. Appl Pathol. 1983;1:251–63.
77. Pucci A, Gagliardotto P, Papandrea C, Di Rosa E, Morello M, di Summa M, Mollo F. An unusual myxoid leiomyosarcoma of the heart. Arch Pathol Lab Med. 1996;120:583–6.
78. Mazzola A, Spano JP, Valente M, Gregorini R, Villani C, Di Eusanio M, Ciocca M, Minuti U, Giancola R, Basso C, Thiene G. Leiomyosarcoma of the left atrium mimicking a left atrial myxoma. J Thorac Cardiovasc Surg. 2006;131:224–6.
79. Read RC, White HJ, Murphy ML, Williams D, Sun CN, Flanagan WH. The malignant potentiality of left atrial myxoma. J Thorac Cardiovasc Surg. 1974;68: 857–68.
80. Kusumi T, Minakawa M, Fukui K, Saito S, Ohashi M, Sato F, Fukuda I, Kijima H. Cardiac tumor comprising two components including typical myxoma and atypical hypercellularity suggesting a malignant change. Cardiovasc Pathol. 2009; 18:369–74.
81. Al-Mateen M, Hood M, Trippel D, Insalaco SJ, Otto RK, Vitikainen KJ. Cerebral embolism from atrial myxoma in pediatric patients. Pediatrics. 2003;112: e162–7.

Other Benign Cardiac Tumors

4

Cristina Basso, Tomaso Bottio, Gaetano Thiene, Marialuisa Valente, and Gino Gerosa

Papillary Fibroelastoma (or Papilloma)

Papillary fibroelastoma (PFE, also known as endocardial fibroelastic papilloma or giant Lambl excrescence) represents the second most frequent benign lesion after cardiac myxoma, excluding pericardial cyst [1, 2]. While in the past it was mostly an incidental autoptic observation, an exponential increase of clinically diagnosed PFEs occurred in the last 20 years due to the widespread use of two-dimensional trans-thoracic and trans-esophageal echocardiography, even in asymptomatic patients [3]. In the Armed Forces Institute of Pathology series, 8% of primary cardiac tumors are represented by PFEs [4].

It is a benign endocardial tumor lined by endothelial cells. Usually small in size (10–20 mm), some PFE can reach greatest dimensions (up to 50 mm) [5]. They are mostly single masses (80–90%), attached to the endocardium, more often valvular than mural. PFE represents the most common primary tumor of cardiac valves, with preferential localization on the semilunar cusps of the aortic valve (Fig. 4.1), followed by the atrio-ventricular (AV) valves (Figs. 4.2 and 4.3) and the pulmonary valve; more rarely, it has been reported on a wide variety of other endocardial locations, including papillary muscles (Figs. 4.4 and 4.5), chordae tendineae, and atrial and ventricular walls [6–10].

At gross examination, it is generally a soft mass, white–gray in color, although not infrequently some brownish areas due to fresh or organizing thrombus superimposition can be observed. With its multiple papillary fronds, the PFE resembles a sea-anemone, particularly when it is immersed under water (Figs. 4.1b, 4.3b, and 4.4b), otherwise the fronds can collapse and the tree-like structure disappears, thus explaining why many PFE are grossly mislabeled as valve myxomas.

At histopathology examination, each frond branching out from the main stalk consists of a single layer of endothelial cells, covering an intermediate myxoid layer rich in proteoglycans and a central avascular core, in which elastic fibers are most prominent [4, 5] (Fig. 4.6). Fibroblasts and occasional inflammatory cells are visible in the inner layers. Acute and organizing thrombi may be found within the fronds, sometimes obscuring the papillary appearance (Fig. 4.2).

At immunohistochemistry, the single layer of endothelial cells covering each frond expresses

C. Basso, M.D., Ph.D. (✉) • G. Thiene, M.D. • M. Valente, M.D.
Pathological Anatomy, Department of Cardiac, Thoracic and Vascular Sciences, Azienda Ospedaliera-University of Padua Medical School, via A. Gabelli, 61, Padua 35121, Italy
e-mail: cristina.basso@unipd.it

G. Gerosa, M.D. • T. Bottio, M.D., Ph.D.
Cardiac Surgery, Department of Cardiac, Thoracic and Vascular Sciences, Azienda Ospedaliera-University of Padua Medical School, via N. Giustiniani, 2, Padua 35128, Italy

C. Basso et al. (eds.), *Cardiac Tumor Pathology*, Current Clinical Pathology,
DOI 10.1007/978-1-62703-143-1_4, © Springer Science+Business Media New York 2013

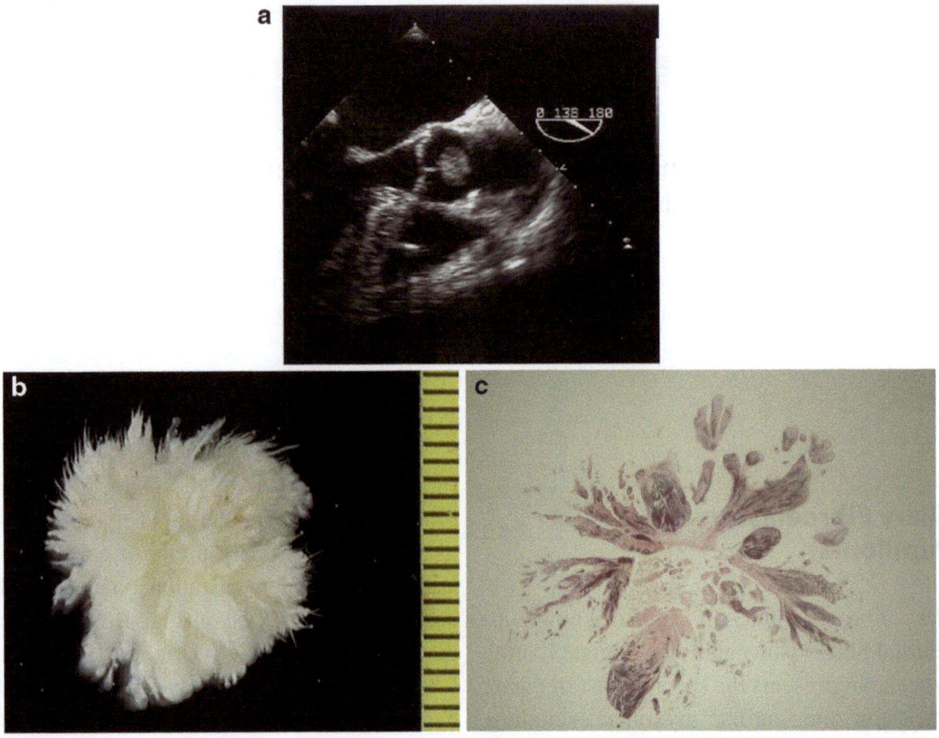

Fig. 4.1 Papillary fibroelastoma of the aortic valve: incidental finding during echocardiographic screening in a 77-year-old asymptomatic woman (from Bottio et al. [7] modified). Reprinted with permission of the Italian Society of Cardiology. (**a**) Trans-oesophageal 2D echocardiography, short axis: a mobile mass attached to the non-coronary cusp with a short pedicle is visible. (**b**) Gross view of the surgically resected mass resembling a sea anemone under water. (**c**) Panoramic histologic section of the resected mass: multiple fronds are branching out from a main stalk, each consisting of a central avascular fibroelastic axis (elastic Van Gieson stain)

vimentin and CD34, but much less CD31 and factor VIII, when compared to the normal endothelium [1, 11]. Some spindle cells in the inner layers may express S100, to support their dendritic origin.

Electron microscopy confirms the connective tissue structure of the central axis, with longitudinally oriented mature collagen and elastic bundles and fibroblasts immersed within the matrix; lining endothelial cells appear hyperplastic and rich in pinocytic vesicles [4, 5].

The real nature of PFE is still a matter of debate, so that it has been variously described as neoplasm, hamartoma, organized thrombus, and iatrogenic lesion; in the latter situation, PFEs are usually multiple and located mostly on the non-valvular endocardium. Some authors consider PFEs as giant Lambl endocardial excrescences (a frequent finding in valvular heart disease), although, the latter occur typically along the line of closure of semilunar cusps, while PFE can occur anywhere on the cusp surface [4–6]. The frequent finding of fibrin within the PFE fronds seems in keeping with the thrombotic or iatrogenic origin of the lesion [1, 4, 12].

Because of its small dimensions, not leading to intracavitary obstruction, and of the consistency of the papillae due to the firm fibroelastic axis, PFE has been frequently an occasional finding at autopsy and later on at echocardiography in asymptomatic patients. However, PFE can be a source of distal embolism, due to the detachment of platelet and fibrin thrombus layered upon the papillary fronds more than to fragmentation

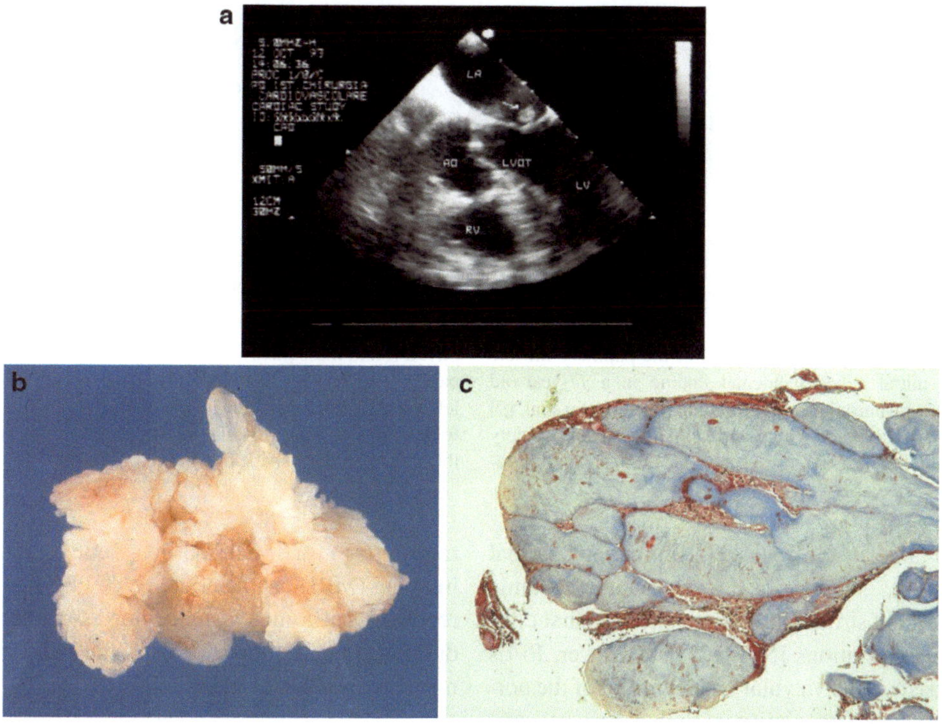

Fig. 4.2 Papillary fibroelastoma of the mitral valve in a 74-year-old woman who underwent coronary artery bypass surgery (from Basso et al. [6] modified). Reprinted with permission of the Italian Society of Cardiology. (**a**) Trans-oesophageal 2D echocardiography: a round mass, 5 mm in diameter, is visible on the atrial side of the anterior mitral valve leaflet (*AO* aorta, *LA* left atrium, *LV* left ventricle, *LVOT* left ventricular outflow tract, *RV* right ventricle). (**b**) Gross view of the resected mass, showing the irregular surface with variable color. (**c**) At histology, a fibrin network is visible within the fibroelastic fronds of the tumor (Heidenhain trichrome stain)

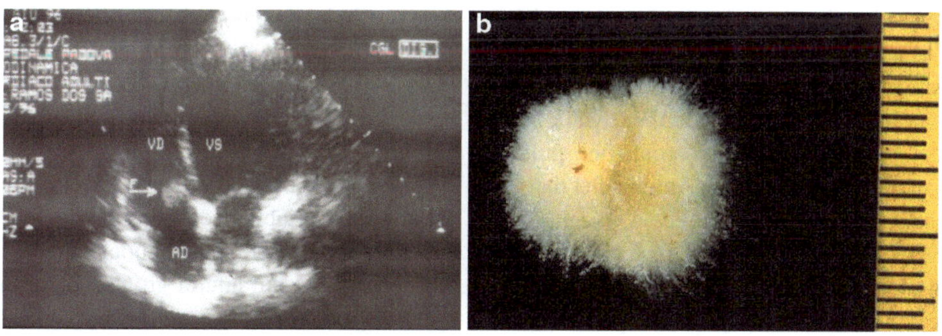

Fig. 4.3 Papillary fibroelastoma of the tricuspid valve in a 40-year-old woman with a history of palpitations and effort dyspnea (from Scalia et al. [10] modified). Reprinted with permission of the Italian Society of Cardiology. (**a**) Trans-thoracic 2D echocardiography, apical four-chamber view: a 10×15 mm mass (F= fibroelastoma) is attached to the septal leaflet of the tricuspid valve with a short pedicle (*arrow*) (*AD* right atrium; *VD* right ventricle; *VS* left ventricle). (**b**) Gross view of the surgically excised mass: note the short fronds of the tumor which resembles a cotton flock

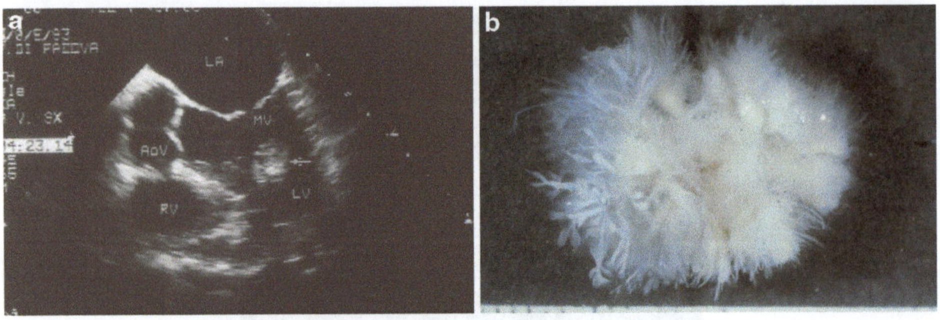

Fig. 4.4 Papillary fibroelastoma of the papillary muscle of the mitral valve: incidental finding in a 77-year-old woman with chronic atrial fibrillation (from Bottio et al. [9] modified). Reprinted with permission of the Italian Society of Cardiology. (**a**) Trans-oesophageal 2D echocardiography: a round mass *(arrow)* appears attached to the anterior papillary muscle of the mitral valve (*AoV* aortic valve, *LA* left atrium, *LV* left ventricle, *MV* mitral valve, *RV* right ventricle). (**b**) Gross examination of the excised mass reveals the usual papillary shape due to multiple fronds

of the tumor itself [5, 6, 11]. Angina, myocardial infarction, sudden death, transient ischemic attacks, and stroke are often reported as first clinical manifestations [5, 14–25]. Moreover, PFEs localized on the valvular endocardium of the aortic semilunar cusps adjacent to the coronary ostia can lead to fatal myocardial ischemia, due to transient tumor wedging into the coronary ostium itself [13].

Nowadays, PFE is a frequent incidental observation at echocardiography performed for routine check-up even in asymptomatic patients. The potential risk of systemic embolism suggests prophylactic surgery for left-sided PFEs, with the majority of patients undergoing tumor excision without the need for valve replacement. On the opposite, the casual finding of right-sided PFEs does not justify surgery, due to the trivial consequences of microembolization into the pulmonary circulation [10, 26, 27]. Antiplatelet therapy must be considered in any case.

PFE is easily detected by transthoracic two-dimensional echocardiography, usually appearing as a small, mobile, irregular, and pedunculated valvular mass [28]. It is quite common to observe the frond-like shape of the endocardial mass, with “shimmering” edges, a feature that can help in differential diagnosis with cardiac myxoma. However, when the fronds are shorter, differential diagnosis can be difficult thus explaining why many PFEs undergo surgery with a wrong diagnosis of cardiac myxoma [4]. Computed tomography (CT) and cardiac magnetic resonance imaging (MRI) characterization of PFE has been reported, but tumor visualization is challenging due to its small dimensions and the rapid movements with cardiac cycles.

Hemangioma (or Angioma)

It is a benign vascular tumor which accounts for up to 4% of primary cardiac tumors in the AFIP series [3]. According to the histopathologic features, three patterns can be identified: (a) *cavernous hemangioma* (multiple dilated thin walled vessels); (b) *capillary hemangioma* (capillary-like smaller vessels); (c) *arterio-venous hemangioma or cirsoid aneurysm* (dysplastic malformed arteries and veins) [1, 4, 29].

At gross examination, cardiac hemangiomas show highly variable size, with a maximum diameter occasionally >8 cm. In about 75% of cases they present an intramural growth, while in the remaining 25% an intracavitary atrial or ventricular growth is observed (Fig. 4.7). Usually, arterio-venous and cavernous hemangiomas are not capsulated and tend to be infiltrative intramural, while capillary hemangiomas are intracavitary to mimic cardiac myxomas.

The histologic structure is similar to that of extracardiac hemangiomas, with the three patterns mentioned above (Fig. 4.7d). The capillary

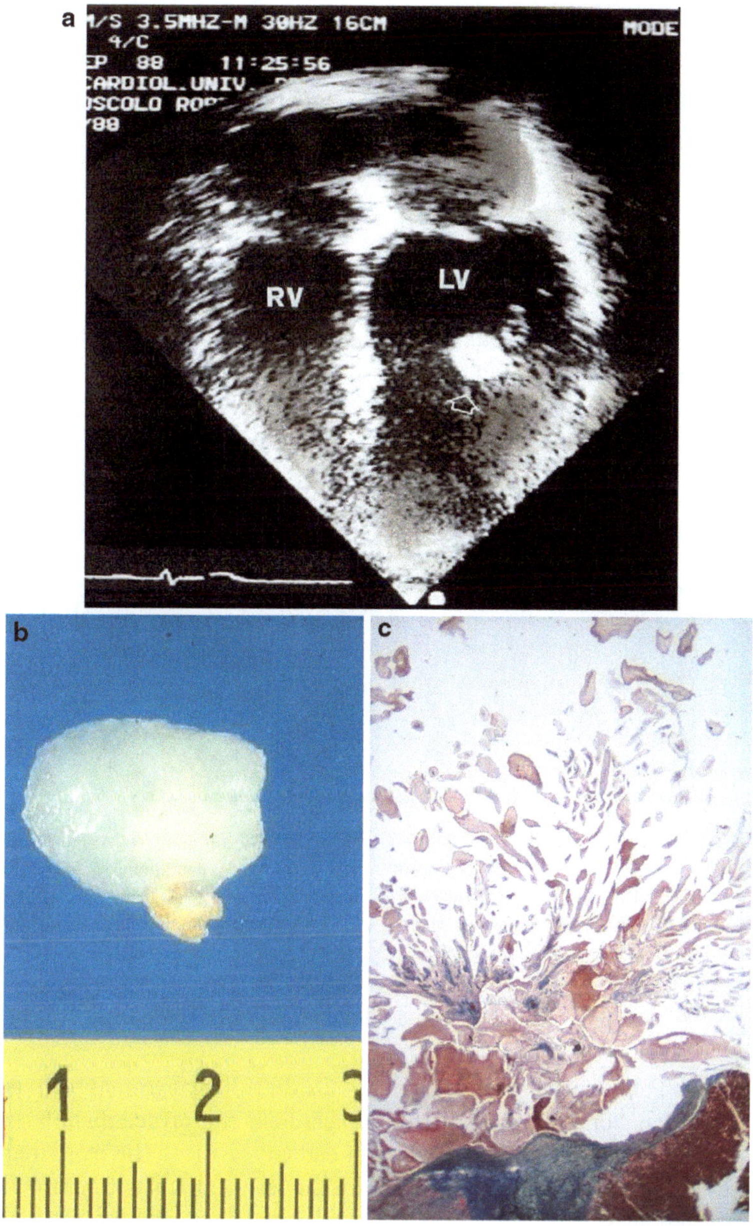

Fig. 4.5 Papillary fibroelastoma of the mitral valve papillary muscle in a 31-year-old man with acute myocardial infarction and normal coronary arteries (from Valente et al. [5] modified). Reprinted with permission of the Italian Society of Cardiology. (**a**) Transthoracic 2D echocardiography, apical four-chamber view: a round mass *(arrow)*, 17×15 mm in size, is attached to the anterior papillary muscle of the mitral valve (*LV* left ventricle, *RV* right ventricle). (**b**) Gross view of the resected mass: note the short pedicle and the apparently smooth surface out of the water. (**c**) Histologic examination reveals the papillary structure of the tumor (Heidenhain trichrome stain)

pattern usually presents a myxoid matrix with immersed nodules of small capillary-size vessels, with endothelial cells, pericytes, and fibroblasts; the cavernous pattern consists of large dilated capillary or venous vascular spaces with either thick or thin walls, full of blood; the arteriovenous pattern is characterized by heterogeneous dysplastic vessel types, with muscularized

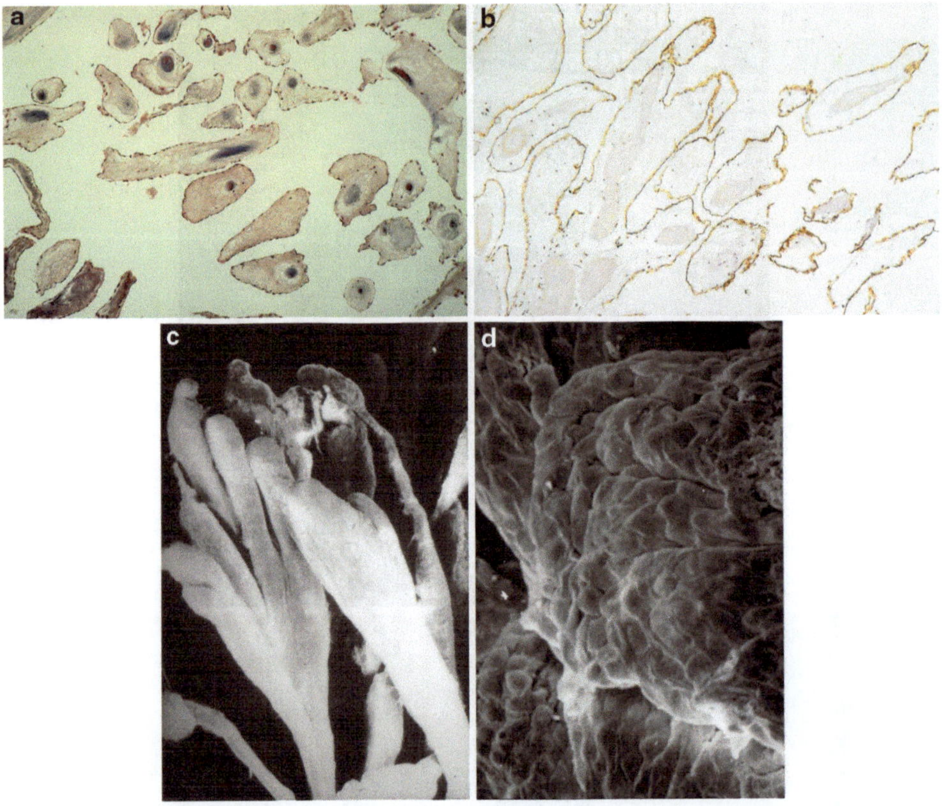

Fig. 4.6 Histologic and ultrastructural features of endocardial papillary fibroelastoma (same case as Fig. 4.5). Reprinted with permission of the Italian Society of Cardiology. (**a**) Each papillary frond consists of a central fibroelastic core and a myxoid matrix, covered by a single layer of endothelial cells (elastic Van Gieson stain). (**b**) At immunohistochemistry, the lining cells express endothelial markers (CD31). (**c**) Scanning electron microscopy confirms the papillary structure of the tumor. (**d**) At higher magnification, the continuous endothelial lining of the papillae is visible

arteries, veins, and capillaries showing irregularly thickened walls, and may contain fibrous tissue and fat. Cardiac hemangiomas have frequently combined features of cavernous, capillary, and arterio-venous hemangiomas.

Papillary hyperplasia of endothelial cells is an unusual finding, probably due to exuberant reactive endothelial proliferation as a part of a process of organizing thrombosis. However, at difference from angiosarcoma, necrosis and nuclear atypia are never observed.

At immunohistochemistry, the cells lining the vascular spaces typically express endothelial markers CD31, CD34, and factor VIII.

Cardiac hemangiomas can arise from the epicardium and myocardium but are also found in cardiac cavities. The most frequent locations are the left ventricular wall, the interventricular septum, the right ventricle, and the atria. They are rare on the epicardium and even exceptional on the valves [2, 4, 29–33].

From the clinical view point, intracavitary hemangiomas can present with obstructive symptoms like myxomas, while the intramural ones with arrhythmias and conduction disturbances, congestive heart failure, myocardial ischemia, pericardial effusion, and exceptionally with cardiac tamponade due to intrapericardial rupture. Most cardiac

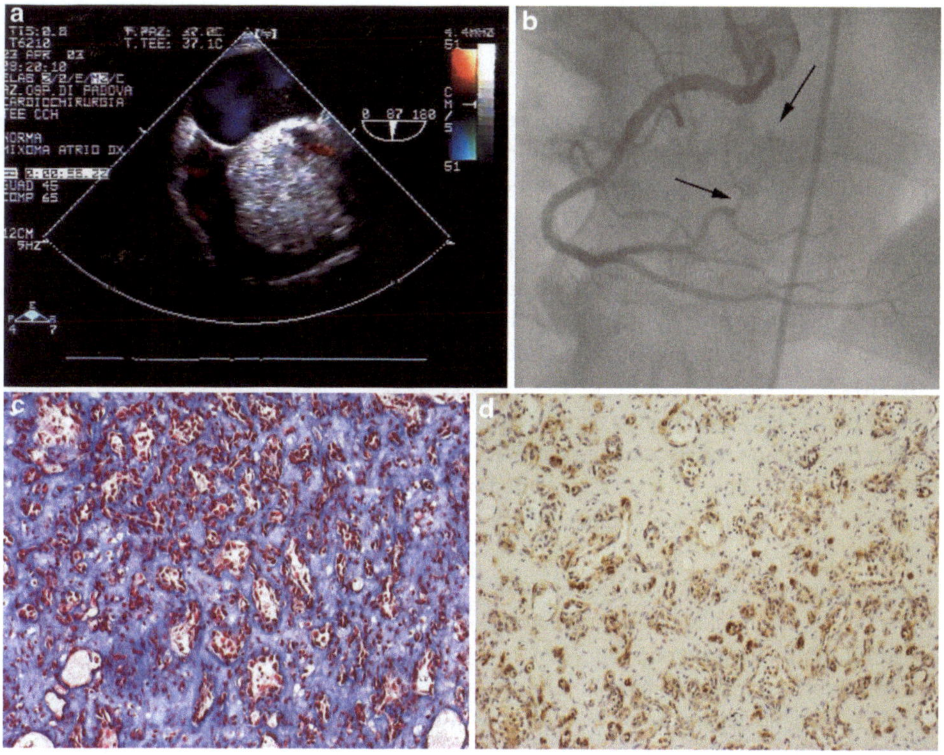

Fig. 4.7 Right atrial hemangioma in a 62 year old woman with effort dyspnea (from Rizzoli et al. [31] modified). Reprinted with permission of the Italian Society of Cardiology. (**a**) Trans-oesophageal 2D echocardiography showing an atrial septal mass protruding into the atrial cavity to interfere with the blood flow: Color Doppler reveals an afferent coronary artery branch. (**b**) Selective coronary angiography confirms that the mass is vascularized from a collateral branch of the right coronary artery. (**c**) At histology, the mass consists of numerous vascular structures full of blood and lined by a single layer of endothelial cells (Heidenhain trichrome stain). (**d**) At immunohistochemistry, the lining cells are positive for endothelial markers (CD31)

hemangiomas are discovered incidentally at autopsy or during echocardiographic screening.

The majority of cardiac hemangiomas are sporadic. However, although rarely, an association with extracardiac hemangiomas of the gastrointestinal tract and port-wine stain of the face has been reported. The Kasabach–Merritt vascular syndrome has been described in the setting of giant cardiac hemangioma, due to thrombosis and coagulopathies [34, 35].

Diagnosis during life can be suspected on the basis of tissue characterization of the mass through echocardiography and MRI, and of vascularization of the mass by a coronary artery branch at angiography or perfusion MRI (Fig. 4.7b) [31].

Among benign vascular tumors, *cardiac lymphangiomas* need to be mentioned. They are usually intrapericardial, although some cardiac variants have been reported [4]. They are soft, spongy masses, with solid fibrotic areas, and a histologic structure similar to that of hemangiomas, where the vascular spaces are filled with lymph instead of blood.

Lipoma

It is a primary benign cardiac tumor composed of mature adipocytes [4]. Lipomas usually do not represent an indication to surgical resection, thus explaining why their prevalence in surgical pathology series is low. Higher estimates up to 10% of heart tumors are reported when lipomatous hypertrophy of the atrial septum, which is a separate entity, is included [1, 4, 36–38].

Cardiac lipomas may occur anywhere in the heart, with a predilection for visceral and parietal pericardium [2, 4, 39]. Other sites are represented by interventricular septum and valves (valve "fibrolipoma") [40].

Histopathologic examination reveals circumscribed masses of mature adipocytes, enmeshed in a thin fibrous collagen network (Fig. 4.8).

As for other primary cardiac tumors, clinical presentation is variable depending on the site and size of lipoma, and many are incidental findings at autopsy or during cardiac imaging investigation. CT and MRI can help in the diagnostic work-up, being able to establish the fatty nature of the mass.

Lipomas should not be confused with lipomatous hypertrophy of the interatrial septum, a non-encapsulated benign lesion characterized by mature adipose cell hyperplasia intermixed with enlarged cardiac myocytes typically located in the atrial septum (Fig. 4.9). A prevalence of 1.1% has been reported in an autoptic series [36]. It is often associated with obesity (about one-third of cases), advanced age, and cardiomegaly, as an intracardiac extension of the subepicardial fat, so that lipomatous hypertrophy has been considered an acquired dysmetabolic process; however, its finding also in nonobese people is in keeping with a hamartomatous origin [36–38].

Palpitations due to atrial arrhythmias (atrial fibrillation or flutter, premature beats) are the usual clinical symptoms. Conduction disturbances may also occur. When the lipomatous hypertrophy is so large as to interfere or obstruct the venae cavae orifices, congestive heart failure may appear to require surgical resection. This nosologic entity has been re-emphasized in the clinical setting after the advent of cardiac imaging

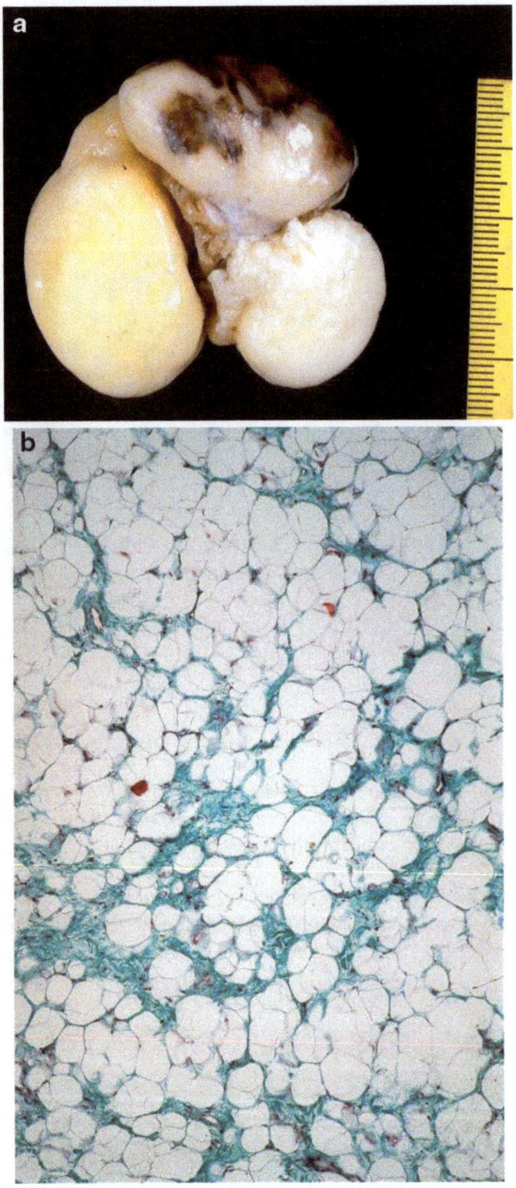

Fig. 4.8 Right atrial lipoma, incidental finding at echocardiography in a 85-year-old woman followed up for ischemic heart disease. Reprinted with permission of the Italian Society of Cardiology. (**a**) Gross view of the surgically resected mass: note the *yellow* appearance of the smooth, round intracavitary mass. (**b**) At histology, mature adipocytes with interspersed connective tissue are visible (Masson trichrome stain)

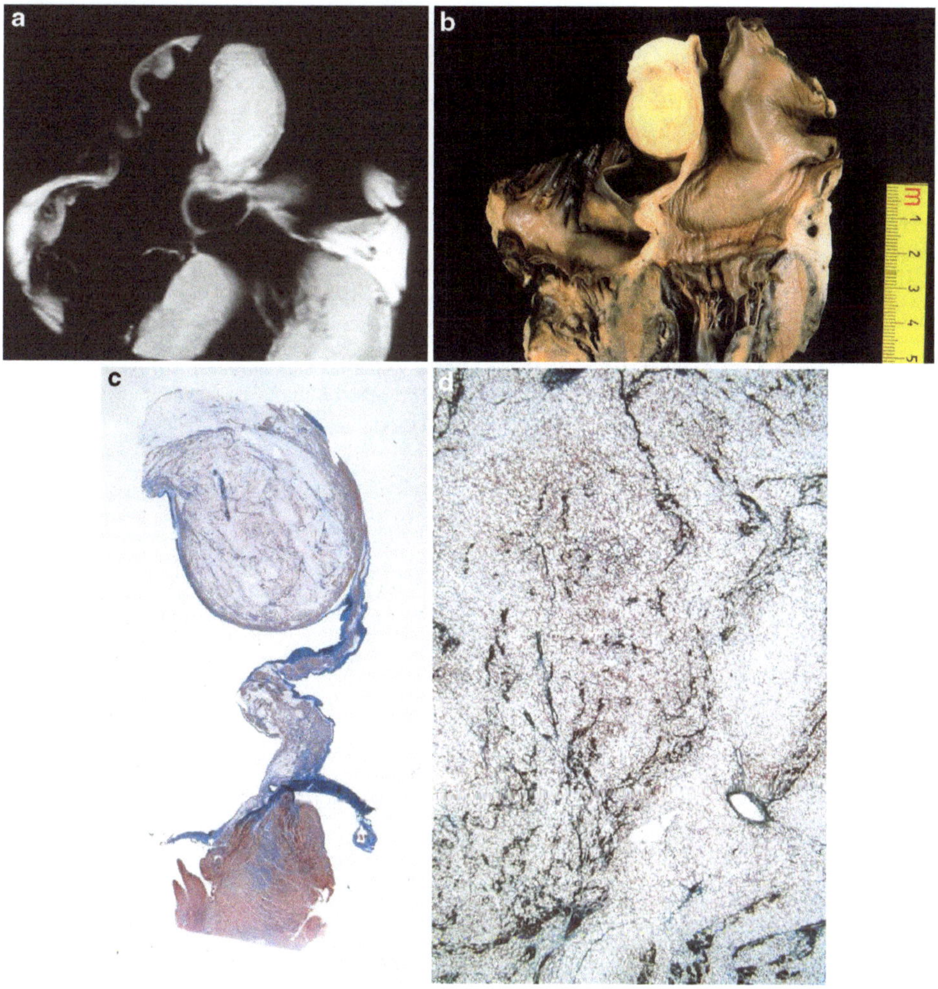

Fig. 4.9 Lipomatous hypertrophy of the atrial septum (atrial septal lipoma) at autopsy in a 74-year-old woman with a history of tuberculosis and diabetes (from Basso et al. [38] modified). Reprinted with permission of the Italian Society of Cardiology. (**a**) Ex vivo cardiac magnetic resonance showing a hyperintense signal similar to that of epicardial fat. (**b**) After longitudinal section of the heart, an oval-shaped lipomatous mass, 3×2 cm in size, is visible in the atrial septum. (**c**) At histology, the non-capsulated mass presents mature adipocytes with tiny interstitial fibrosis and rare cardiac myocytes (Heidenhain trichrome stain). (**d**) Close-up of C (Heidenhain trichrome stain)

modalities with tissue characterization properties such as CT and MRI [41].

Blood Cyst (Valvular)

It is a congenital cyst of the valvular endocardium, small in size and usually without clinical significance. They are usually multiple and typically located along the closure rim of the AV valve leaflets, or more rarely semilunar cusps, in newborns and infants, particularly under 2 months of age [4, 42]. They consist of blood entrapped into leaflet crevices, covered by flat endothelium (Fig. 4.10). They are considered like diverticula of malformative origin, due to the invagination of the valvular endocardium.

The sequestered blood may exceptionally increase so much that the cyst, assuming huge intracavitary dimensions, creates obstructive symptoms and requires surgery [43].

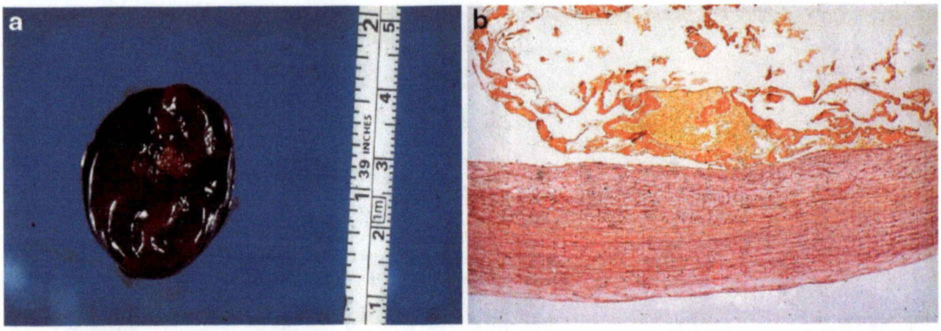

Fig. 4.10 Giant blood cyst in a 4 months infant (Gallucci et al. [43]). Reprinted with permission of the Italian Society of Cardiology. (**a**) Gross view of the surgically resected mass which appears *dark red*. (**b**) At histology, the cyst wall consists of fibrous tissue with rare elastic fibers, covered by endothelium with clots and mural thrombi

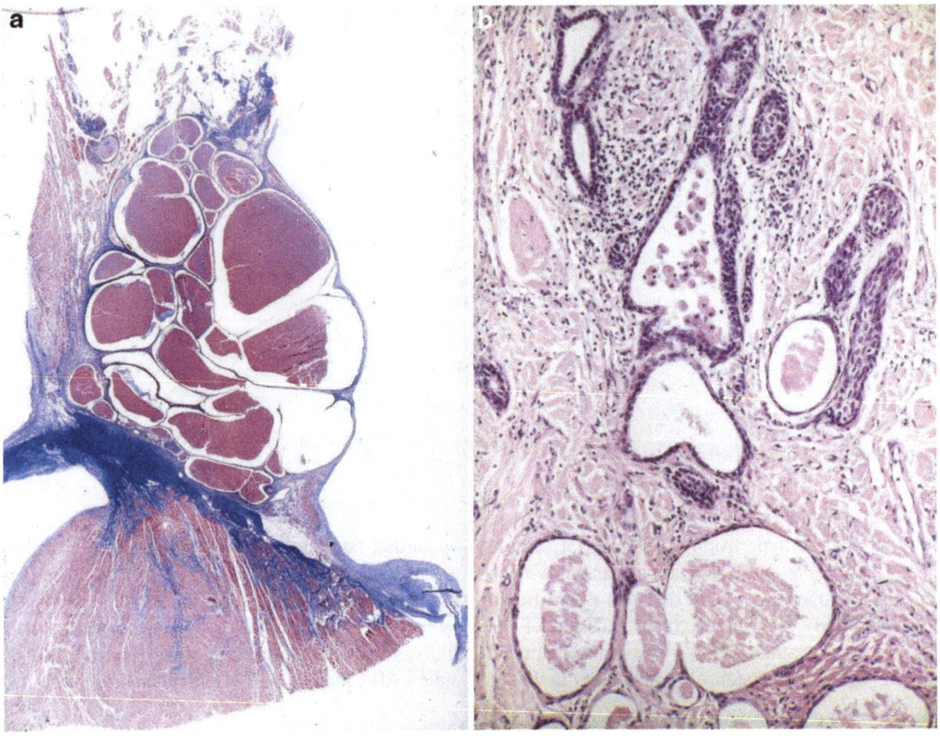

Fig. 4.11 Cystic tumor of the AV node, incidental finding at autopsy in a 78-year-old woman who died of ischemic heart disease. Reprinted with permission of the Italian Society of Cardiology. (**a**) Histologic section at the level of the AV node: note the subendocardial mass consisting of multiple cysts variable in size filled with mucoid material (Alcian PAS). (**b**) The cysts are lined by cuboid and transitional cells (hematoxylin–eosin stain)

Cystic Tumor of the AV Node

It is a benign, multicystic mass, also known as tawarioma (from Tawara, the discoverer of the AV node) or celothelioma (mesothelioma of the AV node, because wrongly considered of possible pericardial dysontogenetic origin). This tumor is located in the triangle of Koch, at the right side of the atrial septum in front of the coronary sinus, exactly at the level of the AV node [44–46]. Tumor histogenesis, whether mesothelial or endodermal, has been debated for a long time

[1, 4]. Immunohistochemistry studies then provided evidence of an origin from "endodermal remnants" (primitive endoderm), thus abandoning the term celothelioma or mesothelioma of the AV node. Since the diagnosis can be reached at any age, the congenital nature is not proven in all.

At gross examination, it appears multicystic even at naked eye, ranging in size from 2 to 20 mm. Histologically, it infiltrates and compresses the AV node, not touching the borders of the central fibrous body and without extension into the ventricular myocardium or valvular tissue (Fig. 4.11). The cysts, which are filled with mucoid substance, are lined by cuboid, squamous, or transitional epithelial cells. At immunohistochemistry, these cells strongly express cytokeratin, epithelial membrane antigen (EMA), carcinoembryonic antigen, and B72.3 [1].

The mean age at presentation is 38 years, with a *F/M* ratio 3/1. Complete AV block is the clinical presentation in about 75% of patients, incomplete AV block in 15%, and sudden death in 10%. Some are rare incidental findings in newborns with congenital heart diseases.

The majority of cases have been diagnosed at autopsy or after cardiac transplantation through histologic investigation of the conduction system, although rare cases of in vivo diagnosis with surgical removal have been reported [46].

Pericardial Cyst

Pericardial cysts are a frequent incidental finding during routine chest x-ray. Most probably disontogenetic in nature (i.e., pericardial diverticula), they consist of uni- or multi-loculated cysts, full of serous liquid, with a thin and smooth wall.

At histology, the pericardial cyst wall consists of highly vascularized connective tissue rich in collagen bundles, with rare elastic fibers and scattered lymphocytic and plasmacellular infiltrates; the cyst wall is lined on both sides by a single layer of flat mesothelial cells, sometimes hyperplastic, which express positivity for cytokeratin [4] (Fig. 4.12).

The most common location is the right cardiophrenic angle, followed by the left one; more rarely, they are located in the anterior, superior, or inferior mediastinal spaces.

Although most probably congenital, pericardial cysts are usually diagnosed in the adult age, without any gender predilection. They are mostly asymptomatic or pauci-symptomatic, despite the huge dimensions they can reach (up to 16 cm) due to increasing storage of fluid within the cystic cavity. Symptoms include chest pain, dyspnea, cough, palpitations, and even congestive heart failure. Once diagnosed, it does not represent "per se" an indication for surgery, except for cases with compressive/obstructive symptoms.

Other Rare Non-myxomatous Benign Cardiac Tumors

These are distinct nosologic entities recently reported as to require an update of the WHO classification of primary cardiac tumors.

Hamartoma of mature cardiac myocytes is a relatively new entity described in young adults, either asymptomatic or with fatal arrhythmias. It consists of single or multiple, non encapsulated, poorly demarcated, firm white masses in the ventricles or atria, resembling normal myocardium. They are formed by mature, hypertrophicied cardiomyocytes with cross striations and large, bizarre nuclei, and spatial disorganization ("myocardial disarray") to mimic focal hypertrophic cardiomyopathy [47].

Adult cellular rhabdomyoma is a quite rare benign neoplasm of striated myocytes [48]. Ranging in size from 2 to 5 cm, it presents as soft, bulging mass, tan to brown, with a pseudo-capsule. At histology, this tumor differs from the pediatric cardiac rhabdomyoma since it is composed of tightly packed, monomorphic, round to polygonal cardiomyocytes with eosinophilic granular cytoplasm and only occasional spider cells. No association with tuberous sclerosis has been reported. The prognosis is unknown but presumably benign.

Inflammatory myofibroblastic tumor (also known as plasma cell granuloma or inflammatory pseudotumor) is a very rare cardiac tumor with an

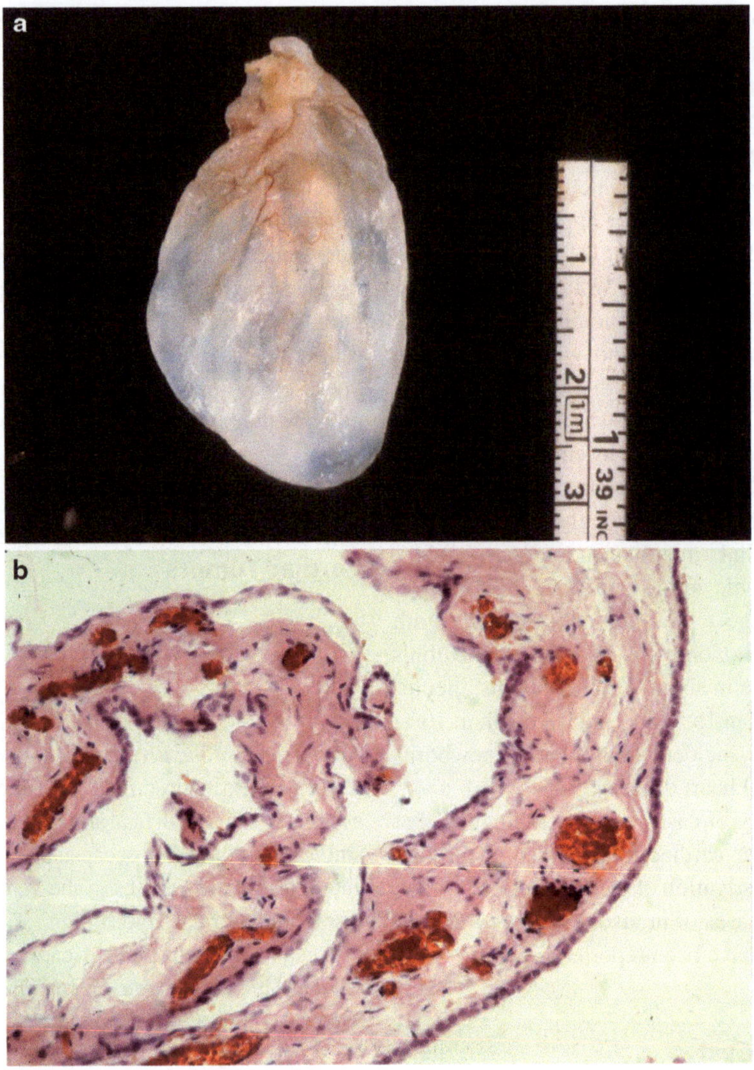

Fig. 4.12 Pericardial cyst, incidental finding in a 52-year-old man during surgery for mitral valve replacement. Reprinted with permission of the Italian Society of Cardiology. (**a**) Gross view of the uni-loculated cyst filled with serous fluid. (**b**) At histology, the cyst wall consists of vascularized connective tissue covered by a single layer of mesothelial cells (hematoxylin–eosin stain)

endocavitary growth that can be found at any endocardial site in the heart, although it prefers the ventricles. Grossly, they can reach large dimensions (up to 8 cm) and show a relatively narrow attachment to the mural endocardium. At histology, the mass consists of spindle myofibroblasts, fibroblasts, and chronic inflammatory cells, such as plasma cells, lymphocytes, macrophages, and few eosinophils [1]. Fibrin thrombus deposition on the surface is a common feature.

Other benign cardiac neoplasms or tumor-like lesions which are not anymore listed in the recent WHO classification, but are still mentioned in the series of the Armed Force Institute of Pathology and in the literature, include granular cell tumor, paraganglioma (or cardiac pheochromocytoma), neurofibroma, leiomyoma, intracardiac bronchogenic cyst, thyroid heterotopy, and mesothelial incidental cardiac excrescences (also known as cardiac MICE) [4].

References

1. Basso C, Valente M, Poletti A, Casarotto D, Thiene G. Surgical pathology of primary cardiac and pericardial tumors. Eur J Cardiothorac Surg. 1997;12:730–7.
2. Burke AP, Veinot JP, Loire R, Virmani R, Tazelaar H, Kaniya H, Araoz PA, Watanabe G. Tumours of the heart. In: Travis WD, Brambilla E, Muller-Hermelink HK, Harris CC, editors. Pathology and genetics of tumours of the lung, pleura, thymus and heart. IARC Press: Lyon; 2004. p. 249–88.
3. Sun JP, Asher CR, Yang XS, Cheng GG, Scalia GM, Massed AG, Griffin BP, Ratliff NB, Stewart WJ, Thomas JD. Clinical and echocardiographic characteristics of papillary fibroelastomas: a retrospective and prospective study in 162 patients. Circulation. 2001;103:2687–93.
4. Burke A, Virmani R. Atlas of tumor pathology. Tumors of the heart and great vessels. Washington, DC: Armed Forces Institute of Pathology; 1996.
5. Valente M, Basso C, Thiene G, Bressan M, Stritoni P, Cocco P, Fasoli G. Fibroelastic papilloma: a not so benign cardiac tumor. Cardiovasc Pathol. 1992;1:161–6.
6. Basso C, Bottio T, Valente M, Bonato R, Casarotto D, Thiene G. Primary cardiac valve tumours. Heart. 2003;89:1259–60.
7. Bottio T, Pittarello D, Bonato R, Thiene G, Gerosa G, Casarotto D, Basso C. Echocardiographic diagnosis of aortic valve papillary fibroelastoma. Tex Heart Inst J. 2004;31:322–3.
8. Mazzucco A, Bortolotti U, Thiene G, Dan M, Stritoni P, Scutari M, Stellin G. Left ventricular papillary fibroelastoma with coronary embolization. Eur J Cardiothorac Surg. 1989;3:471–3.
9. Bottio T, Basso C, Rizzoli G, Casarotto D, Thiene G. Case report: fibroelastoma of the papillary muscle of the mitral valve: diagnostic implications and review of the literature. J Heart Valve Dis. 2002;11:288–91.
10. Scalia D, Basso C, Rizzoli G, Lupia M, Budano S, Thiene G, Venturini A. Should right-sided fibroelastomas be operated upon? J Heart Valve Dis. 1997;6:647–50.
11. Rubin MA, Snell JA, Tazelaar HD, Lack EE, Austenfeld JL, Azumi N. Cardiac papillary fibroelastoma: an immunohistochemical investigation and unusual clinical manifestations. Mod Pathol. 1995;8:402–7.
12. Boone SA, Campagna M, Walley VM. Lambl's excrescences and papillary fibroelastomas: are they different? Can J Cardiol. 1992;8:372–6.
13. Israel DH, Sherman W, Ambrose JA, Sharma S, Harpaz N, Robbins M. Dynamic coronary ostial obstruction due to papillary fibroelastoma leading to myocardial ischemia and infarction. Am J Cardiol. 1991;67:104–5.
14. Basso C, Thiene G, Dalla Volta S. Embolia coronarica: una causa spesso dimenticata di infarto miocardico e morte improvvisa. G Ital Cardiol. 1992;22:751–60.
15. McFadden PM, Lacy JR. Intracardiac papillary fibroelastoma: an occult cause of embolic neurologic deficit. Ann Thorac Surg. 1987;43:667–9.
16. Waltenberger J, Thelin S. Papillary fibroelastoma as an unusual source of repeated pulmonary embolism. Circulation. 1994;89:24–33.
17. Etienne Y, Jobic Y, Houel JF, Barra JA, Boschat J, Meunier M, Penther P. Papillary fibroelastoma of the aortic valve with myocardial infarction: echocardiographic diagnosis and surgical excision. Am Heart J. 1994;127:443–5.
18. Zell DN, Diamond M, Beringer D. Angina and sudden death resulting from papillary fibroelastoma of the aortic valve. Ann Emerg Med. 1985;14:470–3.
19. Mann J. Papillary fibroelastoma of the mitral valve: a rare cause of transient neurological deficits. Br Heart J. 1994;71:6.
20. Fowles RE, Miller DC, Egbert BM, Fitzgerald JW, Popp RL. Systemic embolization from a mitral valve papillary endocardial fibroma detected by two-dimensional echocardiography. Am Heart J. 1981;102:128–30.
21. Lee KS, Topol EJ, Stewart WJ. Atypical presentation of papillary fibroelastoma mimicking multiple vegetations in suspected subacute bacterial endocarditis. Am Heart J. 1993;125:1443–5.
22. Gallo R, Kumar N, Prabhakar G, Awada A, Maalouf Y, Duran CM. Papillary fibroelastoma of mitral valve chordae. Ann Thorac Surg. 1993;55:1576–7.
23. Kasarskis EJ, O'Connor W, Earle G. Embolic stroke from cardiac papillary fibroelastomas. Stroke. 1988;19:1171–3.
24. Topol EJ, Biern RO, Reitz BA. Cardiac papillary fibroelastoma and stroke: echocardiographic diagnosis and guide excision. Am J Cardiol. 1986;80:129–32.
25. Fine G, Pai SR. Cardiac papillary fibroelastoma: a source of coronary artery emboli and myocardial infarction. Henry Ford Hosp Med J. 1984;32:204–8.
26. Frumin H, O'Donnell L, Kerin NZ, Levine F, Nathan Jr LE, Klein SP. Two-dimensional echocardiographic detection and diagnostic features of tricuspid papillary fibroelastoma. J Am Coll Cardiol. 1983;2:1016–8.
27. Wolfe JT, Finck SJ, Safford RE, Persellin ST. Tricuspid valve papillary fibroelastoma: echocardiographic characterization. Ann Thorac Surg. 1991;51:116–8.
28. Shub C, Tajik AJ, Seward JB, Edwards WD, Pruitt RD, Orszulak TA, Pluth JR. Cardiac papillary fibroelastomas. Two dimensional echocardiographic recognition. Mayo Clin Proc. 1981;56:629–33.
29. Burke AP, Johns J, Virmani R. Hemangiomas of the heart: a clinico-pathologic study of 10 cases. Am J Cardiovasc Pathol. 1991;13:283–90.
30. Brizard C, Latremouille C, Jebara VA, Acar C, Fabiani JN, Deloche A, Carpentier AF. Cardiac hemangiomas. Ann Thorac Surg. 1993;56:390–4.
31. Rizzoli G, Bottio T, Pittarello D, Napodano M, Thiene G, Basso C. Atrial septal mass: transesophageal

echocardiographic assessment. J Thorac Cardiovasc Surg. 2004;128:767–9.
32. Chang JS, Young ML, Chiu WM, Lue HC. Infantile cardiac hemangioendotelioma. Pediatr Cardiol. 1992;13:52–5.
33. Palmer TE, Tresch DD, Bonchek LI. Spontaneous resolution of a large, cavernous hemangioma of the heart. Am J Cardiol. 1986;58:184–5.
34. Gengenbach S, Ridkler PM. Left ventricular hemangioma in Kasabach–Merritt syndrome. Am Heart J. 1991;121:202–3.
35. Weston CF, Hayward MW, Seymour RM, Stephens RM. Cardiac hemangioma associated with a facial port-wine stain and recurrent atrial tachycardia. Eur Heart J. 1988;9:668–71.
36. Shirani J, Roberts WC. Clinical, electrocardiographic and morphologic features of massive fatty deposits ("lipomatous hypertrophy") in the atrial septum. J Am Coll Cardiol. 1993;22:226–38.
37. Heyer CM, Kagel T, Lemburg SP, Bauer TT, Nicolas V. Lipomatous hypertrophy of the interatrial septum: a prospective study of incidence, imaging findings, and clinical symptoms. Chest. 2003;124:2068–73.
38. Basso C, Barbazza R, Thiene G. Images in cardiovascular medicine. Lipomatous hypertrophy of the atrial septum. Circulation. 1998;97:1423.
39. Schrepfer S, Deuse T, Detter C, Treede H, Koops A, Boehm DH, Willems S, Lacour-Gayet F, Reichenspurner H. Successful resection of a symptomatic right ventricular lipoma. Ann Thorac Surg. 2003;76:1305–7.
40. Benvenuti LA, Mansur AJ, Lopes DO, Assis RVC. Primary lipomatous tumors of the cardiac valves. South Med J. 1996;89:1018–20.
41. Isner JM, Swan 2nd CS, Mikus JP, Carter BL. Lipomatous hypertrophy of the interatrial septum: in vivo diagnosis. Circulation. 1982;66:470–3.
42. Zimmerman KG, Paplanus SH, Dong S, Nagle RB. Congenital blood cysts of heart valves. Hum Pathol. 1983;14:699–703.
43. Gallucci V, Stritoni P, Fasoli G, Thiene G. Giant blood cyst of tricuspid valve. Successful excision in an infant. Br Heart J. 1976;38:990–2.
44. Rossi L, Piffer R, Turolla E, Frigerio B, Coumel P, James TN. Multifocal Purkinje-like tumor of the heart. Occurrence with other anatomic abnormalities in the atrioventricular junction of an infant with junctional tachycardia, Lown–Ganong–Levine syndrome, and sudden death. Chest. 1985;87:340–5.
45. Nojima Y, Ishibashi-Ueda H, Yamagishi M. Cystic tumour of the atrioventricular node. Heart. 2003;89:122.
46. Paniagua JR, Sadaba JR, Davidson LA, Munsch CM. Cystic tumour of the atrioventricular nodal region: report of a case successfully treated with surgery. Heart. 2000;83:E6.
47. Burke AP, Ribe JK, Bajaj AK, Edwards WD, Farb A, Virmani R. Hamartoma of mature cardiac myocytes. Hum Pathol. 1998;29:904–9.
48. Burke AP, Gatto-Weis C, Griego JE, Ellington KS, Virmani R. Adult cellular rhabdomyoma of the heart: a report of 3 cases. Hum Pathol. 2002;33:1092–7.

Primary Cardiac Tumors in the Pediatric Age

5

Massimo A. Padalino, Cristina Basso, Ornella Milanesi, Gaetano Thiene, and Giovanni Stellin

Introduction

Most of primary cardiac tumors in the pediatric age group are benign. However, they may cause major symptoms because of their intracardiac position and/or dimensions [1–9]. In addition, since up to 10% of cardiac tumors may be malignant, a precise histopathologic diagnosis is of paramount importance for a proper diagnosis and therapeutical plan [3, 7].

Cardiac tumor prevalence in the pediatric age is not easy to assess. Postmortem examination data account for an overall incidence of cardiac tumors in the pediatric population ranging between 0.028 and 0.08% [4], and 14.2% of all tumors occur in patients younger than 16 years of age [5].

Based on recent data from the Cardiovascular Program at Boston Children's Hospital, diagnosis of cardiac tumor was possible in 67 children among 38,952 who were evaluated between 1980 and 1998 (0.17%) [6]. Surely, the real incidence of this disease is greater than previously thought, mostly because of improved cardiac imaging techniques.

Although myxomas are the most common cardiac tumors in adults [7, 8], in the pediatric age the most frequent heart tumors are rhabdomyomas (45%), followed by fibromas (25%), myxomas (10–15%), and intrapericardial teratomas (10%) [4, 6, 9–15]. In addition, rhabdomyomas are the most common cardiac neoplasms in the neonate and infant, while in teenagers myxomas occur more often [3, 6].

Due to the peculiar characteristics of each type of tumor, they will be discussed separately.

Primary Benign Cardiac Tumors

Rhabdomyoma

Rhabdomyomas represent the most common heart neoplasms in pediatric age, with an estimated prevalence of 45–63% [1, 2,15]. Diagnosis may be prenatal (24% in the Boston Children's Hospital experience) [6], but it is often achieved at birth. Children may be asymptomatic or only mildly symptomatic, despite an extensive infiltration of the myocardium, and presenting only with a cardiac murmur at physical examination [4, 9]. Usually, prenatal diagnosis occurs when arrhythmias, hydrops, delayed fetal growth, or family history for tuberous sclerosis have been detected on routine fetal screening [16].

M.A. Padalino, M.D., Ph.D. (✉) • G. Stellin, M.D.
Pediatric Cardiac Surgery, Department of Cardiac, Thoracic and Vascular Science, Azienda Ospedaliera-University of Padua Medical School, Via N. Giustiniani 2, Padua 35128, Italy
e-mail: massimo.padalino@unipd.it

C. Basso M.D., Ph.D. • G. Thiene M.D.
Pathological Anatomy, Department of Cardiac, Thoracic and Vascular Sciences, Azienda Ospedaliera-University of Padua Medical School, via A. Gabelli, 61, Padua 35121, Italy

O. Milanesi M.D.
Pediatric Cardiology, Department of Pediatrics, Azienda Ospedaliera-University of Padua Medical School, via N. Giustiniani, 2, Padua 35128, Italy

C. Basso et al. (eds.), *Cardiac Tumor Pathology*, Current Clinical Pathology,
DOI 10.1007/978-1-62703-143-1_5, © Springer Science+Business Media New York 2013

Rhabdomyomas are usually multiple, well-defined, whitish or grayish nodular masses [2–4, 6]; they are single masses in only 10% of the cases [2, 3]. They may appear everywhere in the heart, more often in the ventricular myocardium [2–4, 9, 13]. Mostly intramural, they may sometimes protrude into the ventricular cavity, or they may appear as pedunculated or sessile masses [17] (Fig. 5.1a).

At histology, rhabdomyomas typically present with enlarged vacuolated cells, with sparse cytoplasm with glycogen deposits and so-called “spider” cell appearance, i.e., cells characterized by cytoplasm radial extensions with contractile myofilaments from the central nucleus to the cell periphery [3, 7, 8] (Fig. 5.1b). Immunohistochemical studies show the typical features of striated muscle cells (myoglobin, desmin, actin, and vimentin positive), thus confirming the diagnosis. At transmission electron microscopy, rhabdomyoma cells look like myocytes with abundant glycogen, rare mitochondria, and intercalated disks sparse all around the periphery of the cell instead of being localized at the cell poles.

Clinical features of rhabdomyomas depend on their localization, number and dimensions [18]: for example, a large intramural or intracavitary mass may cause ventricular outflow obstruction, or atrioventricular or semilunar valve distortion [3, 11, 18]. Congestive heart failure, respiratory distress, or even low cardiac output syndrome may occur in neonates or infants [13, 17–19]. In the most severe cases, the ventricular obstruction may even mimic a severe subvalvar aortic stenosis or hypoplastic left heart syndrome or pulmonary stenosis [20–22]. Exceptionally, the tumoral masses may infiltrate diffusely the myocardium, as to cause a severe contractile and diastolic dysfunction, even mimicking a restrictive cardiomyopathy [12].

In the literature, all the commonest arrhythmias (including sudden death) have been described in association with cardiac rhabdomyomas [1, 2, 12, 19, 23]. Direct compression of the conduction system may account for atrial or supraventricular tachyarrhythmias, such as the Wolff Parkinson White syndrome [19, 23]. Most common electrocardiographic abnormalities are left axial deviation, atrial and/or ventricular enlargement, ST elevation, bundle branch block, various degrees of atrioventricular block [1, 12, 19].

The chest X-ray may be absolutely normal, or show cardiomegaly and pulmonary edema in the most compromised patients [1, 4, 12, 19].

Two-dimensional echocardiography remains the main diagnostic tool. Typically, rhabdomyomas are multiple, well-circumscribed nodular masses, which are highly echogenic, either intramural or pedunculated intracavitary (Fig. 5.1a,b), and localized everywhere in the myocardium [17–23]. Rhabdomyomas present with a homogeneous echogenicity due to the absence of fibrosis, necrosis, calcification, as well as cystic and hemorrhagic areas. This is an important feature to distinguish them from thrombi, myxomas, and other tumors [6]. In addition, pericardial effusion is rarely detected at echocardiographic examination [6].

Rhabdomyomas are frequently associated with tuberous sclerosis (86%) [19, 23], while about 50% of children with tuberous sclerosis have a cardiac rhabdomyoma. Tuberous sclerosis is an autosomal dominant disease, with variable penetrance and expression, which may potentially involve all organs, including the brain, pancreas, kidney, skin, and retina. Usual is the association with epilepsy (due to neurofibromatosis lesions), mental retardation (evident by 1 year of age), and skin lesions.

Almost 50% of patients with rhabdomyoma present with a family history of tuberous sclerosis. Recently, two genes have been found to be associated with tuberous sclerosis: TSC1, which codifies for the protein hamartin (9q34); and TSC2, which codifies for the protein tuberin (16p13.3) [24, 25]. These two proteins are involved in the tumor suppression mechanism, but their precise role in cardiac tumor development remains still unknown.

The natural history of rhabdomyomas is characterized by the possibility of spontaneous regression, which may be partial or complete [3, 4, 7, 11, 14]. For this reason, surgery is reserved only to severely symptomatic patients; when symptoms

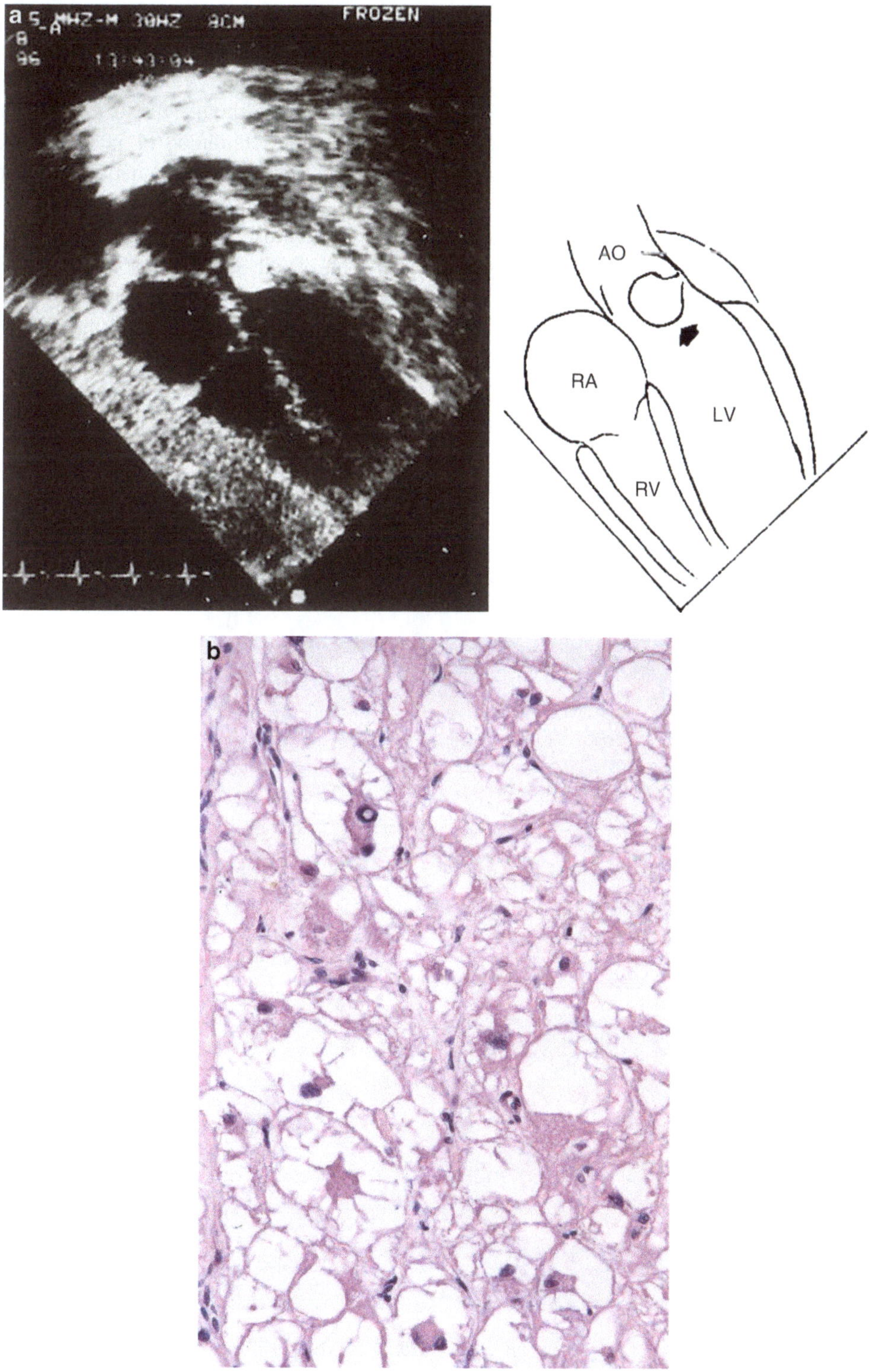

Fig. 5.1 Rhabdomyoma in a 7-month-old child with a systolic murmur due to subaortic stenosis (*modified from De Dominicis et al.* [22]). Reprinted with permission of the Italian Society of Cardiology. (**a**) Two-dimensional echocardiography, subcostal view: note the left ventricular outflow tract obstruction due to an endocavitary mass attached to the anterolateral wall in the subaortic area. (**b**) At histology, the resected mass shows the pathognomonic spider cells with cytoplasmatic myofibrils radiating to the cell periphery (hematoxylin–eosin stain)

are mild or even absent, clinical follow-up, associated with oral medication, is usually indicated [4, 11, 26]. The most common reason for surgical referral is ventricular arrhythmias, which do not respond to drug therapy and obstruction of ventricular outflows. Surgical resection of the tumoral mass aims to remove all tissue causing clinical symptoms/signs and ideally should be as radical as possible. However, the well-known possibility of cardiac mass regression allows to safely perform a partial resection whenever a greater removal of tissue may jeopardize important cardiac structures [3, 4, 10–12, 15, 18–23]. This surgical strategy presents excellent early and long-term outcomes [3, 26].

Fibroma

Cardiac fibroma is the second most frequent type of cardiac tumor in the pediatric age (about 20%) [1–4, 7, 9, 11]. Although the diagnosis is more frequent in late childhood or in teenagers, the tumor may become symptomatic also in early childhood or even in the neonate [27, 28] (Fig. 5.2). Macroscopically at gross examination, the fibroma usually is a single, solid, well-defined, whitish and whorled mass, almost invariably intramural, and usually located in the right or left ventricular free walls, or in the interventricular septum [1–5, 7]. These tumors may reach huge dimensions, even up to 8 cm of diameter, to obstruct the ventricular cavity [27, 28].

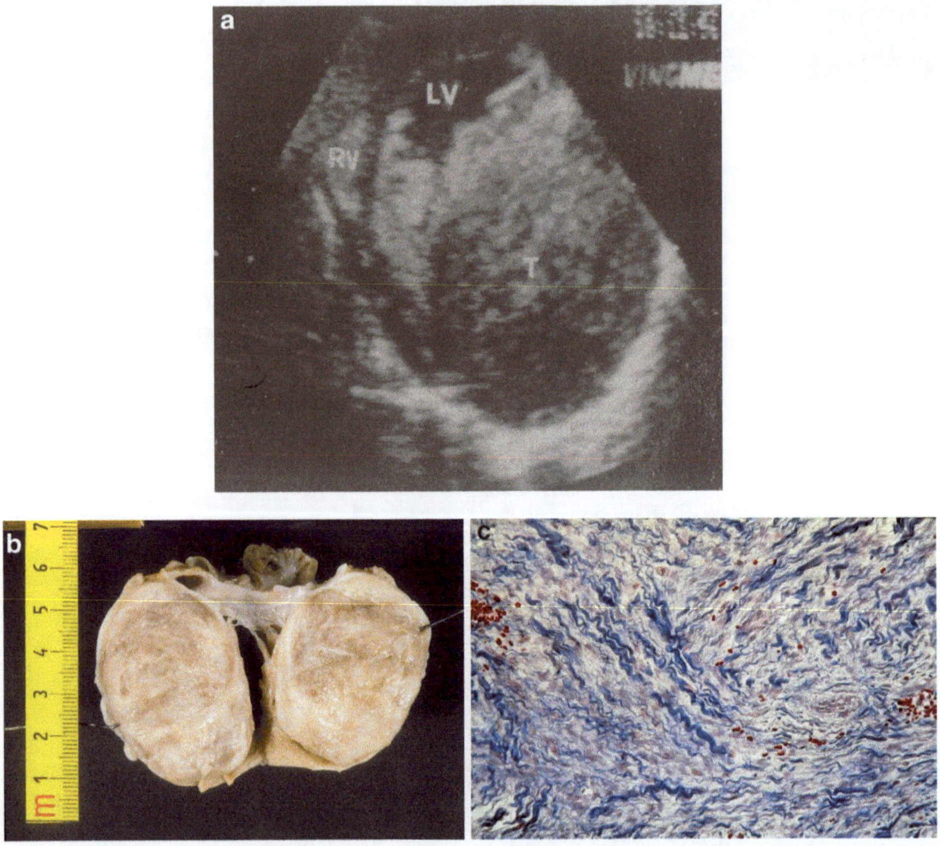

Fig. 5.2 Fibroma in a neonate who underwent heart transplant at 38 days of life, after prenatal echocardiographic diagnosis of left ventrciular mass (*modified from Valente et al.* [27]). Reprinted with permission of the Italian Society of Cardiology. (**a**) Fetal two-dimensional echocardiography of the tumor (T) of the left ventricular free wall (LV). (**b**) Macroscopically, by opening the explanted heart along the obtuse margin, a large intramural oval-shaped, whorled and whitish mass, obstructing the mitral valve orifice, is visible. (**c**) At histology, fibromatous proliferation with abundant collagen fibers (Heidenhain trichrome stain)

At histology, the fibroma consists of a homogeneous mass of fibroblasts mixed with abundant collagen and elastic fibers, and often entrapping some cardiomyocytes. They are not encapsulated and often extend into the surrounding myocardium. The amount of cells decreases during the time, while the collagen content increases [3, 5, 7, 27]. Occasionally, these tumors may present lymphomonocyte aggregates, and areas of calcification which are detected on chest X-ray or CT scan [12]. Spontaneous regression or malignant degeneration has never been described [1, 2, 4, 5, 7, 9].

Clinical symptoms are mostly caused by the dimensions of the mass and from its location. Occasionally, they may be asymptomatic despite large dimensions and be an incidental finding [29]. More commonly, since they can infiltrate the ventricular septum myocardium and the conduction axis, fibromas may cause ventricular arrhythmias and conduction disturbances which may even be lethal causing sudden death [4, 9, 30]. Whenever the mass is large and intramural, it may protrude in the ventricular outflow tract and cause severe mechanical obstruction, together with contractile dysfunction and severe congestive heart failure [1, 3–5, 9, 27, 28].

At echocardiography, fibromas appear as solid single intramural masses, homogeneously dense, with a diameter ranging from few mm to some cm, and usually involving the ventricular free wall or the interventricular septum [3, 4, 9]. Cardiac magnetic resonance imaging (MRI) enables the physician to achieve a better definition of the mass and of its relation with the surrounding structures [28] (Fig. 5.3).

Noteworthy, about 3% of patients with Gorlin syndrome (or nevoid basal cell carcinoma syndrome) show cardiac fibromas [31]. This is an autosomal dominant disorder that affects many areas of the body with an increased risk of developing various tumors and is due to mutations in the *PTCH1,* a tumor suppressor gene.

Surgical referral depends on the presence of clinical symptoms [3, 15]. Although regression has never been described, the asymptomatic patients are usually followed up clinically. Aim of surgical intervention is the resection of the mass, which may be excised completely and safely even if huge [28] (Fig. 5.3). However, whenever a total resection could be potentially dangerous, partial resection is also effective in the early and long term; cavo-pulmonary shunt anastomosis in cases with a very large fibroma of the right ventricle has been even performed [4, 32]. In the most severe cases, with massive infiltration of the myocardium, heart transplant can be the only therapeutic option [15, 27].

Myxoma

Myxoma is the most frequent cardiac tumor in adults [7, 8], but it represents only the 10–15% of cardiac tumors in the pediatric age [1–5]. It is more often diagnosed in teenagers, while it is rare but clinically very dramatic in infants [33] (Fig. 5.4).

Myxoma is usually sporadic, but 10% of patients present an association with the so-called Carney complex, with autosomal dominant inheritance [34, 35].

Intracardiac myxomas are very friable, polypoid, gelatinous masses, sessile or pedunculated, yellowish or reddish. When present, the stalk is typically attached to the endocardium of the fossa ovalis. Although they are usually single masses, multiple or biatrial masses have been reported in the literature [7, 36]. They are more frequently localized in the left atrium, but they have been described everywhere inside the heart [1–5, 7, 8, 33].

Microscopically, myxomas present with a myxoid mucopolysaccharidic matrix containing fusiform, stellate, or polygonal cells, and sometimes aggregated in pseudovascular structures [7] (Fig. 5.5).

Myxomas are benign neoplasms, but they may have a “malignant” behavior because of their dimensions, location, recurrency, or systemic embolization risk [8, 13, 33]. A malignant histologic variant has never been described.

The myxoma usually presents with three types of clinical symptoms and signs, i.e., obstructive, embolic, and constitutional.

Since they are pedunculated and mobile, myxomas in the left or right atrium may impinge into the mitral or tricuspid valve orifice, thus blocking

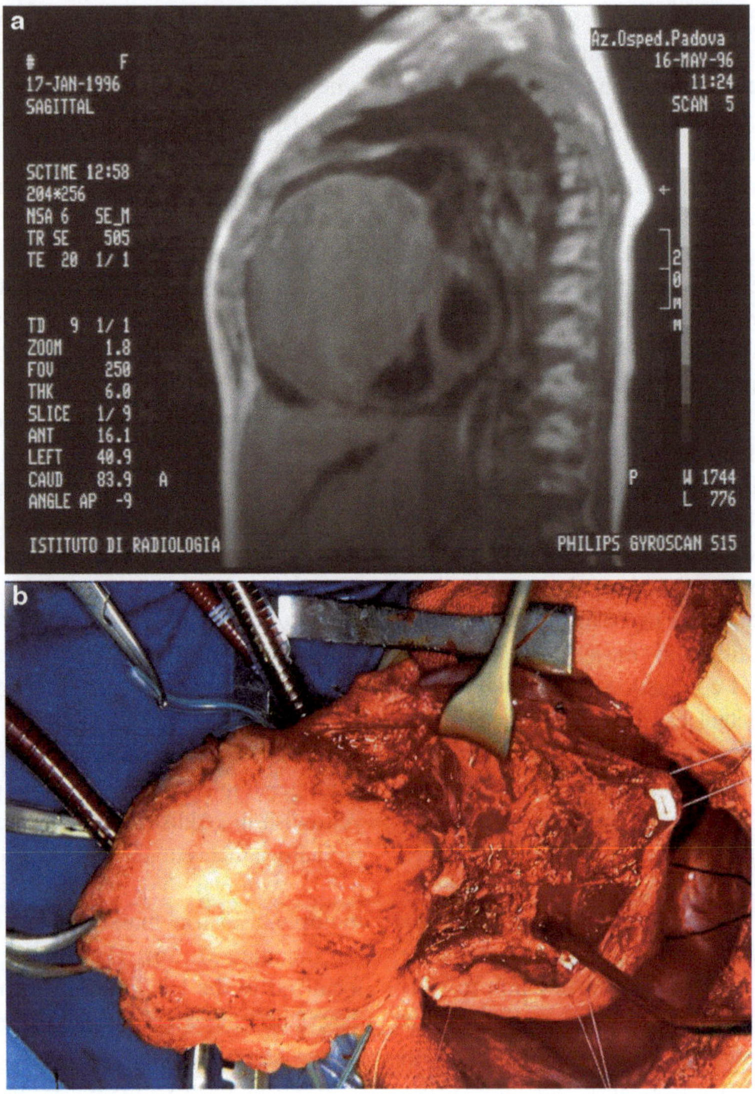

Fig. 5.3 Fibroma in a 5-month-old infant with congestive heart failure and liver enlargement (*modified from Padalino et al.* [28]). Reprinted with permission of the Italian Society of Cardiology. (**a**) Cardiac magnetic resonance imaging in sagittal view: note a large homogeneous mass, 6×4×5 cm, involving the anterior wall of the right ventricle, with an almost complete obliteration of the ventricular cavity and of the pulmonary outflow tract. (**b**) Intraoperative image of the mass involving the right ventricular free wall, which required a ventricular patch plasty after resection

the blood flow during diastole. This hemodynamic block can cause transient heart failure, recurrent syncope (Fig. 5.4b), or even sudden death [8, 13, 32]. Myxomas with a long pedicle may even protrude into the ventricular cavity and cause outflow tract obstruction. At physical examination, a characteristic mesodiastolic murmur or "tumor plop" is often heard, due to mass prolapse into the mitral valve orifice during diastole. These clinical manifestations are often related to the patient position, typically occurring when he or she is standing up; on the contrary, the myxoma moves away from the valve with symptoms relief while lying down. Finally, because of the fast growth of the mass in a small atrial cavity, cardiac myxoma in children usually

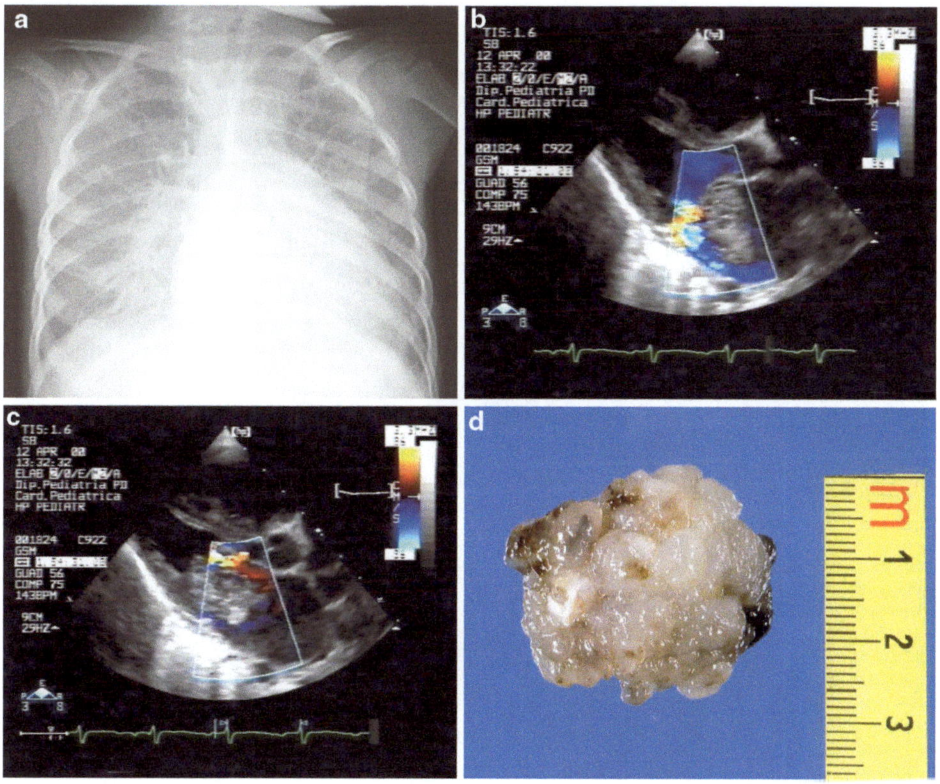

Fig. 5.4 Myxoma in a 6-year-old child with congestive heart failure (*modified from Padalino et al.* [32]). Reprinted with permission of the Italian Society of Cardiology. (**a**) Chest X-ray showing cardiomegaly. (**b**) Two-dimensional color Doppler echocardiography (systole): note the presence of a mass in the left atrium. (**c**) Two-dimensional color Doppler echocardiography (diastole): note the mass prolapse into the mitral valve orifice. (**d**) The resected mass is gelatinous, whitish, with a fine villous surface

presents with severe congestive heart failure and low cardiac output syndrome [3, 33].

The embolic risk is related to the intrinsic friable structure of this tumor, which may embolize either in the systemic or in the pulmonary circulation, depending on its location. Emboli may consist of fragments either of the myxoma or of the thrombus that frequently develop on the surface of the tumor itself. Paradoxical embolism may be caused by a myxoma of the right atrium through a patent foramen ovale [4, 7–9]. Whenever a child presents with embolic manifestations, an accurate two-dimensional echocardiographic examination must be done as soon as possible to rule out a cardiac myxoma.

The so-called "constitutional" symptoms or signs are aspecific and include fever, weight loss, Raynaud's syndrome, anemia, increased C reactive protein, low platelet count, arthralgias, myalgias, mostly due to IL-6 release, which is associated with protein synthesis and production of inflammatory mediators [37]. All these features usually disappear soon after myxoma resection.

At echocardiography, myxoma appears as a lobulated intracavitary mass which is attached with a thin stalk to the endocardium. The color Doppler evaluation enables the estimation of obstruction or regurgitation of the mitral or tricuspid valves. In addition, whenever the myxoma is on the right side of the heart, right ventricular pressure measurement is useful to rule out pulmonary embolism. Ventricular myxoma, although rare, may cause dynamic obstruction of the outflow tract.

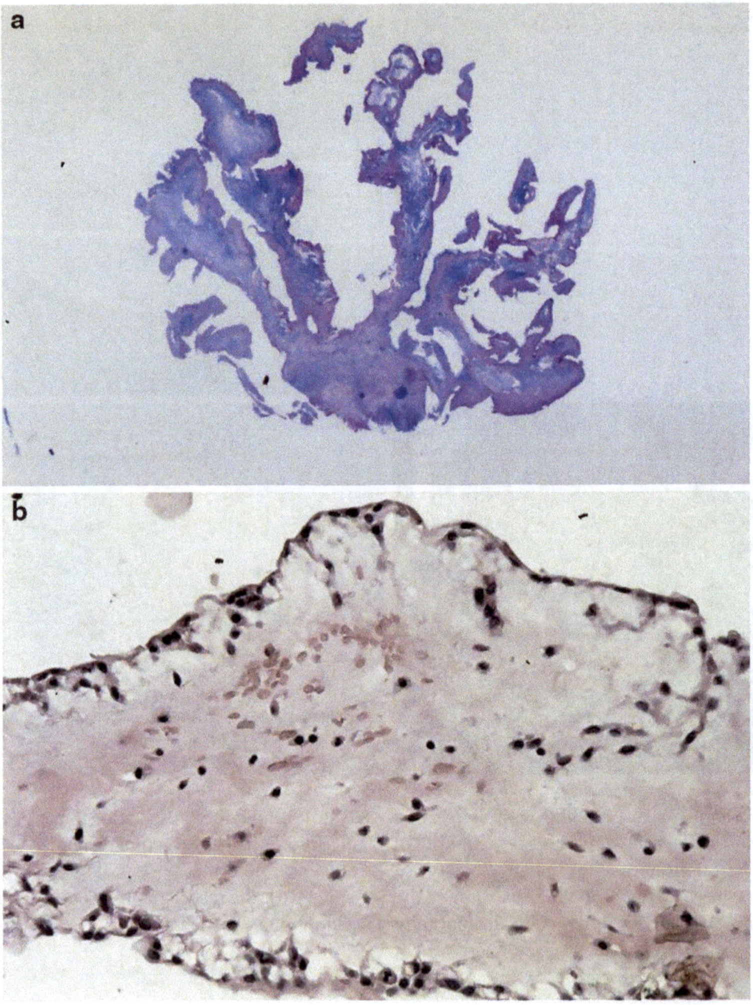

Fig. 5.5 Same case of Fig. 5.4. Reprinted with permission of the Italian Society of Cardiology. (**a**) Histology confirms the villous structure of the tumor, with an abundant myxoid matrix (Alcian PAS ×3). (**b**) At higher magnification, single cells embedded within a myxoid matrix are visible (hematoxylin eosin stain, ×120)

Due to the unpredictable risk of tumor embolization, diagnosis of intracardiac myxoma is by definition an indication to prompt surgical resection of the mass [3, 6, 7, 15, 33]. The surgeon must remove not only the myxoma, but also the endocardial tissue which surrounds the thin stalk of the mass, in order to prevent the well-known risk of myxoma recurrence. Moreover, since the mass is highly friable, it is imperative to avoid manipulation of the heart before the cardio-pulmonary bypass is established and the aorta cross-clamped.

Intrapericardial Teratoma (Germ Cell Tumor)

Germ cells tumors are classified depending on the germ they derive from, such as seminoma (or dysgerminoma), embrional carcinoma, yolk sac tumor, choriocarcinoma, and teratoma [2]. Among more than 100 cases of intrapericardial germ cell tumors reported in the literature, 90% of teratomas involve the pericardium, while only 10% involves the myocardium. Diagnosis occurs typically within the first month of life [38, 39]. They are very rare, usually benign, in contrast

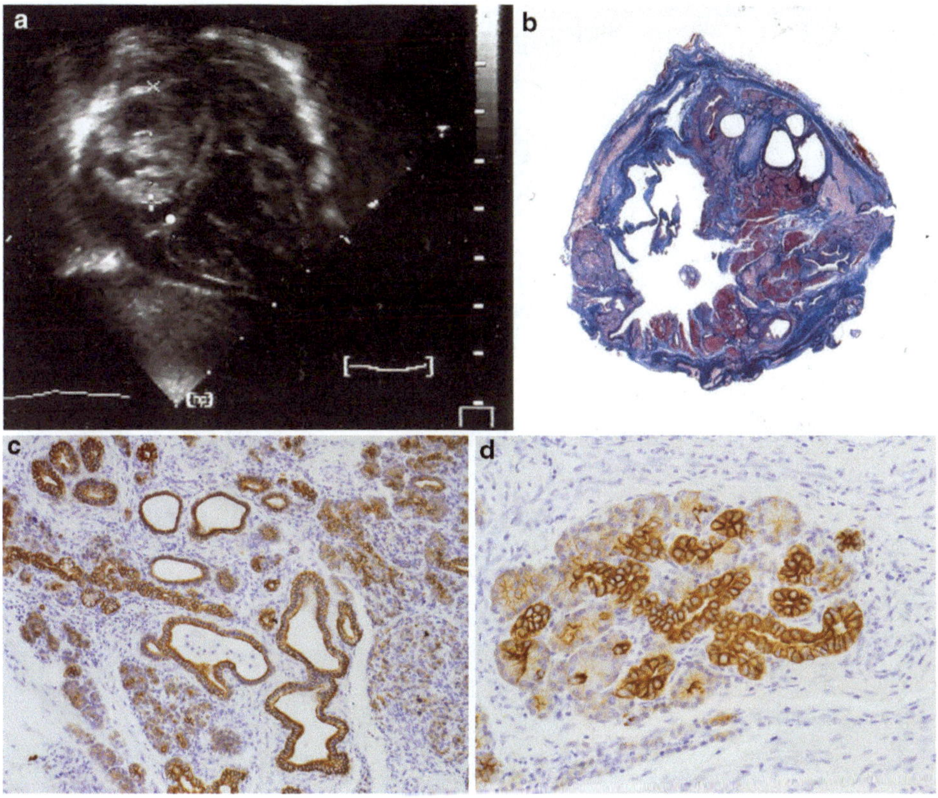

Fig. 5.6 Teratoma in a 12-day-old neonate with pericardial effusion at birth (*modified from Padalino et al.* [3]). Reprinted with permission of the Italian Society of Cardiology. (**a**) Two-dimensional echocardiography, subcostal four-chamber view: note the presence of a dishomogeneous and cystic mass at the root of the great vessels. (**b**) Transverse panoramic histologic section of the resected mass: note the typical cystic structure (Heidenhain trichrome stain). (**c**) At immunohistochemistry, multiple immature elements of different embryonic origin are visible (pan-keratin antibody). (**d**) Close-up of (**c**): note intestinal epithelium (pan-keratin antibody)

with those occurring in adult age which are mostly malignant germ cell tumors.

A teratoma is an encapsulated tumor with tissue or organ components resembling normal derivatives of all three germ layers, although sometimes all three germ layers are not identifiable (and are probably misclassified as bronchogenic cysts). Tissue composition may be highly variable, since teratomas may contain hair, teeth, bone, cartilage, lung or gastroenteric and many other tissues [4, 7–9, 38, 39].

Teratomas are generally solitary, encapsulated cystic masses with intervening solid areas, often connected to the aortic root or to the pulmonary artery by means of a thin vascularized pedicle (Fig. 5.6). They are usually localized at the base of the heart, anterior to the aorta, close to the superior vena cava, and may cause compression of these latter structures but also of the right atrium and ventricle and of the pulmonary artery [40]. They may grow up to reach even 15 cm of diameter, to become even bigger than the heart itself.

The neonate with an intrapericardial teratoma is usually severely symptomatic. In fact, because of the large dimensions and the intrapericardial position, the mass usually compresses the surrounding cardiac and vascular structures, and even the pulmonary parenchyma. Pericardial effusion is commonly associated. This may concur in causing a severe respiratory distress, cardiac tamponade, and low cardiac output syndrome that may be fatal if prompt diagnosis and treatment are not provided [39, 40].

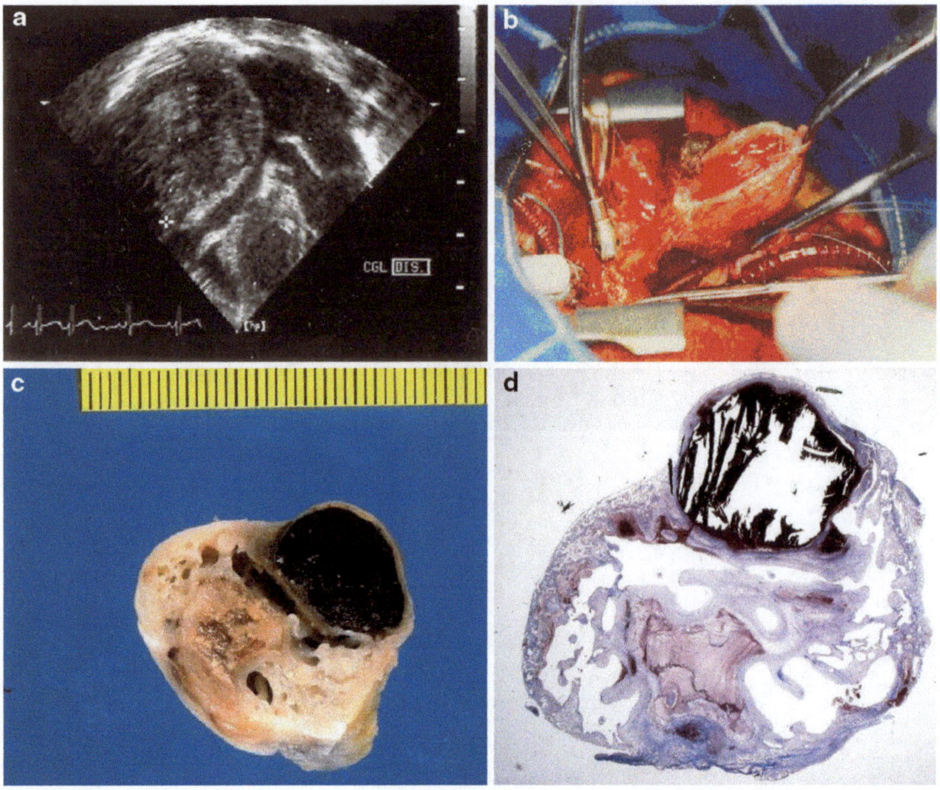

Fig. 5.7 Hemangioma in a 5 days old neonate, with paroxysmal supraventricular tachycardia at birth and a diagnosis of right atrial mass (*modified from Padalino et al.* [32]). Reprinted with permission of the Italian Society of Cardiology. (**a**) Two-dimensional echocardiography, subcostal four-chamber view: note the presence of a dyshomogeneous mass inside the right atrium. (**b**) Surgical view after right atriotomy. (**c**) Macroscopic view of the resected mass: note the multiple vascular spaces filled of blood. (**d**) Histology confirms the diagnosis of benign cavernous hemangioma (Heidenhain trichrome stain)

Diagnosis is usually achieved with two-dimensional echocardiography during both the fetal and the neonatal period [41, 42]. The teratoma looks like a single pedunculated mass, inside the pericardium; it appear as a dyshomogenous mass because of the presence of cystic and calcified areas. Two-dimensional echocardiography allows a precise evaluation of the mass dimensions, location, and associated pericardial effusion, thus guiding the physician for pericardial fluid drainage [40]. Fetal echocardiography enables an early diagnosis to plan a prompt surgical management at birth [40, 41]. Surgical resection of the mass is often lifesaving and effective, since tumor relapse or pericardial effusion recurrence has never been reported [43]. Surgery consists in a complete resection of the mass and of its vascularised pedicle from the ascending aorta, and from the adjacent pericardium. Since the mass is typically extracardiac, cardiopulmonary bypass is not required but a careful dissection and ligation of the aorta and/or pulmonary artery is needed to prevent massive hemorrhage being the blood supply from the root of these vessels [44].

Hemangioma

Cardiac hemangioma and all other tumors derived from vascular tissue (lymphangiomas) are rare benign cardiac tumors which may arise everywhere in the heart. Two-dimensional echocardiography shows multiple echo-transparent masses, often associated with pericardial effusion, which may grow within the myocardium but also intracardiac (Fig. 5.7) [45, 46]. They are frequently clinically silent as to be an incidental finding during routine examination; sometimes they may trigger arrhythmias or cause obstructive symptoms. In asymptomatic patients, clinical and echocardiographic follow-up is usually enough, On the contrary, surgical resection is indicated whenever the mass causes symptoms and is well defined and circumscribed. However, if the mass is diffusely infiltrating the myocardium, cardiac transplantation may be the only therapeutic option [45, 46].

Histiocytoid Cardiomyopathy

This lesion is also known as oncocytic cardiomyopathy, Purkinje cell tumor or hamartoma, focal lipid cardiomyopathy, idiopathic infantile cardiomyopathy [47, 48]. It occurs mostly in the first 2 years of life.

Concerning its pathogenesis, nowadays it is considered a tumor deriving from the cardiomyocyte with some Purkinje cell features, although many other theories have been advanced including viral infections, myocardial ischemia, glycogen storage disease, and mitochondrial cardiomyopathy.

Macroscopically, these masses present as single or multiple subendocardial yellowish nodules or plaques, 1–15 mm in size. The most common locations are the conduction system and the left ventricle, but they may be also found in the right atrium and ventricle. In up to one-third of patients the tumors may be associated with cardiac or extracardiac anomalies such as atrial and ventricular septal defects, hypoplastic left heart syndrome, cleft palate, and anomalies of the eyes, skin, and central nervous system.

Microscopically, these multifocal islands contain large, polygonal, or oval cells, with a coarse granular pale eosinophilic cytoplasm (Fig. 5.8). The cytoplasm is filled with abundant, bizarre looking mitochondria. The term oncocytic cardiomyopathy describes the process of the granules (mitochondria) displacing the working myofibrils. When compared to rhabdomyoma, there are many mitochondria with no T tubules or complex intercellular junctions, and no vacuoles or myofibrils (Fig. 5.8). At immunohistochemistry, tumor cells react with antibodies to desmin, myoglobin, myosin, and muscle-specific actin, whereas there is no expression of histiocyte antigens.

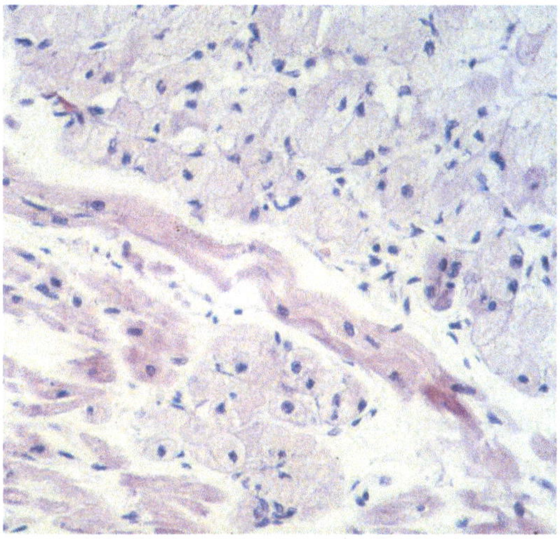

Fig. 5.8 Purkinje cell tumor in a 13-month-old child presenting with cyanosis and dyspnea. Reprinted with permission of the Italian Society of Cardiology. Histology shows focal islands of Purkinje-like cells, clearly distinct from the normal surrounding cardiomyocytes (hematoxylin–eosin stain)

Echocardiography may reveal nodular deposits on the ventricular endocardium or valves. If left untreated, oncocytic cardiomyopathy may have a fatal course in affected infants. Surgical excision or cryoablation of the multiple nodular lesions is required for long-term cure, with a survival rate of 80% [26, 49]. A few cases of cardiac transplantation due to extensive disease have been also reported.

Other Benign Cardiac Tumors

Other types of benign cardiac tumors in infancy are extremely rare and include lipoma and papilloma, which may occur anywhere inside the heart [1, 2, 4, 9].

Finally, a very rare and peculiar type of cardiac tumor is the *inflammatory myofibroblastic tumor* (or inflammatory pseudotumor, plasma cell granuloma), a proliferation of uncertain histogenesis. Histologically, it is composed of spindled myofibroblasts, fibroblasts, and chronic inflammatory cells including lymphocytes, macrophages, plasma cells, and eosinophils [49]. Grossly, they are endocardial lesions which often have a narrow attachment to the endocardium and protrude into the cardiac chambers. There is often organizing fibrin thrombus on the surface. Echocardiographic evaluation shows a homogeneous intracavitary mass that often fills completely the cardiac cavity. It may be silent or can cause obstructive symptoms; surgery is usually indicated [50].

Primary Malignant Cardiac Tumors in the Pediatric Age

Malignant primary cardiac tumors are extremely rare in infancy and pediatric age. There no series in the literature to date. In a review of neonatal and fetal heart tumors published prior to 2004, sarcoma represented 0 and 2% of total cases, respectively [51]. It is suspected that several pediatric heart tumors reported in the medical literature as sarcomas are probably misdiagnosed inflammatory myofibroblastic tumors (see above).

References

1. Fyler DC. Report of the New England regional infant cardiac program. Pediatrics. 1980;65:376–461.
2. Burke AP, Veinot JP, Loire R, Virmani R, Tazelaar H, Kaniya H, Araoz PA, Watanabe G. Tumours of the heart. In: Travis WD, Brambilla E, Muller-Hermelink HK, Harris CC, editors. Pathology and genetics of tumours of the lung, pleura, thymus and heart. Lyon: IARC Press; 2004. p. 249–88.
3. Padalino MA, Basso C, Milanesi O, Vida VL, Svaluto Moreolo G, Thiene G, Stellin G. Surgically treated primary cardiac tumors in early infancy and childhood. J Thorac Cardiovasc Surg. 2005;129:1358–63.
4. Beghetti M, Gow RM, Haney I, Mawson J, Williams WG, Freedom RM. Pediatric primary benign cardiac tumors: a 15 year review. Am Heart J. 1997;134:1107–14.
5. Burke A, Virmani R. Tumors of the heart and great vessels. Atlas of tumor pathology, series 3, fascicle 16. Washington, DC: Armed Force Institute of Pathology; 1995.
6. Marx GA, Moran AM. Cardiac tumors. In: Allen HD, Adams FH, Moss AJ, editors. Moss & Adams's heart disease in infants, children and adolescents: including the fetus and young adult. Philadelphia, PA: Lippincott Williams & Wilkins; 2001. p. 1432–45.
7. Basso C, Valente M, Poletti A, Casarotto D, Thiene G. Surgical pathology of primary cardiac and pericardial tumors. Eur J Cardiothorac Surg. 1997;12:730–8.
8. Bortolotti U, Maraglino G, Rubino M, Santini F, Milano A, Fasoli G, Livi U, Thiene G, Gallucci V. Surgical excision of intracardiac myxomas: a 20 year follow up. Ann Thorac Surg. 1990;49:449–53.
9. Freedom RM, Lee KJ, MacDonald C, Taylor G. Selected aspects of cardiac tumors in infancy and childhood. Pediatr Cardiol. 2000;21:299–316.
10. Jacobs JP, Anastasios KK, Holland FW, Hershowitz K, Ferrer PL, Perryman RA. Surgical treatment for cardiac rhabdomyomas in children. Ann Thorac Surg. 1994;58:1552–5.
11. Becker AE. Primary heart tumors in the pediatric age group: a review of salient pathologic features relevant for clinicians. Pediatric Cardiol. 2000;21:317–23.
12. Bini RM, Westaby S, Bargeron Jr LM, Pacifico AD, Kirklin RW. Investigation and management of primary cardiac tumors in infants and children. J Am Coll Cardiol. 1983;2:351–7.
13. Sallee D, Spector ML, van Heeckeren DW, Patel CR. Primary pediatric cardiac tumors: 17 year experience. Cardiol Young. 1999;9:155–62.
14. Chan HSL, Sonley MJ, Moes F, Daneman A, Smith CR, Martin DJ. Primary and secondary tumors of childhood involving the heart, pericardium and great vessels. Cancer. 1985;56:825–36.
15. Padalino MA, Vida VL, Boccuzzo G, Tonello M, Sarris GE, Berggren H, Comas JV, Di Carlo D, Di Donato RM, Ebels T, Hraska V, Jacobs JP, Gaynor JW, Metras D, Pretre R, Pozzi M, Rubay J, Sairanen H, Schreiber C, Maruszewski B, Basso C, Stellin G. Surgery for primary cardiac tumors in children: early and late results in a multicenter European congenital heart surgeons association study. Circulation. 2012;126:22–30.
16. Deeg KH, Voigt HJ, Hofbeck M, Singer H, Kraus J. Prenatal ultrasound diagnosis of multiple cardiac rhabdomyomas. Pediatr Radiol. 1990;20:291–2.
17. Fischer DR, Beerman LB, Park SC, Bahnson HAT, Fricker FJ, Mathews RA. Diagnosis of intracardiac rhabdomyoma by two dimensional echocardiography. Am J Cardiol. 1984;53:978–97.
18. Roberts WC. Primary and secondary neoplasms of the heart. Am J Cardiol. 1997;80:671–82.
19. Shaher RM, Mintzer J, Farina M, Alley R, Bishop M. Clinical presentation of rhabdomyoma of the heart in infancy and childhood. Am J Cardiol. 1972;30:95–103.
20. Abdel-Rahman U, Ozaslan F, Esmaeili A, Moritz A. A giant rhabdomyoma with left ventricular inflow occlusion and univentricular physiology. Thorac Cardiovasc Surg. 2005;53:259–60.
21. Friedberg M, Silverman NH. Right ventricular outflow tract obstruction in an infant. Heart. 2005;91:748.
22. De Dominicis E, Frigiola A, Thiene G, Menicanti L, Bozzola L, Finocchi G. Subaortic stenosis by solitary rhabdomyoma. Successful excision in an infant following 2D echocardiogram and Doppler diagnosis. Chest. 1989;95:470–2.
23. Bosi G, Lintermans JP, Pellegrino PA, Svaluto Moreolo G, Vliers A. The natural history of cardiac rhabdomyoma with and without tuberous sclerosis. Acta Pediatr. 1996;85:928–31.

24. Povey S, Burley MW, Attwood J, Benham F, Hunt D, Jeremiah SJ, Franklin D, Gillett G, Malas S, Robson EB. Two loci for tuberous sclerosis: one on 9q34 and one on 16p13. Ann Hum Genet. 1994;58:107–27.
25. van Slegtenhorst M, de Hoogt R, Hermans C, Nellist M, Janssen B, Verhoef S, Lindhout D, van den Ouweland A, Halley D, Young J, Burley M, Jeremiah S, Woodward K, Nahmias J, Fox M, Ekong R, Osborne J, Wolfe J, Povey S, Snell RG, Cheadle JP, Jones AC, Tachataki M, Ravine D, Sampson JR, Reeve MP, Richardson P, Wilmer F, Munro C, Hawkins TL, Sepp T, Ali JB, Ward S, Green AJ, Yates JR, Kwiatkowska J, Henske EP, Short MP, Haines JH, Jozwiak S, Kwiatkowski DJ. Identification of the tuberous sclerosis gene TSC1 on chromosome 9q34. Science. 1997;277:805–8.
26. Takach TJ, Reul GI, Ott DA, Cooley DA. Primary cardiac tumors in infants and children: immediate and long term operative results. Ann Thorac Surg. 1996;62:559–64.
27. Valente M, Cocco P, Thiene G, Casula R, Poletti A, Milanesi O, Fasoli G, Livi U. Cardiac fibroma and heart transplantation. J Thorac Cardiovasc Surg. 1993;106:1208–12.
28. Padalino MA, Basso C, Thiene G, Stellin G. Giant right ventricular fibroma in an infant. Circulation. 2002;106:386.
29. Takahashi K, Imamura Y, Ochi T, Hamanda M, Ito T, Hiwada K, Kokubu T. Echocardiographic demonstration of an asymptomatic patient with left ventricular fibroma. Am J Cardiol. 1984;53:981–2.
30. Filiatrault M, Beland MJ, Neilson KA, Paquet M. Cardiac fibroma presenting with clinically significant arrhythmias in infancy. Pediatr Cardiol. 1991; 12:118–20.
31. Vaughan CJ, Veugelers M, Basson CT. Tumors and the heart: molecular genetic advances. Curr Opin Cardiol. 2001;16:195–200.
32. Beghetti M, Haney I, Williams WG, Mawson J, Freedom RM, Gow RM. Massive right ventricular fibroma treated with partial resection and a cavopulmonary shunt. Ann Thorac Surg. 1996;62:882–4.
33. Padalino MA, Basso C, Svaluto Moreolo G, Thiene G, Stellin G. Left atrial myxoma in a child. Case report and review of literature. Cardiovasc Pathol. 2003;12:233–6.
34. Carney JA, Gordon H, Carpenter PC, Shenoy BV, Go VL. The complex of myxomas, spotty pigmentation, and endocrine overactivity. Medicine. 1985;64:270–83.
35. Carney JA, Hruska LS, Beauchamp GD, Gordon H. Dominant inheritance of the complex of myxomas, spotty pigmentation, and endocrine overactivity. Mayo Clin Proc. 1986;61:165–72.
36. Cilliers AM, van Unen H, Lala S, Vanderdonck KH, Hartman E. Massive biatrial myxomas in a child. Pediatr Cardiol. 1999;20:150–1.
37. Kanda T, Umeyama S, Sasaki A, Nakazato Y, Morishita Y, Imai S, Suzuki T, Murata K. Interleukin-6 and cardiac myxoma. Am J Cardiol. 1994;74:965–7.
38. Sumner TE, Crowe JE, Klein A, McKone RC, Weaver RL. Intrapericardial teratoma in infancy. Pediatr Radiol. 1980;10:51–3.
39. Agozzino L, Vosa C, Arciprete P, de Leva F, Cotrufo M. Intrapericardial teratoma in the newborn. Int J Cardiol. 1984;5:21–8.
40. Benatar A, Vaughan J, Nicolini U, Corrin B, Licoln C. Prenatal pericardiocentesis: its role in the management of intrapericardial teratoma. Obstet Gynecol. 1992;79:856–9.
41. Cyr DR, Guntheroth WG, Nyberg DA, Smith JR, Nudelman SR, Ek M. Prenatal diagnosis of an intrapericardial teratoma. A cause for non immune hydrops. J Ultrasound Med. 1988;7:87–90.
42. Farooki ZQ, Arciniegas E, Hakimi M, Clapp S, Jackson W, Green EW. Real time echocardiographic features of intrapericardial teratoma. J Clin Ultrasound. 1982;10:125–8.
43. Banfield F, Dick II M, Behrendt DM, Rosenthal A, Pescheria A, Scott W. Intrapericardial teratoma: a new and treatable cause of hydrops fetalis. Am J Dis Child. 1980;134:1174–5.
44. Paw PT, Jamieson SW. Surgical management of intrapericardial teratoma diagnosed in utero. Ann Thorac Surg. 1997;64:552–4.
45. Tabry IF, Nassar VH, Rizk G, Touma A, Dagher IK. Cavernous hemangioma of the heart: case report and review of literature. J Thorac Cardiovasc Surg. 1975;69:415–20.
46. Grenadier E, Margulis T, Palant A, Safadi T, Merin G. Huge cavernous hemangioma of the heart: a completely evaluated case report and review of the literature. Am Heart J. 1989;117:479–81.
47. Rossi L, Piffer R, Turolla E, Frigerio B, Coumel P, James TN. Multifocal Purkinje-like tumor of the heart. Occurrence with other anatomic abnormalities in the atrioventricular junction of an infant with junctional tachycardia, Lown–Ganong–Levine syndrome, and sudden death. Chest. 1985;87:340–5.
48. Ferrans VJ, McAllister Jr HA, Haese WH. Infantile cardiomyopathy with histiocytoid change in cardiac muscle cells. Report of six patients. Circulation. 1976;53:708–19.
49. Garson A, Smith RT, Moak JP, Kearney DL, Hawkins EP, Titus JL, Cooley DA, Ott DA. Incessant ventricular tachycardia in infants: myocardial hamartomas and surgical cure. J Am Coll Cardiol. 1987;10:619–26.
50. Rose AG, McCormick S, Cooper K, Titus JL. Inflammatory pseudotumor (plasma cell granuloma) of the heart. Report of two cases and literature review. Arch Pathol Lab Med. 1996;120:549–54.
51. Burke A, Virmani R. Pediatric heart tumors. Cardiovasc Pathol. 2008;17:193–8.

Primary Malignant Tumors of the Heart

6

Marialuisa Valente, Stefania Rizzo, Ornella Leone, and Cristina Basso

Introduction

Primary malignant tumors of the heart are rare and are represented by sarcomas, primary lymphomas, and malignant pericardial tumors.

According to the "WHO histological classification of the tumors of the heart" [1] primary cardiac malignancies include:

- Angiosarcoma
- Epithelioid hemangioendothelioma
- Pleomorphic malignant fibrous histiocytoma (MFH)/undifferentiated pleomorphic sarcoma
- Fibrosarcoma and myxoid fibrosarcoma
- Rhabdomyosarcoma
- Leiomyosarcoma
- Synovial sarcoma
- Liposarcoma
- Cardiac lymphoma
- Primary malignant pericardial tumors (solitary fibrous tumor, malignant mesothelioma, germ cell tumor)

M. Valente, M.D. (✉) • S. Rizzo, M.D.
• C. Basso, M.D., Ph.D.
Pathological Anatomy, Department of Cardiac, Thoracic and Vascular Sciences,
Azienda Ospedaliera-University of Padua Medical School, via A. Gabelli, 61, Padua 35121, Italy
e-mail: marialuisa.valente@unipd.it

O. Leone, M.D.
Department of Pathology, S. Orsola-Malpighi Hospital, Via Massarenti, 9, Bologna 40138, Italy

There are a few differences in this recent WHO classification compared to the previous one utilized by the Armed Forces Institute of Pathology [2] (a) epithelioid hemangioendothelioma has been introduced; (b) malignant fibrous histiocytoma (MFH) and undifferentiated pleomorphic sarcoma are regarded as synonyms and cases reported in the past as osteosarcomas are now considered as MFH with osseous differentiation; (c) myxosarcoma is thought to be a myxoid variant of fibrosarcoma. Finally, other very rare primary cardiac tumors, like malignant schwannoma, malignant rhabdoid tumor [2], and carcinosarcoma [3] are not mentioned by the WHO classification.

There is no TNM classification for primary malignant cardiac tumors, and, due to their low frequency, there is no specific grading scheme for sarcomas. Thus, the general criteria proposed for grading malignant tumors of the soft tissues are utilized also for the cardiac ones [4].

The two most widely used grading systems for soft tissue sarcomas are those proposed by the United States National Cancer Institute (NCI) [5] and by the Fédération Nationale des Centres de Lutte Contre le Cancer (FNCLCC) [6]. According to the latter, a histological score from 1 to 3 is assigned to each of three parameters, i.e., tumor differentiation, mitotic rate, and amount of necrosis in untreated primary soft tissue sarcomas. The final grade is obtained by adding the three scores. The grade has been demonstrated to be the main predictive factor for metastases in soft tissue

C. Basso et al. (eds.), *Cardiac Tumor Pathology*, Current Clinical Pathology,
DOI 10.1007/978-1-62703-143-1_6, © Springer Science+Business Media New York 2013

pleomorphic sarcoma, undifferentiated sarcoma and synovial sarcoma [7].

The prognosis for cardiac sarcomas firstly depends on complete surgical resection. This is only rarely achieved, so adjuvant chemotherapy and more rarely radiotherapy are also given. Orthotopic heart transplantation [8] or even autotransplantation [9] is an option in selected cases.

Angiosarcoma

This sarcoma with endothelial differentiation is the most frequent primary malignant cardiac tumor [10–14]. It has been reported with several synonyms such as hemangioendothelioma, malignant hemangioendothelioma, hemangiosarcoma, hemangioendothelial sarcoma, malignant hemangioma, malignant angioendothelioma, and hemangioendotheliosarcoma.

Epidemiology. Primary cardiac angiosarcomas can occur at any age (from 36 months to 80 years), but they are more frequently diagnosed in the fourth decade [15, 16]. There is no sex predilection.

Localization. Angiosarcomas are usually located within the right atrium, close to the atrio-ventricular sulcus, but they have been seldom reported also in the other cardiac chambers and in the pericardium.

Clinical presentation. The diagnosis of angiosarcoma is usually difficult and late, as the clinical picture, including constitutional symptoms (fever, arthralgias, weakness and loss of weight) is nonspecific. The most common symptom is chest pain [15], followed by right heart failure, haemorrhagic pericardial effusion and supraventricular arrhythmias. Metastases to the lungs are frequently present at diagnosis [17]; coagulation abnormalities are also observed [18].

The diagnosis may be achieved through an endomyocardial biopsy due to frequent right heart localization of the tumor [19], as well as through an open pericardial biopsy in case of pericardial infiltration with hemorrhagic effusion. Cardiac rupture has been rarely described.

Imaging. Two-dimensional echocardiography demonstrates an echogenic mass (Fig. 6.1a) in the right atrium associated with pericardial effusion and/or infiltration [20]. Cardiovascular magnetic resonance imaging (MRI) reveals a nodular and heterogeneous mass with focal areas of increased signal intensity related to hemorrhage. Enhancement along the vascular channels gives a "sunray" appearance [21]. Moreover, MRI allows to distinguish between pericardial neoplasm and pericardial effusion. On computed tomography (CT) angiosarcoma appears as an inhomogeneous mass, with high attenuation caused by hemorrhage, and low attenuation in necrotic areas [20].

Gross features. Angiosarcoma is usually a cauliflower-like dark-red mass, projecting into the right atrial cavity, with variable size and poorly defined borders, infiltrating the pericardium and causing hemorrhagic pericardial effusion. Obstruction of the venae cavae, tricuspid valve, right ventricle, and rarely the pulmonary artery may occur.

Histopathological features. In two thirds of the cases, angiosarcoma is well differentiated; irregularly shaped and anastomotic vascular channels are visible, admixed with papillary proliferation of bizarre endothelial cells, with large hyperchromatic nuclei (Fig. 6.1b, c). In one third of the cases, tumor is poorly differentiated, composed of solid clusters of oval and spindle-shaped cells with eosinophilic cytoplasm and hyperchromatic nuclei furnished with prominent nucleoli. Mitosis and scattered extravascular red blood cells are frequently seen; areas of tumor necrosis and hemorrhage may be present. The immunohistochemical profile reflects the endothelial nature of the malignant cells, which are strongly positive for CD31, CD34, and factor VIII (Fig. 6.1d). Ultrastructural studies rarely contribute to the diagnosis, because Weibel-Palade bodies, the ultrastructural markers of normal endothelial cells, are very rare in the cells of angiosarcoma. However, other features such as pinocytic vesicles, intermediate filaments, prominent rough endoplasmic reticulum, Golgi apparatus, and association with pericytes are present.

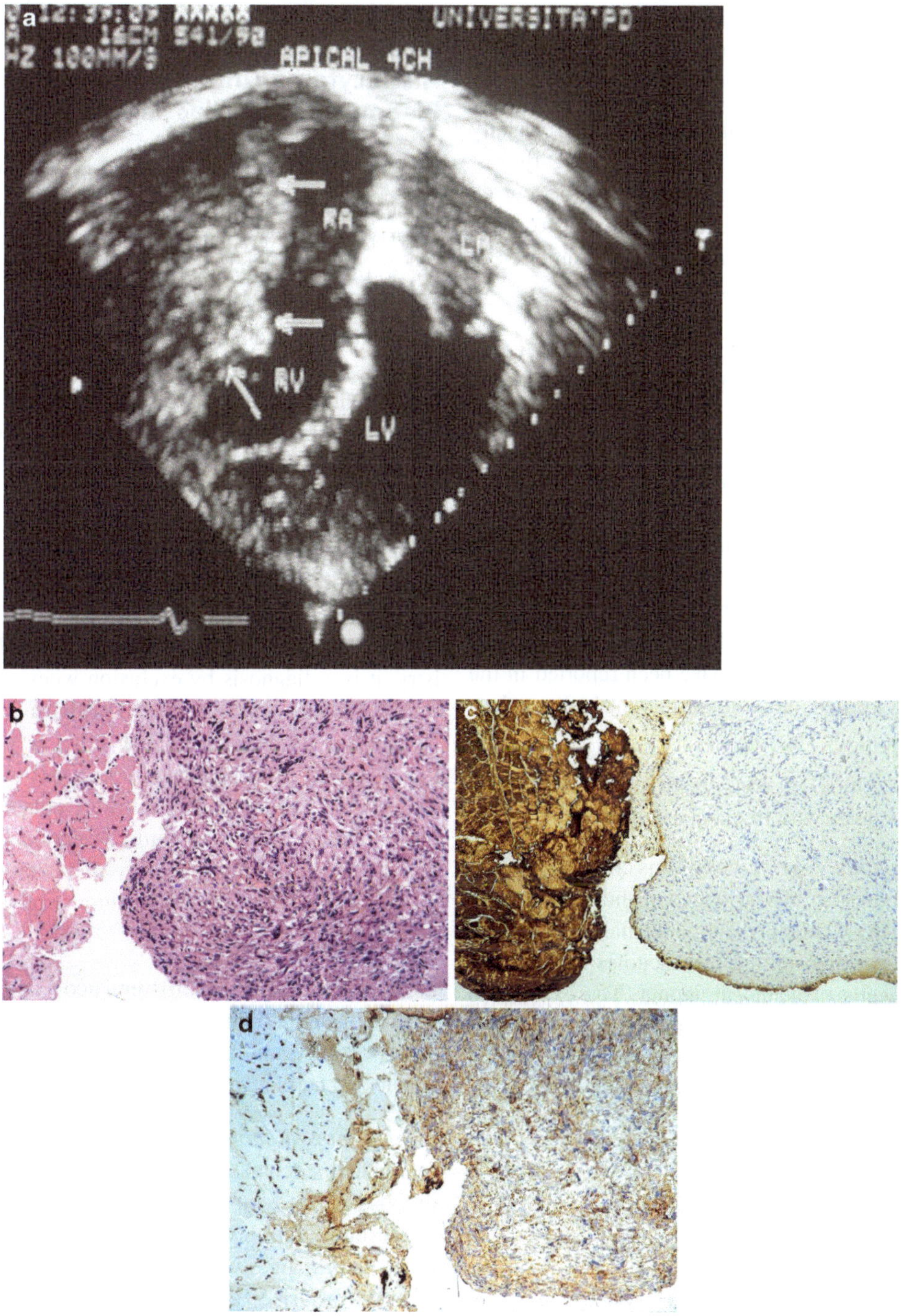

Fig. 6.1 Angiosarcoma in 36-year-old woman, suffering from dyspnea and fever (modified from Poletti et al. [19]). Reprinted with permission of the Italian Society of Cardiology. (**a**) Two-dimensional echocardiogram, apical four-chamber view, showing an irregular, both endocavitary and intramural large mass *(arrows)* in the right atrium (*RA*), extending into the right ventricle (*RV*), 6×8 cm in size. (**b**) Histology of the transvenous endomyocardial biopsy of the mass: the myocardium appears infiltrated by pleomorphic spindle cells with hyperchromatic nuclei forming vascular channels (hematoxylin–eosin stain). (**c**) Immunostaining against myoglobin is strongly positive in the normal myocardium but not in the neoplastic proliferation. (**d**) The tumor cells arranged in vascular channels are positive to factor VIII (*LV* left ventricle)

Genetic studies on angiosarcoma are extremely limited. K-ras alterations [22] and clonal polyploidy [23] have been identified.

Prognosis. Prognosis is extremely poor, usually because of delayed diagnosis, when metastases, in particular to the lungs, have already occurred [24]. Median survival is less than 1 year from the first operation [25]. Cardiac transplantation does not provide long-term survival [8].

Epithelioid Hemangioendothelioma

Epidemiology and localization. Epithelioid hemangioendothelioma is a rare tumor that has been described in the soft tissues of the limbs, usually occurring inside a medium-sized vein, in the lungs (originally considered as an intravascular bronchioalveolar tumor) and in the liver, where it seems to be related to oral contraceptive use. Only a few cases have been reported in the heart, located close to atrio-ventricular sulcus [26] or in the valves [27].

Gross features. It consists grossly of small, reddish nodules with frequent calcifications.

Histopathological features. It is characterized by round or oval cells, arranged in short strands and nests; these cells present with small intracellular lumina, which mimic the vacuoles observed in some cells of adenocarcinoma. The expression of vascular endothelial markers, such as factor VIII, CD31, and CD34, by cells of epithelioid hemangioendothelioma, rules out metastatic adenocarcinoma.

A chromosomal translocation involving chromosomes 1 and 3 has been detected by cytogenetic analysis in 2 out of 3 cases of soft tissue epithelioid hemangioendothelioma [28, 29].

Prognosis. The occurrence of systemic metastases has been described in 10% of the extra-cardiac cases. Cardiac epithelioid hemangio-endothelioma can produce systemic metastases. In the medical literature only a case of epithelioid hemangioendothelioma originating from the heart with systemic metastases has been reported [30].

Pleomorphic Malignant Fibrous Histiocytoma/Undifferentiated Pleomorphic Cardiac Sarcoma

According to the recent WHO classification of soft tissue tumors [4] malignant fibrous histiocytoma (MFH) and undifferentiated pleomorphic sarcoma, previously considered as separate entities, are now regarded as synonyms. They are malignant undifferentiated mesenchymal tumors. Three different subtypes have been described (1) high grade MFH/undifferentiated pleomorphic sarcoma; (2) giant cells MFH/undifferentiated pleomorphic sarcoma; (3) MFH/undifferentiated pleomorphic sarcoma with prominent inflammation.

Epidemiology. Undifferentiated pleomorphic sarcoma was by far the most frequent primary cardiac malignancy (about 50%) in the past [31], but actually, thanks to the use of immunohistochemistry, it is a diagnosis by exclusion when all the immunohistochemical stains fail to give evidence of specific differentiation and it is very rare [32–34]. The Atlas of Armed Force Institute of Pathology [2] reports still a high frequency of these tumors (24% of all cardiac sarcomas), but this is due to the unavailability of material for immunohistochemical/ultrastructural analysis in most cases.

Localization. Most undifferentiated sarcomas arise in the left atrium (posterior wall and/or interatrial septum), and have an intracavitary growth, mimicking cardiac myxoma [35] (Fig. 6.2a).

Clinical presentation. Patients with MFH/undifferentiated sarcomas present with constitutional or obstructive symptoms, including pulmonary congestion, mitral valve obstruction, dyspnea, chest pain, congestive heart failure, or arrhythmias. Metastasis to the lymph nodes, lungs, skin, and systemic organs occurs early.

Echocardiography is helpful in demonstrating a cardiac mass, but CT and MRI are required to assess local extent or metastases for preoperative planning when curative management is contemplated and postoperatively to identify if excision

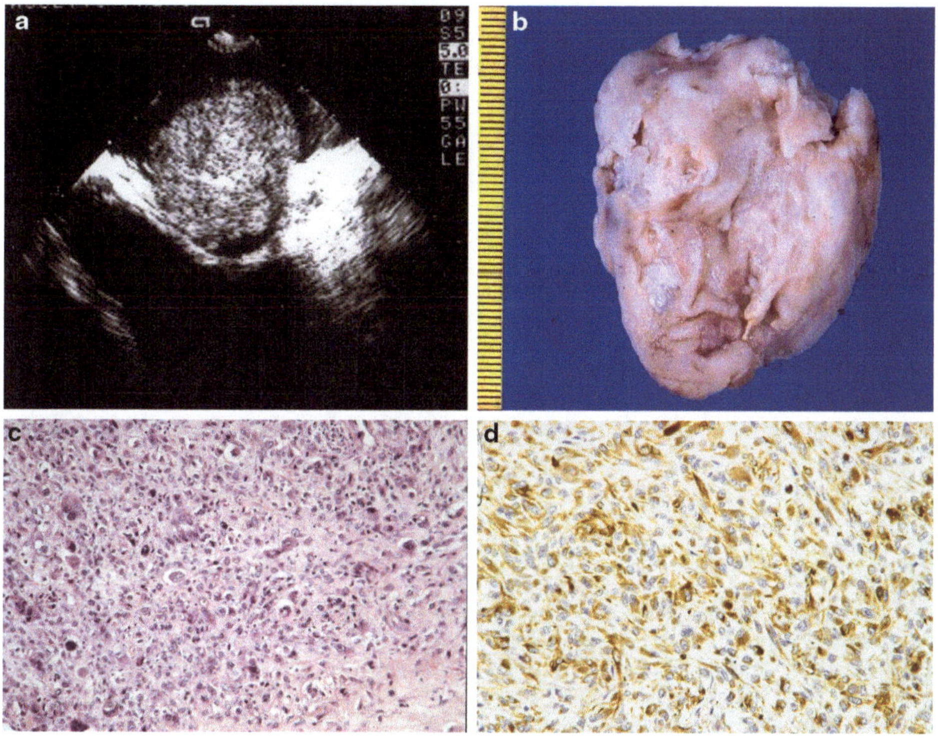

Fig. 6.2 Left atrial malignant fibrous histiocytoma in a 68-year-old man, presenting with fever and increased serum inflammatory markers. Reprinted with permission of the Italian Society of Cardiology. (**a**) Two-dimensional echocardiography: an endoluminal round mass is visible in the left atrium, simulating a myxoma. (**b**) Grossly, the surgical resected mass showed a rough and irregular surface. (**c**) At histology, bizarre cells with pleomorphic nuclei admixed to giant cells and spindle-shaped cells, with high mitotic rate are seen (hematoxylin–eosin stain). (**d**) At immunohistochemistry, the tumor cells are positive to vimentin

is complete and tumor recurrence in the follow-up.

Gross features. Tumor may appear as a yellowish–white polypoid mass, pedunculated or sessile, with areas of necrosis and hemorrhage (Fig. 6.2b). Unlike cardiac myxoma, it may present as multiple intracavitary cardiac masses [36].

Histopathological features. MFH/undifferentiated pleomorphic sarcoma is characterized by a proliferation of bizarre spindle-shaped or epithelioid cells with pleomorphic nuclei, often admixed with giant cells in a storiform pattern. Mitotic figures are usually abundant (Fig. 6.2c, d). The tumor is diagnosed as a pleomorphic MFH/undifferentiated pleomorphic sarcoma when histology and immunohistochemistry fail to give evidence of myogenic or other specific differentiation (endothelial, cardiomyocytes, smooth muscle cells, fibroblasts, adipose, nerves, epithelial cells). Histogenesis of tumor cells is still debated; a histiocytic origin has been suggested due to immunostaining positive for $\alpha 1$ antichymotrypsin, complement receptors, and Ig [37], but the histiocytic markers, including CD15 and CD14, are negative.

Genetic alterations, in particular in chromosome 13, have been reported in soft tissue sarcomas MFH [38–40], but cytogenetic analysis on cardiac tumors is still lacking.

The prognosis of cardiac MFH is very poor, because surgical resection is often incomplete. Chemotherapy and radiotherapy give only temporary improvement. Heart or heart/lung transplantation [8, 35, 41, 42] as well as autotransplantation [43] might be an alternative.

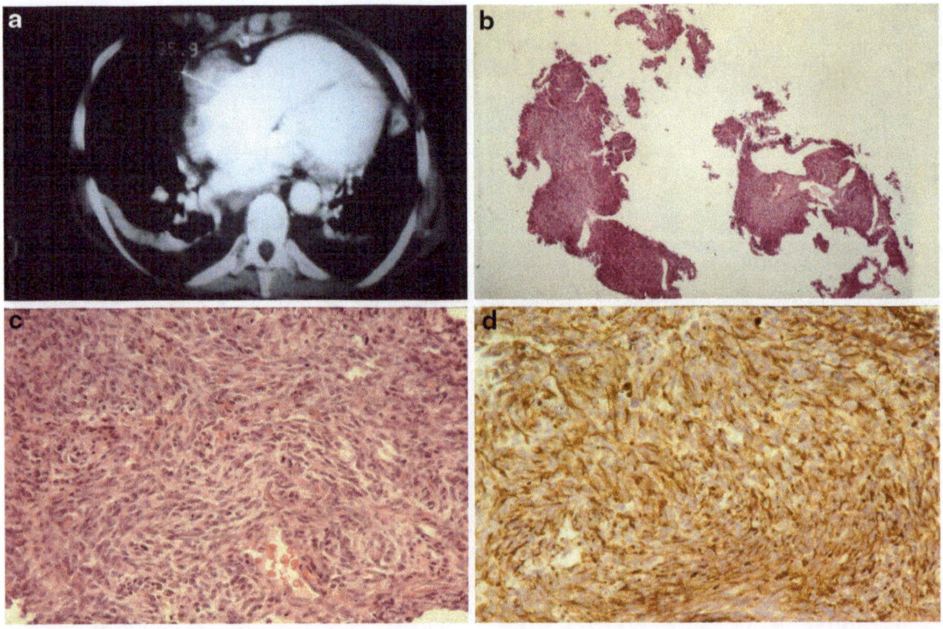

Fig. 6.3 Fibrosarcoma of the right atrium in a 62-year-old woman, suffering from weakness and effort dyspnea. Reprinted with permission of the Italian Society of Cardiology. (**a**) CT showing a mass infiltrating the right atrial free wall. (**b**) Transvenous endomyocardial biopsy: panoramic view of bioptic specimens (hematoxylin–eosin stain). (**c**) At higher magnification, note atypical spindle cells within a fibrous stroma (hematoxylin–eosin stain). (**d**) At immunohistochemistry, the tumor cells are positive for vimentin

Survival of patients ranges from 5 [2] to 18 months [35]. Most patients ultimately die of metastasis or local recurrence.

Heterologous elements such as bone are identified in 15% of MFH. In the past these variants were diagnosed as primary cardiac osteosarcomas, which are almost invariably located in the left atrium [44, 45]; only a case has been described in the right ventricle [46].

Fibrosarcoma and Myxosarcoma

Cardiac fibrosarcoma consists of a malignant proliferation of mesenchymal cells with fibroblastic features [1, 2, 47].

Epidemiology, localization, and clinical presentation. These rare tumors represent about 5–10% of cardiac sarcomas. The most frequent location is in the atria (particularly the left), with both intracavitary and mural (Fig. 6.3a) growth; congestive heart failure due to pulmonary congestion and mitral stenosis are the most common clinical presentations. More rarely, it originates from the pericardium.

Gross features. It is usually a soft, lobulated, polypoid mass projecting into the cardiac chamber.

Histopathological features. Fibrosarcoma is composed of monomorphic spindle cells, with variable mitotic activity (Fig. 6.3b-d) arranged in fascicles with a storiform, "herring-bone"pattern within a collagen stroma. Immunohistochemically, the tumor cells are positive for vimentin and focally for α-smooth muscle actin [48]. Ultrastructural examination reveals features of fibroblasts (spindle morphology and prominent rough endoplasmic reticulum) or myofibroblasts (spindle morphology and prominent rough endoplasmic reticulum together with focal presence of basal lamina, myofilaments, and "dense bodies").

Prognosis. In spite of surgery, survival is poor, about 5 months [2].

According to the WHO classification [1], myxosarcoma is the myxoid variant of cardiac fibrosarcoma, showing ovoid or stellate-shaped cells enmeshed within a myxoid stroma. Neither cellular pleomorphism nor prominent vascular component is present in fibrosarcoma and in myxofibrosarcoma.

In the past, myxosarcoma was thought to be the malignant transformation of myxoma [48]. Nowadays, it is considered the equivalent to the extracardiac soft tissue myxo-fibrosarcoma and fibromyxoid sarcoma at a low grade of malignancy, which are grouped among fibroblastic/myofibroblastic neoplasms [2].

Rhabdomyosarcoma

Rhabdomyosarcoma is a malignant mesenchymal tumor with striated muscle differentiation. In the past, before the use of immunohistochemical stains, it was thought to be the most common primary cardiac sarcoma; nowadays, it is considered very rare, accounting for around 5% of primary malignancies. Probably it is still the most common sarcoma in children [49]. Recently, Donsbech et al. [50] revalued 24 tumors by immunohistochemistry previously diagnosed as rhabdomyosarcomas by simple histological stains; the diagnosis was not confirmed in any case. Noteworthy, no rhabdomyosarcoma has been reported among Mayo Clinic cases [51].

Cardiac rhabdomyosarcomas typically involve the myocardium and show no chamber predilection, although they more often occur in the ventricles than other type of sarcomas.

Gross features. These tumors are large, bulky, infiltrative masses, either gelatinous or soft and necrotic (Fig. 6.4) and rarely present with an endocavitary growth [52].

Histopathological features. In soft tissues, rhabdomyosarcoma is divided into three subtypes, i.e., embryonal (including botryoid variant),

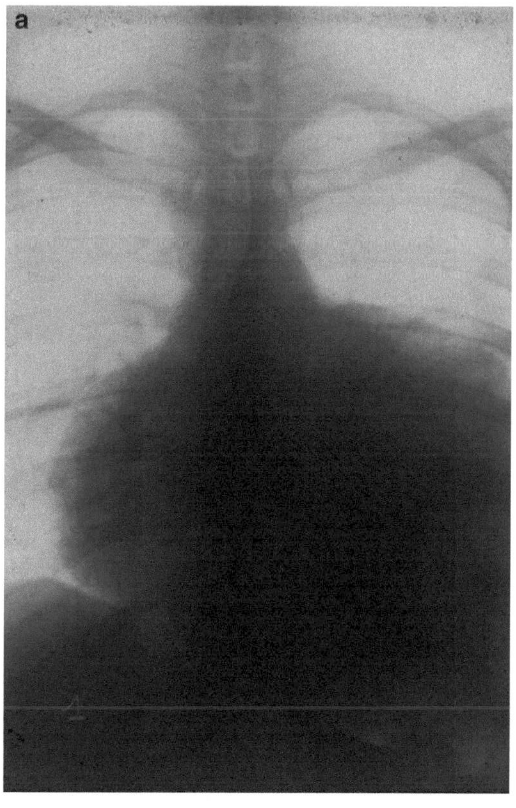

Fig. 6.4 Rhabdomyosarcoma in a 36-year-old patient at autopsy. Reprinted with permission of the Italian Society of Cardiology. (**a**) Chest X-ray shows pericardial and right pleural effusion. (**b**) At ECG, atrio-ventricular dissociation is present. (**c**) At autopsy, the tumor appears as a bulky mass infiltrating the left atrial posterior wall. (**d**) At histology, tumor cells appear pleomorphic and tadpole-like, with small transverse bands in the cytoplasm (hematoxylin–eosin stain)

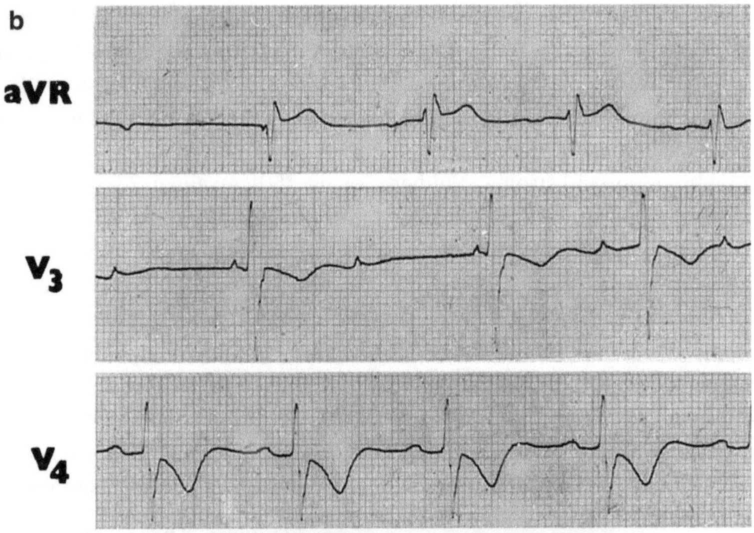

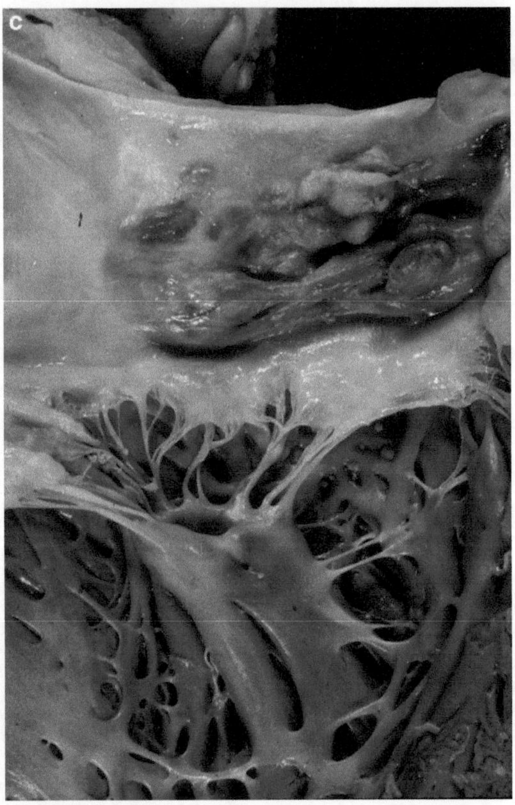

Fig. 6.4 (continued)

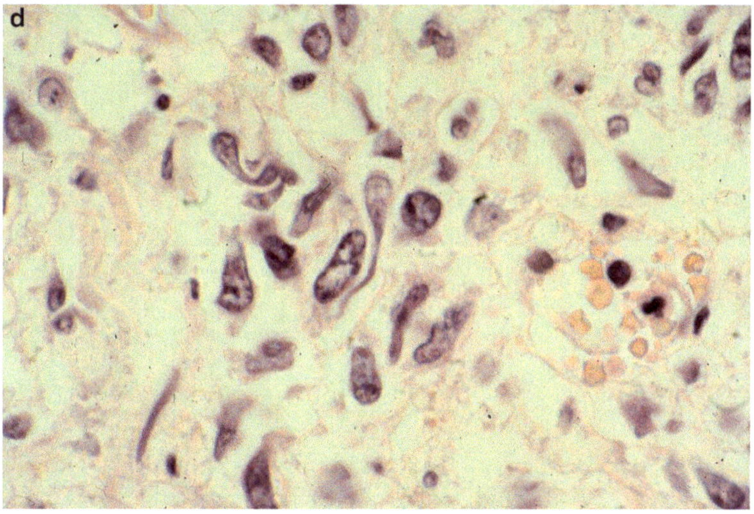

Fig. 6.4 (continued)

alveolar, and pleomorphic. Primary cardiac rhabdomyosarcomas are virtually all of the embryonal subtype. In the heart the botryoid variant has been reported only in two cases [53, 54] and the alveolar subtype only as metastatic [55]. Embryonal rhabdomyosarcoma is composed of small-sized round cells with hyperchromic nuclei and high mitotic rate, and rhabdomyoblasts with eosinophilic and PAS positive cytoplasm, described as "tadpole cells" (Fig. 6.4d). The more the myoblasts, the greater the differentiation.

Positive nuclear immunostaining with antibodies to myogenin [56] and positive cytoplasmic staining with antibodies to desmin allow the diagnosis.

Sarcoma botryoid is a multilobated grape-like mass, histologically showing cambium layer cells in a myxomatous stroma.

Electron microscopy reveals thin and thick filaments and structure resembling Z lines. Cytogenetic analysis shows mutation in exon 1 of K-ras gene [57].

Treatment. Surgical resection is often palliative due to local and distant metastasis, and response to adjuvant radiation and chemotherapy is dismal. In selected cases, cardiac transplantation has been even considered [58].

Leiomyosarcoma

Leiomyosarcoma is a malignant mesenchymal tumor with smooth muscle differentiation.

Epidemiology. Leiomyosarcoma represents about 10% of primary cardiac sarcomas, usually affecting patients during the fourth decade [1, 2], without any sex predilection.

Localization. There are two usual sites of origin. One is the left atrium, where it may present as a single or multinodular endocavitary mass, mimicking the left atrial myxoma, although it is mostly attached to the posterior wall and infiltrates the pulmonary veins [59] (fig 6.5). The second location is the pulmonary infundibulum and artery, where it may present abruptly to mimic pulmonary embolism (Fig. 6.6) [1, 2].

Gross features. It appears like a gray–white, solid sessile, intraluminal mass (Fig. 6.5a, b). In 30% of cases tumor may present as multiple nodules.

Histopathological features. Leiomyosarcoma consists of compacted fascicles of spindle cells with blunt-ended nuclei and eosinophilic cytoplasm (Figs. 6.5c and 6.6b), containing glycogen and perinuclear vacuoles. There are areas of necrosis and high mitotic activity. The spindle cells show positive

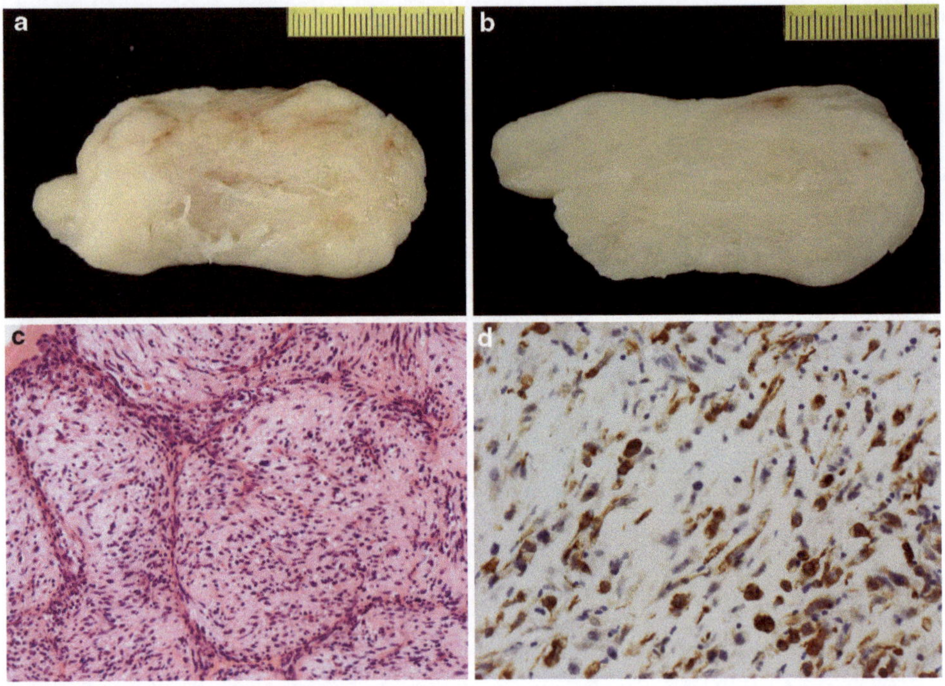

Fig. 6.5 Leiomyosarcoma of the left atrium in a 21-year-old woman with acute pulmonary edema and a preoperative diagnosis of left atrial myxoma. Reprinted with permission of the Italian Society of Cardiology. (**a**) Gross features of the mass resected at surgery, showing a rough and irregular surface. (**b**) Cut-surface of the mass with a *whitish*, lardaceous appearance. (**c**) At histology, pleomorphic cells arranged in a storiform pattern within a myxoid background (hematoxylin–eosin stain). (**d**) Immunohistochemical staining showing tumor cells positivity for desmin

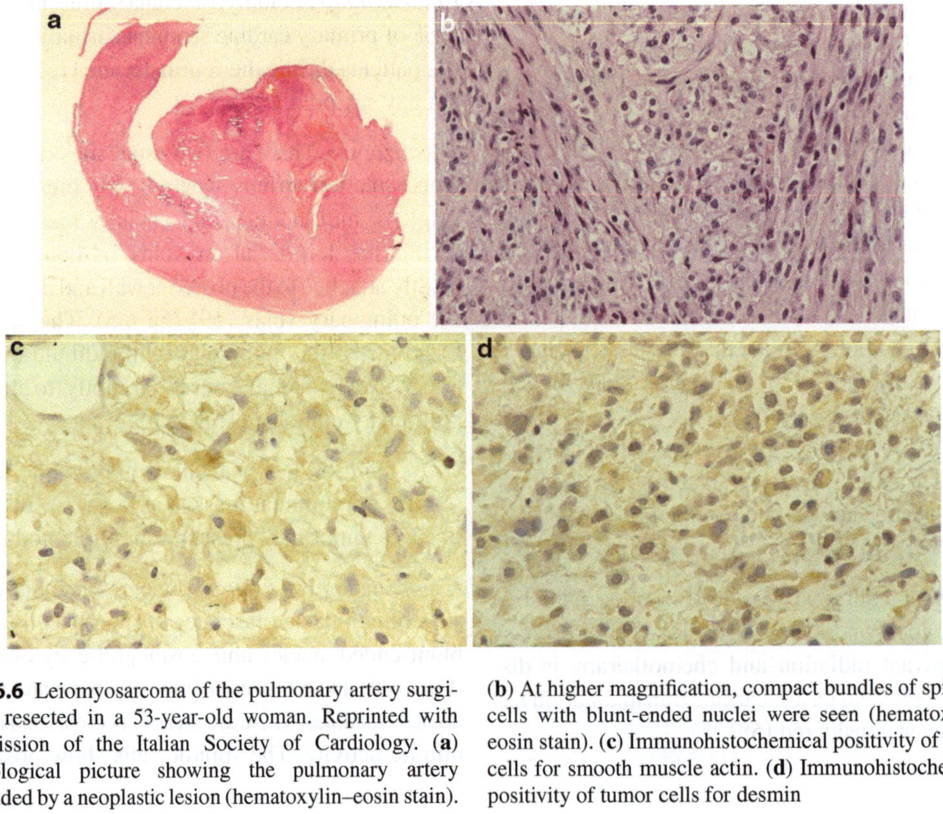

Fig. 6.6 Leiomyosarcoma of the pulmonary artery surgically resected in a 53-year-old woman. Reprinted with permission of the Italian Society of Cardiology. (**a**) Histological picture showing the pulmonary artery occluded by a neoplastic lesion (hematoxylin–eosin stain). (**b**) At higher magnification, compact bundles of spindled cells with blunt-ended nuclei were seen (hematoxylin–eosin stain). (**c**) Immunohistochemical positivity of tumor cells for smooth muscle actin. (**d**) Immunohistochemical positivity of tumor cells for desmin

reactivity for α-smooth muscle actin (Fig. 6.6c) and desmin (Fig. 6.5d and 6.6d).

Prognosis. Surgical resection, usually associated with adjuvant chemotherapy and radiation, is considered palliative, and the mean survival time being about 1 year. Nevertheless, one case survived more than 7 years after surgical resection and radio/chemotherapy, one patient underwent to cardiac transplantation after tumor eradication by chemotherapy, and finally a 21-year-old patient was still alive 24 months after the diagnosis has been reported [60].

Synovial Sarcoma

Synovial sarcoma is a malignant tumor which most commonly arises in the soft tissue near the joints of the arm and leg, but may be found in many organs, including the heart.

Because this characteristic location near the joints and the microscopic similarity to synovia, in the past it was erroneously thought to have a synovial origin. It is a biphasic tumor composed of two kinds of cells, spindle-shaped and epithelioid cells; monomorphic variant, composed only by spindle-shaped cells may occur and is the variant more frequently described in the heart. In all cases a reciprocal translocation t(x; 18)(p11.2; q11.2) is present.

In the literature, 14 cases of synovial sarcoma have been reported that originated in the heart or pericardium. The patients' age range is 13–53 years [61].

There is a predilection for the atria and pericardial surfaces. Clinically, patients present symptoms related to intracardiac obstruction, embolism, or cardiac tamponade.

Gross features. The tumor is whitish, infiltrative, and accompanied by necrosis and hemorrhage.

Histopathological features. Synovial sarcomas are classified into a biphasic type, which is composed of a spindle cell component and an epithelial cell component, proliferating in a nodular or glandular fashion; and a monophasic type, the most common in the heart, consisting of only a uniform spindle cell component. The presence of edema between bundles of spindle cells allows the differential diagnosis with fibrosarcoma.

Immunohistochemical staining shows that the spindle cells are diffusely positive for vimentin, and also focally positive for α-smooth muscle actin and calretinin; instead, epithelioid component is positive for cytokeratins and epithelial membrane antigen (EMA). The cells are negative for CD34, and this feature in association with dense cellular distribution and high grade malignancy helps to distinguish this tumor from solitary fibrous tumor of the pericardium. Differential diagnosis includes also sarcomatoid malignant mesothelioma that grossly proliferates diffusely and covers the surface of the heart; moreover, synovial sarcoma histologically is composed of more uniform tumor cells. Detection of SS18-SSX(SYT-SSX) or t(X; 18)(p11.2; q11.2) chromosomal translocation by molecular genetic analysis using reverse transcription polymerase chain reaction (RT-PCR), performed also in paraffin-embedded tissue blocks [62, 63], is extremely useful for reaching a definitive diagnosis of synovial sarcoma.

Liposarcoma

Liposarcoma is a mesenchymal malignant tumor that contains lipoblasts.

In the literature, about 20 cases have been reported [64]. Liposarcoma usually develops in adulthood, arises in the atria, and has an endoluminal growth, simulating cardiac myxoma [65], but may involve also the pericardium causing effusion or cardiac tamponade [2, 66].

Gross features. On gross examination liposarcomas are generally yellowish masses, sometimes myxoid, flaccid, and multilobulated [2].

Histopathological features. Two main subtypes arise in the heart: pleomorphic liposarcoma, simulating malignant fibrous histiocytoma, and myxoid liposarcoma.

The histological hallmark of liposarcoma is lipoblast, the precursor cell for adipocytes, which in the pleomorphic subtype presents with centrally located nucleus and multiple cytoplasmic small lipid droplets, while in the myxoid subtype it appears as a cell containing a unique large lipid droplet, which displaces the nucleus giving the cell a signet ring shape. In addition a plexiform capillary pattern and a myxoid matrix are present. Mixed forms have been described. Immunohistochemical staining shows S100 positivity in tumor cells. At electron microscopic examination, lipid droplets do not exhibit a discrete membrane.

Sarcomas Not Included in the WHO Classification

Malignant mesenchymoma is defined as a malignant tumor that consists of two or more different mesenchymal components in addition to poorly differentiated mesenchymal cells, as seen in MFH/undifferentiated pleomorphic sarcoma. "Triton's tumors" are rare, malignant tumor made up of both malignant schwannoma cells and malignant rhabdomyoblasts.

Malignant peripheral nerve sheath tumor (MPNST), also called neurofibrosarcoma or malignant schwannoma, is a malignant tumor composed of spindle cells, irregular nuclei, arranged in a plexiform pattern and positive for S100 at immunohistochemistry.

Malignant rhabdoid tumor is characterized ultrastructurally by perinuclear prominent intermediate filaments, positive for vimentin. In the WHO classification [1] it is considered as a subtype of MFH/undifferentiated pleomorphic sarcoma, which sometimes shows similar cells.

Kaposi's sarcoma has been described in the heart as a multifocal tumor in immunocompromised patients [2].

Carcinosarcoma is a high grade malignancy composed of epithelial and mesenchymal cells, showing features of both rhabdomyosarcoma and adenocarcinoma [3].

Cardiac Lymphoma

Primary cardiac lymphoma (PCL) is an extranodal non-Hodgkin's lymphoma exclusively located in the heart and/or pericardium. Primary cardiac lymphomas are very rare, representing 1.3% of primary cardiac tumors [2, 67–69].

They may occur in both immunodeficient and immunocompetent people. The median age of patients with PCL is 62 years (range 5–90), and it occurs three times more frequently in men than in women. The prognosis is poor with median survival of 7 months.

Initial signs and symptoms include shortness of breath, palpitations, chest pain, syncope, arrhythmia, congestive heart failure, or pericardial effusion.

Gross features. It presents as a whitish intramural infiltrating mass which may involve also the pericardium causing massive effusion. The right atrium is the most common site of origin (two third of cases), but any chamber may be involved.

Histopathological features. Almost 80% of PCLs are diffuse large B-cell lymphomas (Fig. 6.7) which at immunohistochemistry reveal expression of CD45 and of the B-cell marker CD20 (Fig. 6.7d), whereas the remaining 20% are CD3 positive T-cell lymphomas.

Immunocompromised HIV-positive individuals and patients affected by Kaposi sarcoma may develop so-called "primary effusion lymphoma" (PEL), that is pericardial effusion without the evidence of neoplastic mass, in which large B-cells present with co-infection by HHV-8/KSHV and EBV.

Cytology of pericardial effusion and molecular techniques may be of help for diagnosis to differentiate B and T-cell lymphomas from reactive lymphocyte hyperplasia.

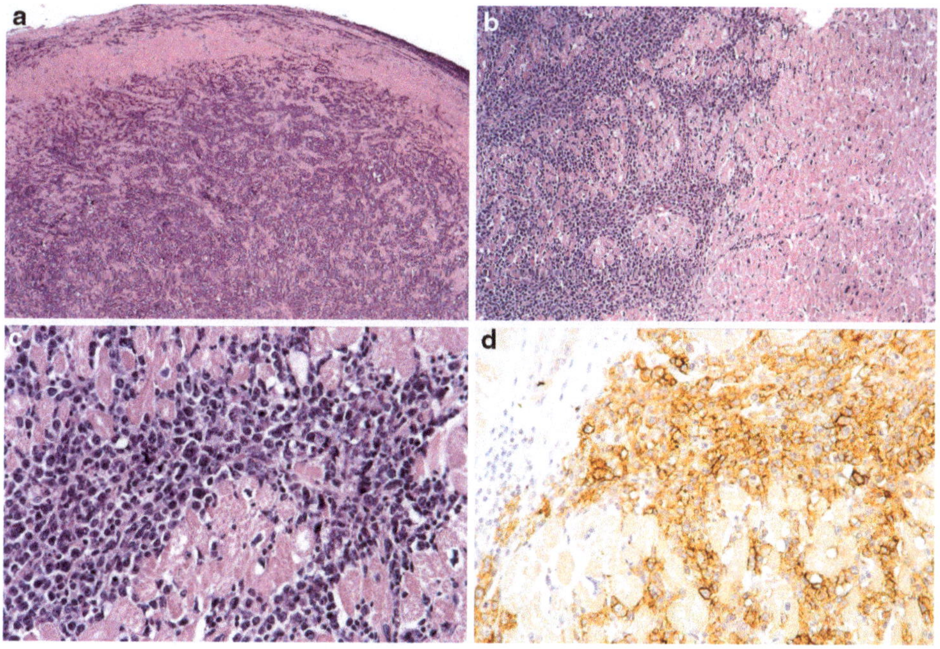

Fig. 6.7 Primary cardiac lymphoma in a 36-year-old man, drug abuser and HIV infected, with echocardiographic finding of a mass infiltrating the right atrial free wall. Reprinted with permission of the Italian Society of Cardiology. (**a**) The myocardium is diffusely infiltrated by proliferating neoplastic cells (hematoxylin–eosin stain). (**b**) Border area between the neoplastic infiltration and normal myocardium (hematoxylin–eosin stain). (**c**) At higher magnification, the tumor cells are large with large nuclei (hematoxylin–eosin stain). (**d**) At immunohistochemistry, tumor cells are positive for CD20, a B-cell marker

Primary Malignant Tumors of the Pericardium

Solitary fibrous tumor. This is a rare spindle cell tumor that occurs most commonly in the pleura, where is known as benign mesothelioma, although may be present also in other locations such as the pericardium [70–72].

Grossly, the tumor is firm, well circumscribed. Histologically spindle cell or hemangiopericytoma-like patterns are observed and fibrous or myxoid areas may be present. The neoplastic cells are CD34 positive [72]. The differential diagnosis includes malignant mesothelioma, low grade fibrosarcoma, and monophasic synovial sarcoma: immunohistochemical stain with CD34 is vital in identifying solitary fibrous tumor.

Prognosis is good, but local recurrence has been reported.

Malignant mesothelioma. Primary pericardial malignant mesothelioma arises from the pericardial mesothelial cell layer. It is a rare tumor, accounting for only about 1% of all mesotheliomas. Mesothelioma development has been correlated with exposure to asbestos or after direct application of asbestos and fiber glass as a treatment for angina pectoris [73, 74], and with radiation therapy for breast and mediastinal malignancies [75]. It affects individuals of any age (mean 45 years). Clinical manifestations are hemorrhagic pericardial effusion, constrictive pericarditis or, more rarely, cardiac tamponade [76].

Imaging techniques such as MRI and CT can be helpful to achieve diagnosis, identifying the pericardial thickening or the pericardial mass and the effusion.

Grossly, pericardial mesothelioma may present as nodules which may become confluent

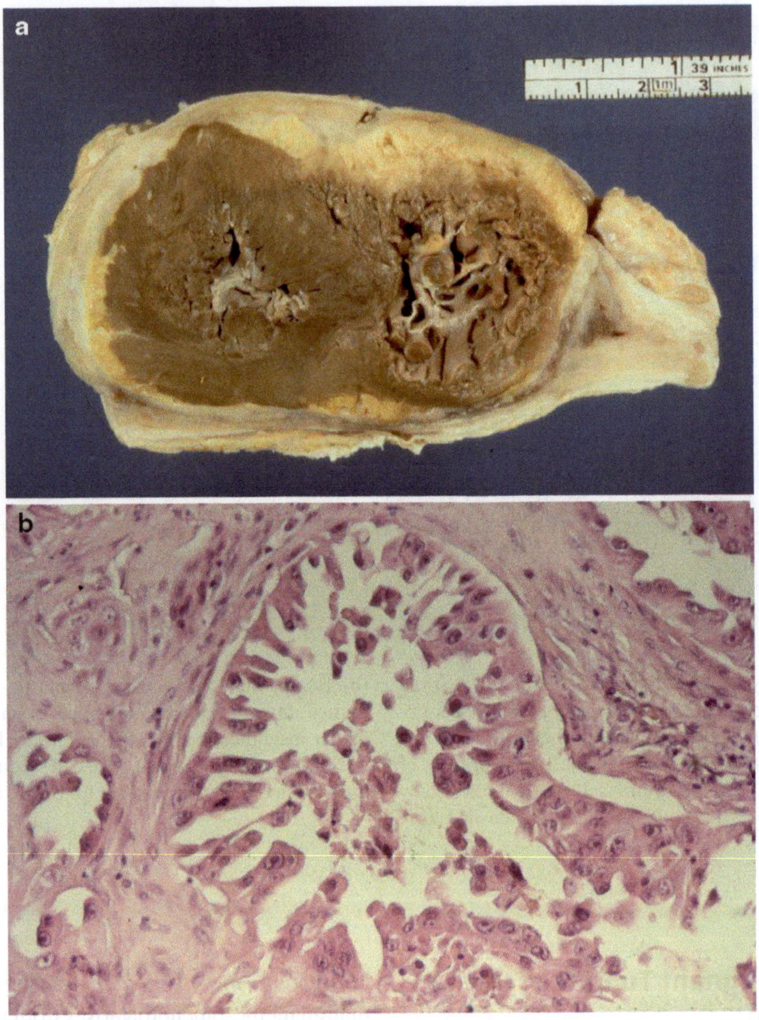

Fig. 6.8 Primary malignant mesothelioma of the pericardium in a 47-year-old man presenting with pericardial effusion. Reprinted with permission of the Italian Society of Cardiology. (**a**) At autopsy, transverse cut of the heart shows the whitish mass encasing both ventricles. (**b**) At histology, tumor cells form characteristic tubulo-papillary structures (hematoxylin–eosin stain)

encasing the heart and the root of the great vessels (Fig. 6.8).

Histologically, the tumor cells may have two distinct patterns i.e., epithelioid, with papillary or tubular configuration, or sarcomatoid. Immunohistochemistry shows calretinin and cytokeratin 5/6 positivity and CEA negativity, at difference from metastatic adenocarcinoma. Presence of cell microvilli at electron microscopy is also diagnostic [2].

The outcome is poor, with a median life expectancy very low, approximately 6 months from diagnosis.

Germ cell tumors. The intrapericardial germ cell tumors are generally benign teratomas. Pathologic evaluation may reveal areas of malignant degeneration with features of a yolk sac tumor [77] secreting alpha-fetoprotein [78]. The prognosis depends upon the extension of these malignant areas.

Yolk sac tumor rarely involves the pericardium; a true "Yolk sac tumor" of the pericardium has been reported only in one case [79].

References

1. Trawis WD, Brambilla E, Muller-Hermelink HK, Harris CC, editors. World Health Organization classification of tumors: pathology and genetics of tumours of the lung, pleura, thymus and heart. Lyon: IARC Press; 2004. p. 250.
2. Burke AP, Virmani R. Tumors of the heart and great vessels. 3rd ed. Washington, DC: Armed Forces Institute of Pathology; 1996.
3. Ramnarine IR, Davidson L, van Doorn CA. Primary cardiac carcinosarcoma: a rare, aggressive tumor. Ann Thorac Surg. 2001;72:927–9.
4. Fletcher CDM, Unni KK, Mertens F. World Health Organization classification of tumors: tumours of soft tissue and bone. Lyon: IARC Press; 2002.
5. Costa J. The grading and staging of soft tissue sarcomas. In: Fletcher CD, McKee PH, editors. Pathobiology of soft tissue tumors. Edinburg: Churchill Livingstone; 1990. p. 221–38.
6. Trojani M, Contesso G, Coindre JM, Rouesse J, Bui NB, de Mascarel A, Goussot JF, David M, Bonichon F, Lagarde C. Soft tissue sarcomas of the adults; study of pathological prognostic variables and definition of a histopathological grading system. Int J Cancer. 1984;33:37–42.
7. Coindre JM, Terrier P, Gouillou L, Le Doussal V, Collin F, Ranchere D, Sastre X, Vilain MO, Bonichon F, N'Guiyen Bui B. Predictive value of grade for metastasis development in the main histologic types of adult soft tissue sarcomas: a study of 1240 patients from the French Federation of Cancer Centers Sarcoma Group. Cancer. 2001;91:1914–26.
8. Uberfuhr P, Meiser B, Fuchs A, Schulze C, Reichenspurner H, Falk M, Weiss M, Wintersperger B, Issels R, Reichart B. Heart transplantation: an approach to treating primary cardiac sarcoma? J Heart Lung Transplant. 2002;21:1135–9.
9. Reardon MJ, Walkes JC, Benjamin R. Therapy insight: malignant primary cardiac tumors. Nat Rev Cardiol. 2006;3:548–53.
10. Butany J, Yu W. Cardiac angiosarcoma: two cases and a review of the literature. Can Cardiol. 2000;16:197–205.
11. Hamidi M, Moody JS, Weigel TL, Kozak KR. Primary cardiac sarcoma. Ann Thorac Surg. 2010;90:176–81.
12. Yu K, Liu Y, Wang H, Hu S, Long C. Epidemiological and pathological characteristics of cardiac tumors: a clinical study of 242 cases. Interact Cardiovasc Thorac Surg. 2007;6:636–9.
13. Simpson L, Kumar SK, Okuno SH, Schaff HV, Porrata LF, Buckner JC, Moynihan TJ. Malignant primary cardiac tumors: review of a single institution experience. Cancer. 2008;112:2440–6.
14. Mayer F, Aebert H, Rudert M, Königsrainer A, Horger M, Kanz L, Bamberg M, Ziemer G, Hartmann JT. Primary malignant sarcomas of the heart and great vessels in adult patients–a single-center experience. Oncologist. 2007;12:1134–42.
15. Glancy DL, Morales Jr JB, Roberts WC. Angiosarcoma of the heart. Am J Cardiol. 1968;21:413–9.
16. Rosenkranz ER, Murphy Jr DJ. Diagnosis and neonatal resection of right atrial angiosarcoma. Ann Thorac Surg. 1994;57:1014–5.
17. Adem C, Aubry MC, Tazelaar HD, Myers JL. Metastatic angiosarcoma masquerading as diffuse pulmonary hemorrhage: clinicopathologic analysis of 7 new patients. Arch Pathol Lab Med. 2001;125:1562–5.
18. Afzal MN, Alguacil-Garcia A. Primary cardiac angiosarcoma: clinical and pathological diagnostic problems. Can J Cardiol. 1997;13:293–6.
19. Poletti A, Cocco P, Valente M, Fasoli G, Chioin R, Thiene G. In vivo diagnosis of cardiac angiosarcoma by endomyocardial biopsy. Cardiovasc Pathol. 1993;2:89–91.
20. Araoz PA, Mulvagh SL, Tazelaar HD, Julsrud PR, Breen JF. CT and MR imaging of benign primary cardiac neoplasms with echocardiographic correlation. Radiographics. 2000;20:1303–19.
21. Economides EG, Singh A. Case of tumor neovascularization demonstrated by cardiac catheterization. Cathet Cardiovasc Diagn. 1998;43:451–3.
22. Garcia JM, Gonzalez R, Silva JM, Dominguez G, Vegazo IS, Gamallo C, Provencio M, Espana P, Bonilla F. Mutational status of K-ras and TP53 genes in primary sarcomas of the heart. Br J Cancer. 2000;82:1183–5.
23. Zu Y, Perle MA, Yan Z, Liu J, Kumar A, Waisman J. Chromosomal abnormalities and p53 gene mutation a cardiac angiosarcoma. Appl Immunohistochem Mol Morphol. 2001;9:24–8.
24. Kim MP, Correa AM, Blackmon S, Quiroga-Garza G, Weilbaecher D, Bruckner B, Ramlawi B, Rice DC, Vaporciyan AA, Reardon MJ. Outcomes after right-side heart sarcoma resection. Ann Thorac Surg. 2011;91:770–6.
25. Hermann MA, Shankerman RA, Edwards WD, Shub C, Schass HV. Primary cardiac angiosarcoma: a clinicopathologic study of six cases. J Thorac Cardiovasc Surg. 1992;103:655–64.
26. Burke AP, Tazelaar H, Butany JW, El-Demellawy D, Loire R, Geva T, Bonilla F, Galvin JR, Veinot JP, Virmani R, Kamiya H, Watanabe G, Grandmougin D, Horimoto M, Hiraga H. Cardiac sarcomas. In: Trawis WD, Brambilla E, Muller-Hermelink HK, Harris CC, editors. World Health Organization classification of tumors: pathology and genetics of tumours of the lung pleura thymus and heart. Lyon: IARC Press; 2004. p. 273–81.

27. Van Bernal JF, Garcia Alberdi E, Gutierrez JA, Garijo MF. Incidental in vivo detection of an epitheliod hemangioendothelioma of the mitral valve. Pathol Int. 2005;55:644–8.
28. Boudousquie AC, Lawce HJ, Sherman R, Olson S, Magenis RE, Corless CL. Complex translocation (7; 22) identified in an epithelioid hemangioendothelioma. Cancer Genetic Cytogenet. 1996;92:116–21.
29. Mendlick MR, Nelson M, Pickering D, Johansson SL, Seemayer TA, Neff JR, Vergara G, Rosenthal H, Bridge JA. Translocation t(1; 3)(p36.3; q25) is a nonrandom aberration in epithelioid hemangioendothelioma. Am J Surg Pathol. 2001;25:684–7.
30. Marchiano D, Fisher F, Hofstetter S. Epithelioid hemangioendothelioma of the heart with distant metastases: A case report and literature review. J Cardiovasc Surg. 1993;34:529–33.
31. Whorton CM. Primary malignant tumors of the heart. Cancer. 1949;2:245–60.
32. Bear PA, Moodie DS. Malignant primary cardiac tumors. The Cleveland Clinic experience, 1956 to 1986. Chest. 1987;92:860–2.
33. Molina JE, Edwards JE, Ward HB. Primary cardiac tumors: experience at the University of Minnesota. Thorac Cardiovasc Surg. 1990;38:183–91.
34. Basso C, Valente M, Poletti A, Casarotto D, Thiene G. Surgical pathology of primary cardiac and pericardial tumors. Eur J Cardiothorac Surg. 1997;12:730–7.
35. Okamoto K, Kato S, Katsuki S, Wada Y, Toyozumi Y, Morimatsu M, Aoyagi S, Imaizumi T. Malignant fibrous histiocytoma of the heart: case report and review of 46 cases in the literature. Intern Med. 2001;40:1222–6.
36. Laya MB, Mailliard JA, Bewtra C, Levin HS. Malignant fibrous histiocytoma of the heart. A case report and review of the literature. Cancer. 1987;59:1026–31.
37. Terashima K, Aoyama K, Nihei K, Nito T, Imai Y, Takahashi K, Daidoji S. Malignant fibrous histiocytoma of the heart. Cancer. 1983;52:1919–26.
38. Mairal A, Terrier P, Chibon F, Sastre X, Lecesne A, Aurias A. Loss of chromosome 13 is the most frequent genomic imbalance in malignant fibrous histiocytoma. A comparative genomic hybridization analysis of a series of 30 cases. Cancer Genet Cytogenet. 1999;111:134–8.
39. Chibon F, Mairal A, Freneaux P, Terrier P, Coindre JM, Sastre X, Aurias A. The RB1 gene is the target of chromosome 13 deletions in malignant fibrous histiocytoma. Cancer Res. 2000;60:6339–45.
40. Simons A, Schepens M, Jeuken J, Sprenger S, van de Zande G, Bjerkehagen B, Forus A, Weibolt V, Molenaar I, van den Berg E, Myklebost O, Bridge J, van Kessel AG, Suijkerbuijk R. Frequent loss of 9p21 (P16(INK4A)) and other genomic imbalances in human malignant fibrous histiocytoma. Cancer Genet Cytogenet. 2000;118:89–98.
41. Gowdamarajan A, Michler RE. Therapy for primary cardiac tumors: is there a role for heart transplantation? Curr Opin Cardiol. 2000;15:121–5.
42. Talbot SN, Taub RN, Keohan ML, Edwards N, Galantowicz ME, Schulman LL. Combined heart and lung transplantation for unresectable primary cardiac sarcoma. J Thorac Cardiovasc Surg. 2002;124:1145–8.
43. Reardon MJ, De Felice CA, Sheinbaum R, Baldwin JC. Cardiac autotransplant for surgical treatment of a malignant neoplasm. Ann Thorac Surg. 1999;67:1793–5.
44. Reynard JS, Gregoratos G, Gordon MJ, Bloor CM. Primary osteosarcoma of the heart. Am Heart J. 1985;109:598–600.
45. Burke A, Virmani R. Osteosarcomas of the heart. Am J Surg Pathol. 1991;15:289–95.
46. Yamagishi M, Bando K, Furuichi S, Ishibashi-Ueda H, Yutani C, Miyatake K. Images in cardiovascular medicine: primary cardiac osteosarcoma in right ventricular outflow tract. Circulation. 2000;101:2220–1.
47. Basso C, Stefani A, Calabrese F, Fasoli G, Valente M. Primary right atrial fibrosarcoma diagnosed by endocardial biopsy. Am Heart J. 1996;131:399–402.
48. Okada M, Ohta T, Yasuoka S, Matsuda S, Shida T, Nakamura K, Asada S. Surgical management of intracavitary tumors. A review of fifteen patients and current status in Japan. J Cardiovasc Surg. 1986;27:641–9.
49. Hui KS, Green LK, Schmidt WA. Primary cardiac rhabdomyosarcoma: definition of a rare entity. Am J Cardiovasc Pathol. 1988;2:19–29.
50. Donsbeck AV, Ranchere D, Coindre JM, Le Gall F, Cordier JF, Loire R. Primary cardiac sarcomas: an immunohistochemical and grading study with long-term follow-up of 24 cases. Histopathology. 1999;34:295–304.
51. Tazelaar HD, Locke TJ, McGregor CG. Pathology of surgically excised primary cardiac tumors. Mayo Clin Proc. 1992;67:957–65.
52. Thiene G, Miraglia G, Menghetti L, Nava A, Rossi L. Multiple lesions of the conduction system in a case of cardiac rhabdomyosarcoma with complex arrhythmias. An anatomic and clinical study. Chest. 1976;70:378–81.
53. Hajar R, Roberts WC, Folger Jr GM. Embryonal botryoid rhabdomyosarcoma of the mitral valve. Am J Cardiol. 1986;57:376.
54. Scott RS, Jagirdar J. Right atrial botryoid rhabdomyosarcoma in an adult patient with recurrent pleomorphic rhabdomyosarcomas following doxorubicin therapy. Ann Diagn Pathol. 2007;11:274–6.
55. Orsmond GS, Knight L, Dehner LP, Nicoloff DM, Nesbitt M, Bessinger Jr FB. Alveolar rhabdomyosarcoma involving the heart. An echocardiographic, angiographic and pathologic study. Circulation. 1976;54:837–43.
56. Quintanilla-Martinez L, Wilkins Jr EW, Choi N, Efird J, Hug E, Harris NL. Thymoma. Histologic subclassification is an independent prognostic factor. Cancer. 1994;74:606–17.
57. Garcia JM, Gonzalez R, Silva JM, Dominguez G, Vegazo IS, Gamallo C, Provencio M, Espana P, Bonilla

F. Mutational status of K-ras and TP53 genes in primary sarcomas of the heart. Br J Cancer. 2000;82:1183–5.
58. Grandmougin D, Fayad G, Decoene C, Pol A, Warembourg H. Total orthotopic heart transplantation for primary cardiac rhabdomyosarcoma: factors influencing long-term survival. Ann Thorac Surg. 2001;71:1438–41.
59. Mazzola A, Spano JP, Valente M, Gregoriani R, Villani C, Di Eusanio M, Ciocca M, Minuti U, Giancola R, Basso C, Thiene G. Leiomyosarcoma of the left atrium mimicking a left atrial myxoma. J Thorac Cardiovasc Surg. 2006;131:224–6.
60. Pessotto R, Silvestre G, Luciani GB, Anselmi M, Pasini F, Santini F, Mazzucco A. Primary cardiac leiomyosarcoma: seven-year survival with combined surgical and adjuvant therapy. Int J Cardiol. 1997;60:91–4.
61. Hazelbag HM, Szuhai K, Tanke HJ, Rosenberg C, Hogendoorn PC. Primary synovial sarcoma of the heart: a cytogenetic and molecular genetic analysis combining RT-PCR and COBRA-FISH of a case with a complex karyotype. Mod Pathol. 2004;17:1434–9.
62. Guillou L, Coindre JM, Bonichon F, Nguyen BB, Terrier P, Collin F, Vilain MO, Mandard AM, le Doussal V, Benhattar J. Detection of the synovial sarcoma translocation t(X;18) (SYT; SSX) in paraffin-embedded tissues using reverse transcriptase-polymerase chain reaction. A reliable and powerful diagnostic tool for pathologists. A molecular analysis of 221 mesenchymal tumors fixed in different fixatives. Hum Pathol. 2001;32:105–12.
63. Amary MF, Berisha F, Bernardi Fdel C, Herbert A, James M, Reis-Filho JS, Fisher C, Nicholson AG, Tirabosco R, Diss TC, Flanagan AM. Detection of SS18-SSX fusion transcripts in formalin-fixed paraffin-embedded neoplasms: analysis of conventional RT-PCR, qRT-PCR and dual color FISH as diagnostic tools for synovial sarcoma. Mod Pathol. 2007;20:482–96.
64. Paraf F, Bruneval P, Balaton A, Deloche A, Mikol J, Maitre F, Scholl JM, De Saint Maur PP, Camilleri JP. Primary liposarcoma of the heart. Am J Cardiovac Pathol. 1990;3:175–80.
65. Nzayinambaho K, Noel H, Cosyns J, Sonnet J, Chalant C. Primary cardiac liposarcoma simulating a left atrial myxoma. Thorac Cardiovasc Surg. 1985;33:193–5.
66. Can C, Arpaci F, Celasum B, Gunham O, Finci R. Primary pericardial liposarcoma presenting with cardiac tamponade and multiple organ metastates (Letter). Chest. 1993;103:328.
67. Cairns P, Butany J, Fulop J, Ralowski H, Hassaram S. Cardiac presentation of non-Hodgkin's lymphoma. Arch Pathol Lab Med. 1987;111:80–3.
68. Petrich A, Cho SI, Billett H. Primary cardiac lymphoma: an analysis of presentation, treatment, and outcome patterns. Cancer. 2011;117:581–9.
69. Rolla G, Bertero MT, Pastena G, Tartaglia N, Corradi F, Casabona R, Motta M, Caligaris-cappio F. Primary lymphoma of the heart. A case report and review of the literature. Leuk Res. 2002;26:117–20.
70. Bortolotti U, Calabro F, Loy M, Fasoli G, Altavilla G, Marchese D. Giant intrapericardial solitary fibrous tumor. Ann Thorac Surg. 1992;54:1219–20.
71. Corgnati G, Drago S, Bonamini R, Trevi GP, Carra R, Di Summa M. Solitary fibrous tumor of the pericardium presenting itself as a pericardial effusion and right ventricular obstruction. J Cardiovasc Surg. 2004;45:393–4.
72. Hanau CA, Miettinen M. Solitary fibrous tumor: histological and immunohistochemical spectrum of benign and malignant variants presenting at different sites. Hum Pathol. 1995;26:440–9.
73. Krismann M, Muller KM. Malignant mesothelioma of the pleura, pericardium and peritoneum. 1: Etiology, pathogenesis, pathology. Chirurg. 2000; 71:877–86.
74. Churg A, Warnock ML, Bensch KG. Malignant mesothelioma arising after direct application of asbestos and fiber glass to the pericardium. Am Rev Respir Dis. 1978;118:419–24.
75. Small GR, Nicolson M, Buchan K. Pericardial malignant mesothelioma: a latent complication of radiotherapy? Eur J Cardiothor Sur. 2008;33:745–7.
76. Loire R, Tabib A. Malignant mesothelioma of the pericardium. An anatomo-clinical study of 10 cases. Arch Mal Coeur Vaiss. 1994;87:255–62.
77. McKenney H. Congenital teratomas. Am J Surg Pathol. 2005;29:29–38.
78. Carachi R, Campbell PE, Chow CW, Mee BB. Alpha-feto-protein-(AFP-)-secreting intra-pericardial teratoma–report of a case diagnosed on CT scanning. Z Kinderchir. 1986;41:369–70.
79. Liang TC, Lu MY, Chen SJ, Lu FL, Lin KH. Cardiac tamponade caused by intrapericardial yolk sac tumor in a boy. J Formos Med Assoc. 2002;101:355–8.

Echocardiographic Approach to the Diagnosis of Cardiac Tumors

7

Paolo Voci and Francesco Pizzuto

Introduction

Before the clinical introduction of echocardiography, the in vivo diagnosis of cardiac tumors was virtually impossible, and almost exclusively done at autopsy [1].

Echocardiography has definitely changed the diagnostic work-up of cardiac tumors, allowing an easy, early, fast, low-cost, and accurate diagnosis [2–12]. As a result, the prognosis improved too. In fact, before the introduction of echocardiography the prognosis was poor not only for malignant, but also for benign neoplasms, such as myxomas, fibromas, and fibroelastomas, which could not be recognized until progressive obstruction of cardiac chambers, severe arrhythmias, and/or embolic events occurred.

The ultrasound diagnosis of cardiac tumors depends on the technological level of the instrumentation and on the operator's skill and experience, which is particularly true for small and unusual lesions. The cardiologist performing the examination should know the clinical history of the patient and should be expert on the wide spectrum of cardiac masses which may be incidentally encountered during a routine examination.

Very often cardiac tumors are asymptomatic at an early stage, and in about 12% of the cases they are occasionally found during ultrasound examination requested for other reasons [13]. They often produce mild clinical signs, but sometimes their first clinical presentation is dramatic with life-threatening arrhythmias, atrioventricular block, pericardial effusion or tamponade, cardiac failure [14], severe valvular regurgitation, pulmonary hypertension secondary to left ventricular inflow obstruction, and embolic events. Sometimes general signs as fever and artralgia may also occur [15].

Prevalence

Primary cardiac tumors are much rarer than metastatic tumors (prevalence at autopsy of 0.001–0.28% and 1.5–21%, respectively) [16–18]. The "3/4 rule" may be a useful mnemonic aid: more than 3/4 of primary tumors are benign and 3/4 of those are atrial myxomas, which therefore are the most common cardiac tumors; 3/4 of malignant cardiac tumors are sarcomas [19].

P. Voci, M.D. (✉)
Department of Internal Medicine,
Section of Cardiology, Tor Vergata University,
Viale Oxford 81, Via Merulana 13, Rome 00185, Italy
e-mail: paolovoci@gmail.com

F. Pizzuto, M.D.
Department of Internal Medicine,
Section of Cardiology, Tor Vergata University,
Viale Oxford 81, Via Nomentana 186, Rome 00185, Italy

C. Basso et al. (eds.), *Cardiac Tumor Pathology*, Current Clinical Pathology,
DOI 10.1007/978-1-62703-143-1_7, © Springer Science+Business Media New York 2013

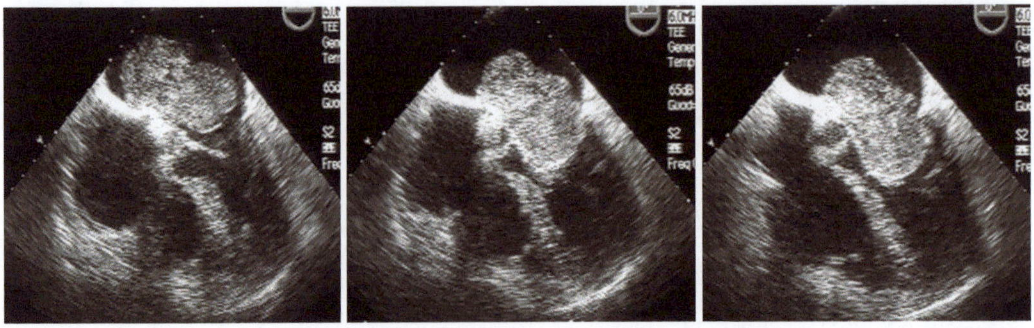

Fig. 7.1 Transesophageal echocardiography. Reprinted with permission of the Italian Society of Cardiology. Large left atrial myxoma attached to the interatrial septum, prolapsing in diastole through the mitral valve

How to Distinguish a Malignant from a Benign Lesion

The histological differentiation of cardiac masses or even the ability to simply distinguish between a malignant and a benign mass is still very difficult with ultrasound, and sometimes even at surgical inspection. Therefore, the histological diagnosis at surgery is deemed necessary to make a correct and definitive diagnosis and to optimize therapy. Despite these important limitations, some ultrasound characteristics as the number of masses, their location, their ultrasound texture, and the presence of calcification, may help suggesting the histological type.

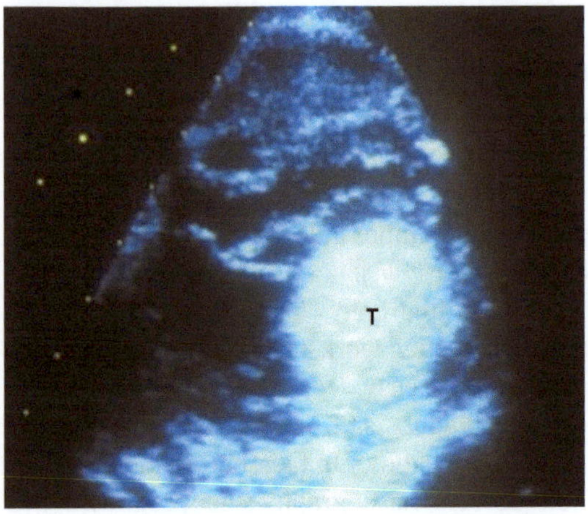

Fig. 7.2 Fetal echocardiography. Reprinted with permission of the Italian Society of Cardiology. Large right ventricular fibroma (T) occasionally seen in a fetus without signs of heart failure

Number. Myxomas are the most frequent cardiac tumors. They are usually made of a single intracardiac mass (Fig. 7.1) but very rarely, and particularly in young patients, they are multiple. Fibromas are made of a single mass too, but they are usually found well before the adolescence when compared to myxomas, and sometimes, albeit very rarely, even in utero (Fig. 7.2). Rhabdomyomas are often multiple (Figs. 7.3 and 7.4), they are associated with tuberous sclerosis, and may regress spontaneously.

Dimensions. Fibromas are usually very large (Fig. 7.2) whereas rhabdomyomas are of variable dimensions (Figs. 7.3 and 7.4), but most often small, and may regress spontaneously. Fibroelastoma is usually small (Fig. 7.5) and other tumors may be very different in size. Obviously, a big mass always derives from the growth of a small mass, therefore, this criterion may have a limited value.

Location. Myxomas are generally found in the atria, particularly in the left atrium, and almost always originate from the atrial septum (Fig. 7.1), whereas rarely involve the valvular or subvalvular apparatus [10]. They are almost never found on the posterior wall of the left atrium, which may help differentiating them from atrial thrombi or leiomyosarcomas. Fibroelastomas are almost always attached to a cardiac valve, mostly to the aortic valve (Fig. 7.5), then to the mitral valve and very rarely the tricuspid valve and the endocardial wall. Rhabdomyomas have a typical intramyocardial distribution. Lipomas are found

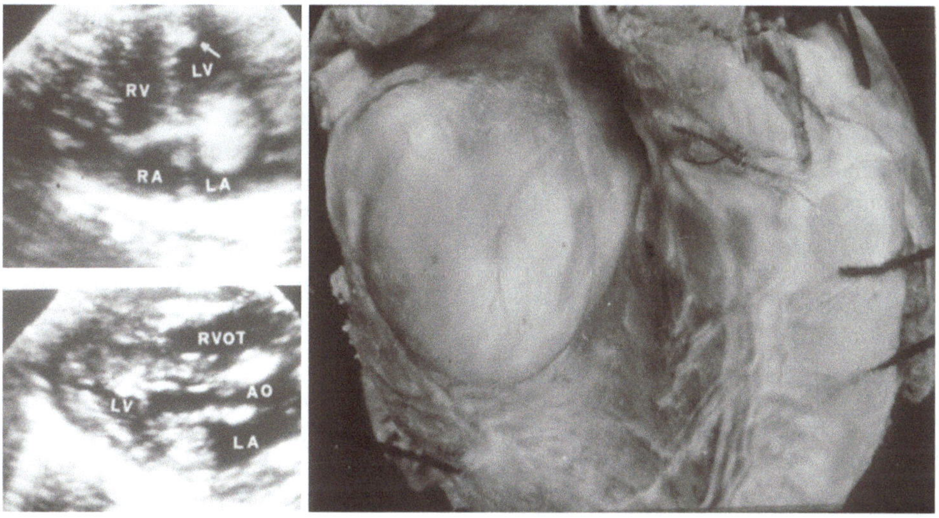

Fig. 7.3 Neonatal echocardiography. Reprinted with permission of the Italian Society of Cardiology. Two rhabdomyomas, the smaller at the apical segment of the interventricular septum (*arrow*) and the larger in the left atrium in a newborn with heart failure, confirmed at autopsy. *AO* aorta, *LA* left atrium, *LV* left ventricle, *RA* right atrium, *RV* right ventricle, *RVOT* right ventricular outflow tract

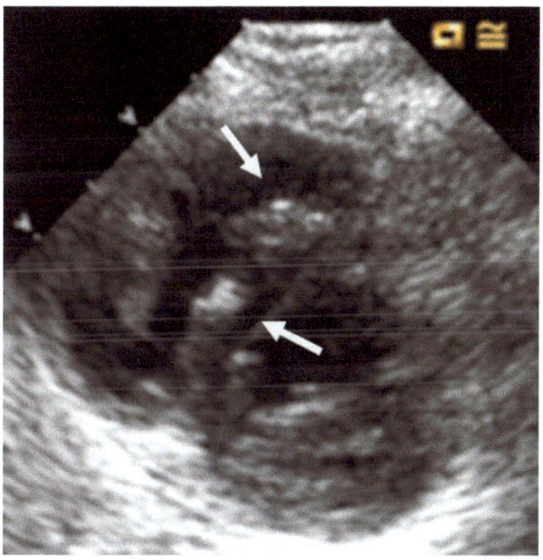

Fig. 7.4 Two-dimensional echocardiography. Reprinted with permission of the Italian Society of Cardiology. Left ventricular short-axis view in a 12-year-old child with tuberous sclerosis. *Arrows* indicate rhabdomyomas in regression

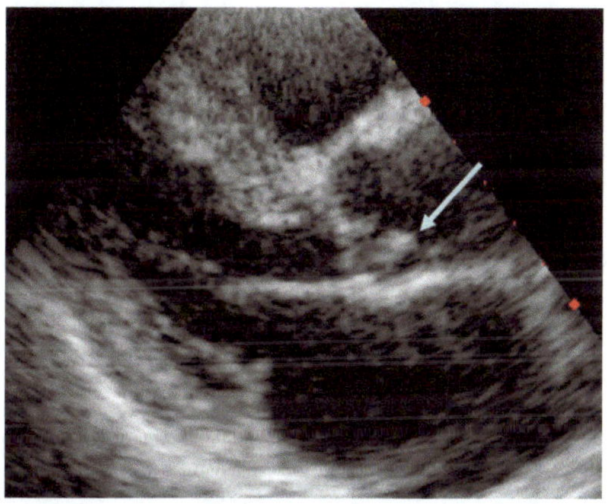

Fig. 7.5 Color-Doppler transthoracic echocardiography. Fibroelastoma of the aortic valve (*arrow*)

in the interatrial septum, they are round or they may produce a diffuse septal infiltration known as septal lipomatosis, but they may be observed in other structures, included the pericardium. Sarcomas (Figs. 7.6 and 7.7) may be found in any part of the heart.

Ultrasound structure. The ultrasound "texture" and some peculiar characteristics of cardiac tumors may help in the differential diagnosis. Teratomas and hamartomas are often non-homogeneous and may have spotty calcifications, whereas rhabdomyomas are homogeneous (Figs. 7.3 and 7.4). Left atrial thrombi can be differentiated from myxomas when a multi-layered structure is detected. Echo-lucent or transparent areas, corresponding to hemorrhagic or necrotic spots at histology, may be also be detected in myxomas, (Fig. 7.1) but exceptionally in vegetations and thrombi. Lipomas are homogeneous and markedly hyper-reflective masses.

Vascularization. A rich vascularization may suggest the diagnosis of malignancy. However, the paraganglioma, which is also called cardiac pheochromocytoma independently from its ability to produce catecholamines, is an exception. In this tumor, which is most often benign, the vascularization is so developed (Fig. 7.8) that coronary steal and even angina may occur [12]. Cardiac hemangioma, which is benign too, is also highly vascularized [5]. Lastly, the presence of vessels in a cardiac mass is not typical of tumors: in fact, old thrombi may be perfused by neovessels which can be imaged by high-resolution ultrasound (Fig. 7.9) [20].

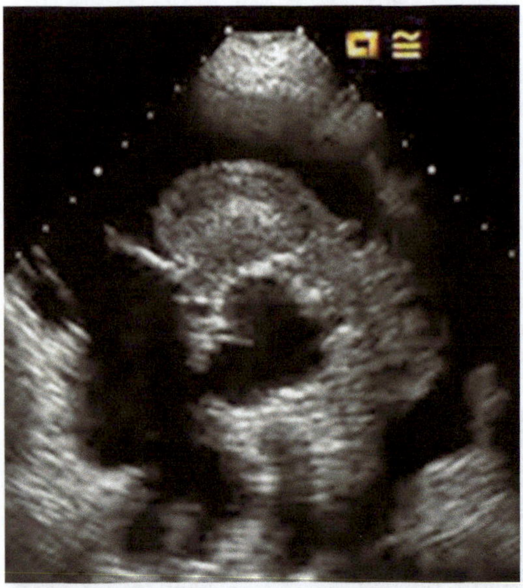

Fig. 7.6 Transthoracic echocardiography. Reprinted with permission of the Italian Society of Cardiology. Short-axis view at the level of the great arteries. Sarcoma infiltrating the right ventricular outflow tract and the pulmonary artery

Cardiac myxoma, the great mimic. The case of myxoma demonstrates how many exceptions may have these diagnostic tips. The cardiac myxoma is a mobile mass attached to the left side of the fossa ovalis by a peduncle allowing wide back and forth excursion in the left atrial chamber. The mass may obstruct in diastole the atrioventricular inflow (Fig. 7.1) thus clinically mimicking mitral stenosis, and similar to mitral stenosis it may produce embolic events secondary to fragmentation of the fragile mass. In 10% of the cases the mass is sessile.

The site of attachment, dimensions, and structure of myxomas may be very heterogeneous. In the large study of Goswami et al. [3] 84% originated from the left atrium, 12% from the right atrium, and the remaining 4% from both atria. Sixty-nine percent of left atrial myxoma originated from the fossa ovalis, 28% from the inferior

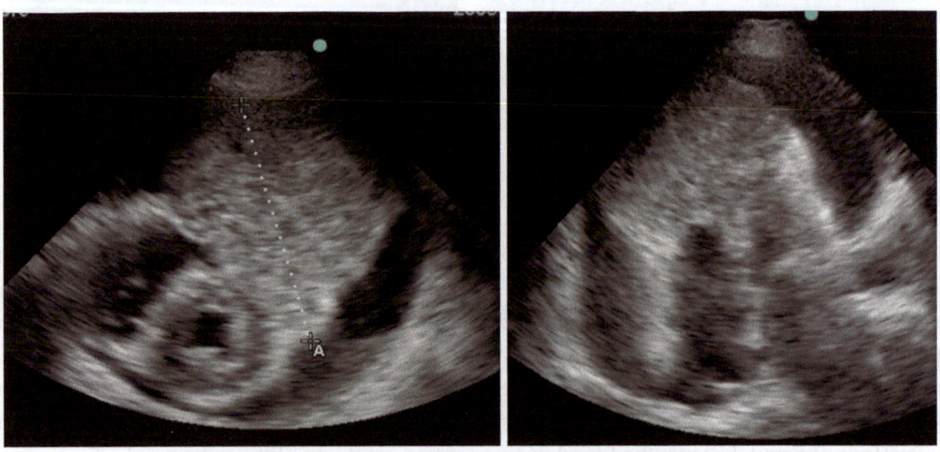

Fig. 7.7 Transthoracic echocardiography. Large sarcoma infiltrating the anteroseptal and apical wall of both left and right ventricles, with massive pericardial effusion

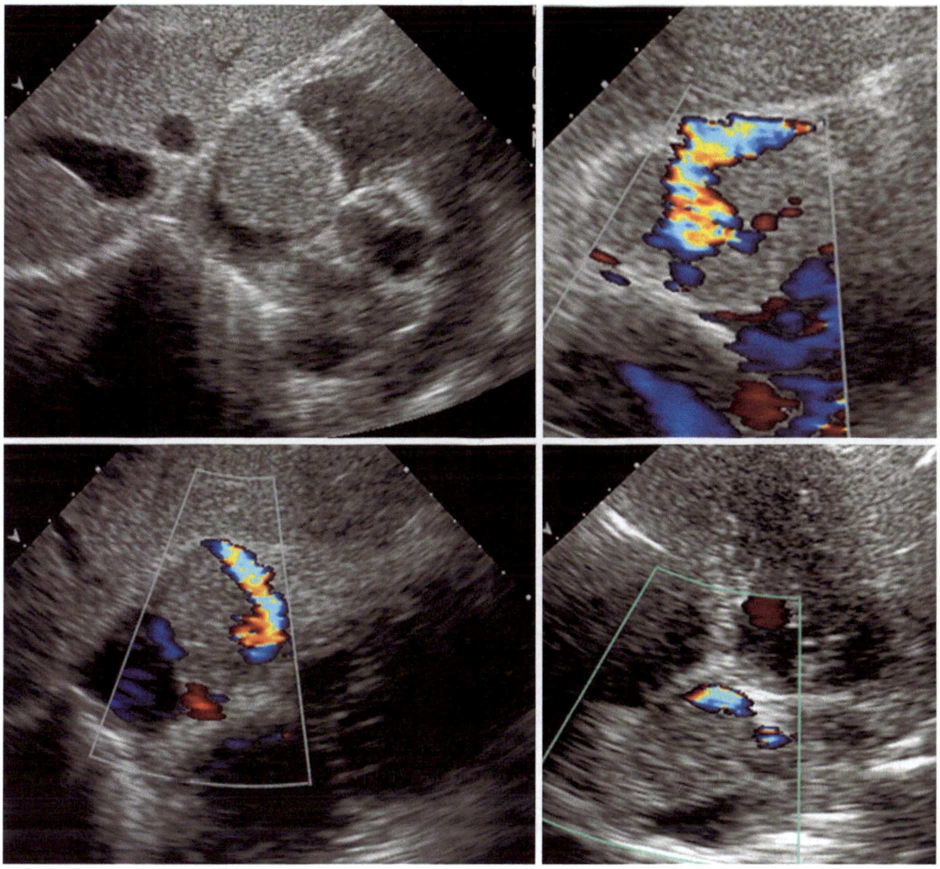

Fig. 7.8 Transthoracic color-Doppler echocardiography. Reprinted with permission of the Italian Society of Cardiology. Richly vascularized right atrial paraganglioma

border of the septum, and the remaining 3% from the lateral wall. Similarly, the great majority of right atrial myxomas originated from the right side of the fossa ovalis. All biatrial myxomas in this large series straddled the fossa ovalis. Very rarely myxomas may be found in both the right and left ventricle. The surface is most often smooth and globular, but in 15% of the cases it may be papillary and friable. Echo-lucent areas within the myxoma can be found in 70% of the cases, often as large as 1 cm [2]. In about 10% of the cases, calcifications may be also observed.

When the diagnosis is made in a young patient, one should always consider the presence of multiple and relapsing lesions and a familiar distribution.

Which Role for Transesophageal Echocardiography?

Transthoracic echocardiography has greatly improved in the last decade allowing better detection of structures in the far field, as the atria. In a recent review of 149 primary cardiac tumors in China [1] transthoracic echocardiography was diagnostic in 93.3% of the cases. In the 10 remaining cases missed at transthoracic echocardiography the mass was in the pericardium (eight cases), in the left atrium (one case), and on the posterior surface of the heart (one case).

Of course, transesophageal echocardiography [5–8] has a better resolution than transthoracic echocardiography, because the acoustic

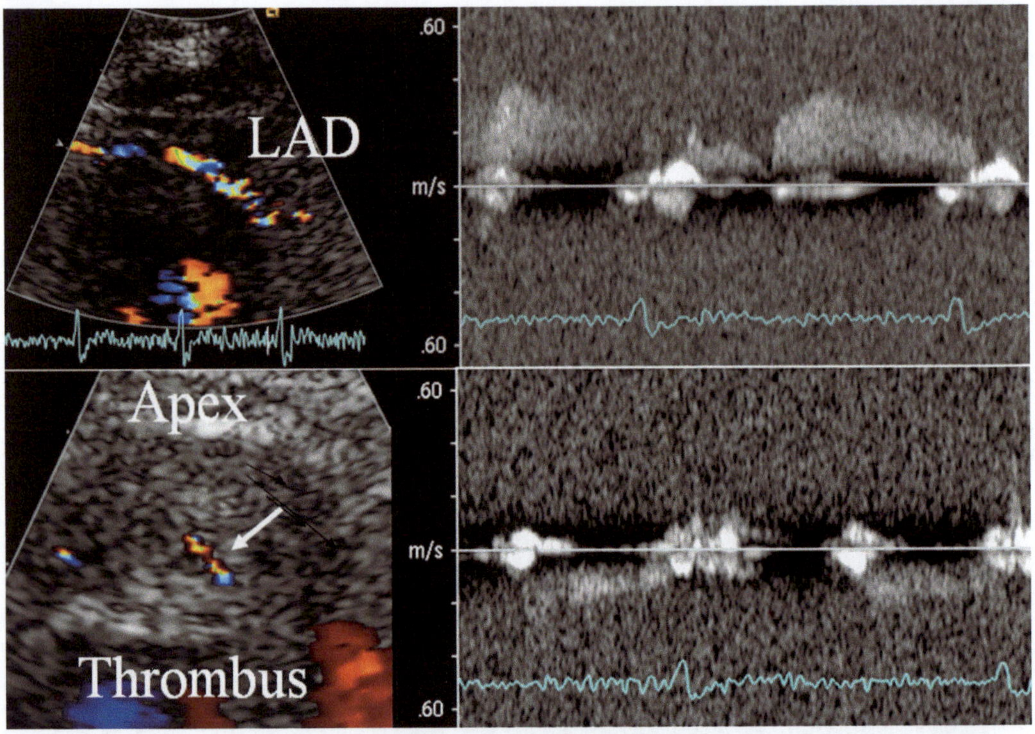

Fig. 7.9 Transthoracic color-Doppler echocardiography. Vascularized apical thrombus. *Upper panel*: epicardial tract of the left anterior descending (LAD) coronary artery visualized by color-Doppler and the corresponding pulsed Doppler tracing with the characteristic anterograde systolic and diastolic flow. *Lower panel*: vascularized apical thrombus with flow directed away from the transducer (*modified from Voci et al.* [20])

impedance is lower and the transducers have a higher spatial resolution. Despite this advantage, transesophageal echocardiography not often brings additional information over transthoracic echocardiography, relevant for surgical referral of the patient [3]. However, the superior wall of the right atrium and the right atrial appendage are only incompletely seen by transthoracic echocardiography and anatomical details of the inferior and superior vena cava may be better seen by transesophageal echocardiography [7].

Intraoperative transesophageal echocardiography is useful to guide surgery and to evaluate the results of valve repair in case of infiltration of the atrioventricular valves or to confirm the absence of intracardiac shunts after septal repair. Lastly, transesophageal echocardiography monitors weaning from cardiopulmonary bypass, particularly patients undergoing partial ventricular resection for infiltrating tumors. Sometimes transesophageal echocardiography may help guiding transvenous biopsy of right chamber masses particularly of inoperable malignant tumors, when the histology is necessary to guide chemotherapy.

Metastatic tumors

The prevalence of cardiac metastasis from tumors originated in the lung, breast, kidney, skin, and colon is 100–1,000 times higher compared to primary cardiac tumors [1]. Cardiac metastases represent a social problem, because paradoxically the improvement in chemo- and radiotherapy, prolonging the life expectancy of these patients also increased the prevalence of cardiac metastasis, from 0.2 to 6% before 1996 to more than 10% in 2003 [2]. Cardiac metastases can be intramyocardial (Fig. 7.10) and/or pericardial (Fig. 7.11) and produce pericardial effusion and tamponade. Lymphoma may compress the cardiac chambers (Fig. 7.12) or produce the superior vena cava syndrome (Fig. 7.13). Kidney tumors may infiltrate the inferior vena cava and reach the right atrium (Fig. 7.14), even causing pulmonary neoplastic embolism.

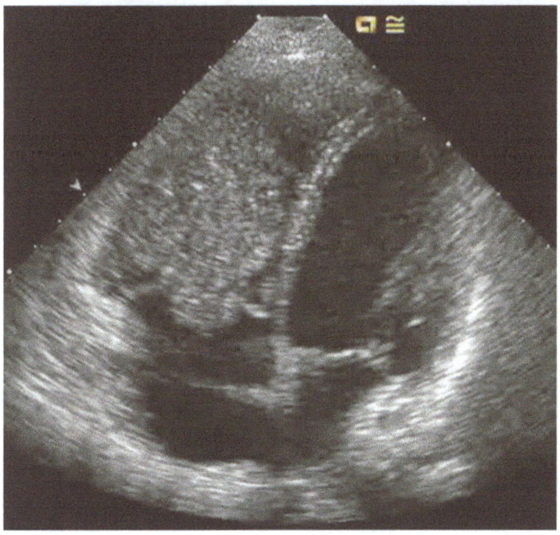

Fig. 7.10 Two-dimensional echocardiography, apical four-chamber projection. Reprinted with permission of the Italian Society of Cardiology. Metastatic melanoma infiltrating almost entirely the right ventricle, and prolapsing in systole through the tricuspid valve

Conclusions

Nowadays, the diagnosis of cardiac tumors is based mainly on transthoracic echocardiography which allows to visualize a cardiac mass and to roughly predict its nature. Transesophageal echocardiography is indicated in the rare cases when transthoracic echocardiography is non-diagnostic, and in the perioperative monitoring of complex lesions.

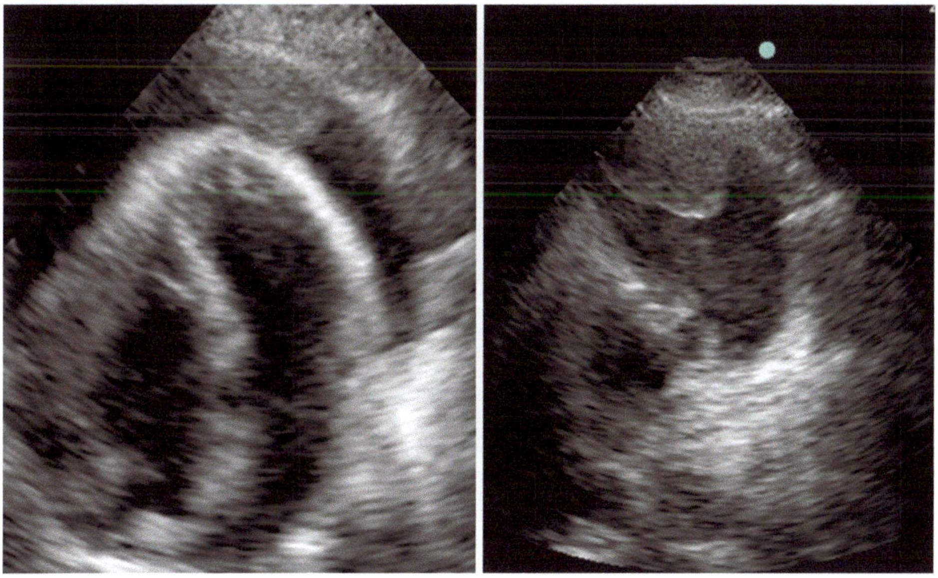

Fig. 7.11 Two-dimensional echocardiography. Pericardial metastasis secondary to a colon carcinoma. The off-axis projection in the *right panel* clearly shows that the mass is attached to the parietal pericardium and does not infiltrate the myocardium, being therefore suitable for surgical resection

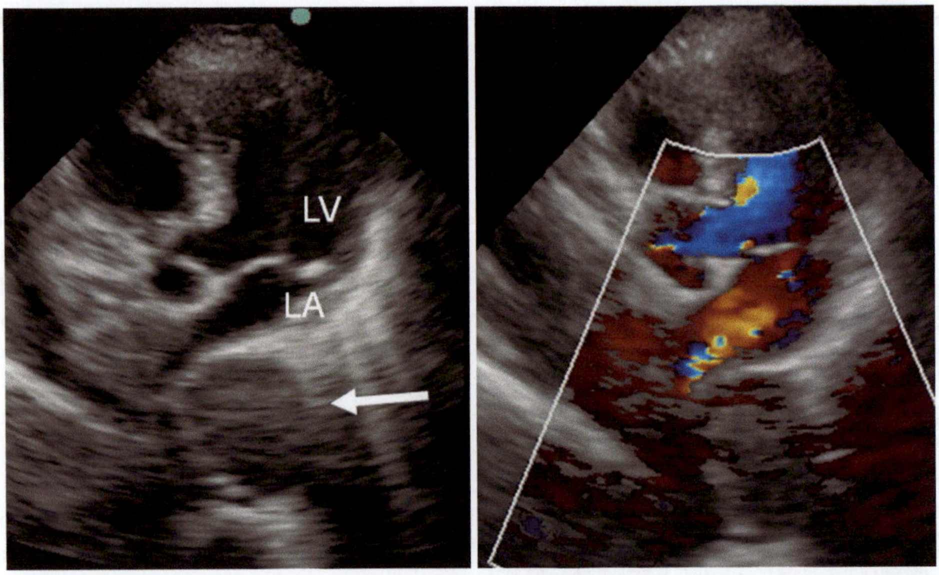

Fig. 7.12 Mediastinal lymphoma compressing the left atrium (LA). *LV* left ventricle

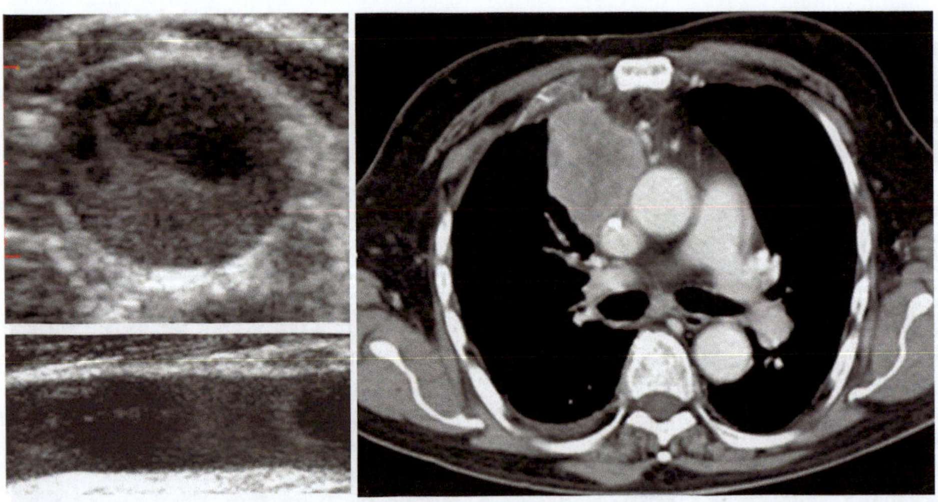

Fig. 7.13 Intrathoracic lymphoma (CT scan, *right panel*) leading to superior vena cava syndrome with marked stagnation of flow in the jugular vein (*left panel*)

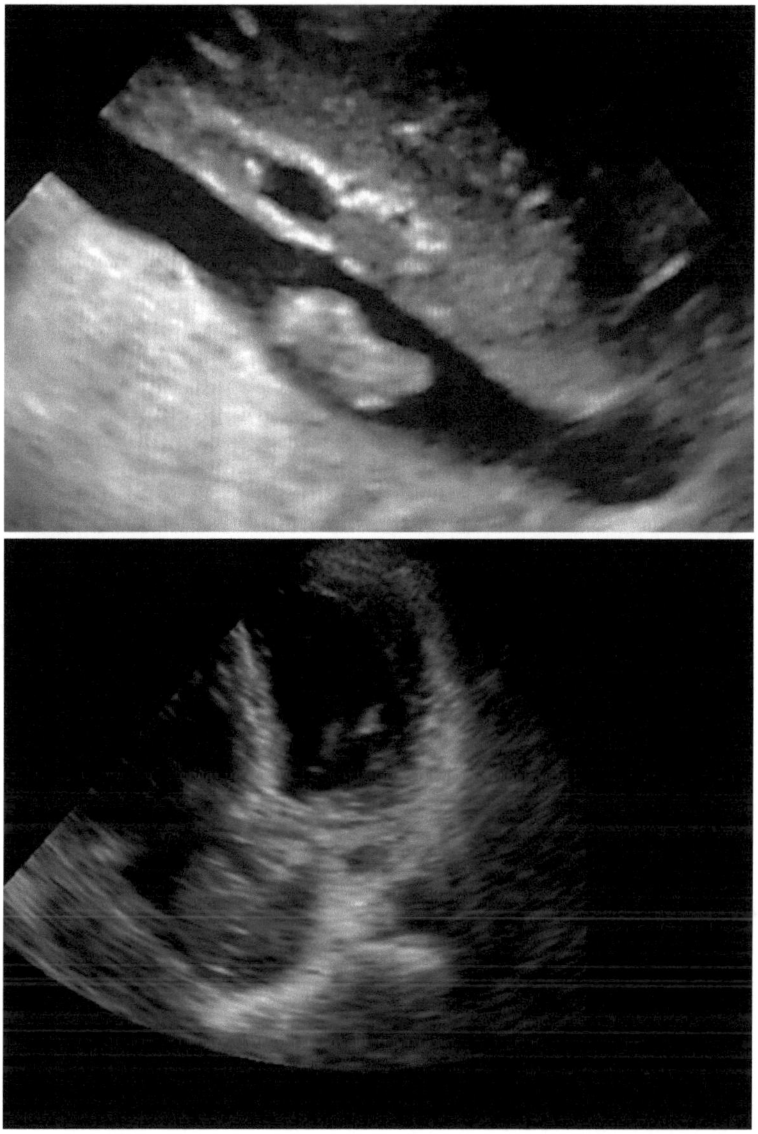

Fig. 7.14 Right kidney tumor producing a mobile mass in the inferior vena cava (*upper panel*) and right atrial metastasis (*lower panel*)

References

1. Meng Q, Lai H, Lima J, Tong W, Qian Y, Lai S. Echocardiographic and pathologic characteristics of primary cardiac tumors: a study of 149 cases. Int J Cardiol. 2002;84:69–75.
2. Butany J, Nair V, Naszemuddin A, Nair GM, Cotton C, Yau T. Cardiac tumors: diagnosis and treatment. Lancet Oncol. 2005;6:219–28.
3. Goswami K, Shirivasta S, Bahl VK, Saxena A, Manchanda SC, Wasir HS. Cardiac myxomas: clinical and echocardiographic profile. Int J Cardiol. 1998;63:251–9.
4. Padalino MA, Basso C, Svaluto Moreolo G, Thiene G, Stellin G. Left atrial myxoma in a child. Case report and review of the literature. Cardiovasc Pathol. 2003;12:233–6.
5. Rizzoli G, Bottio T, Pittarello D, Napodano M, Thiene G, Basso C. Atrial septal mass: transesophageal

echocardiographic assessment. J Thorac Cardiovasc Surg. 2004;128:767–9.
6. Perez de Isla L, De Castro R, Zamorano JL, Almeria C, Moreno R, Moreno M, Lima P, Garcia Fernandez MA. Diagnosis and treatment of cardiac myxomas by transesophageal echocardiography. Am J Cardiol. 2002;90:1419–21.
7. Leibowitz G, Keller NM, Daniel WG, Freedberg RS, Tunica PA, Stottmeister C, Kronzon I. Transesophageal versus transthoracic echocardiography in the evaluation of right atrial tumors. Am Heart J. 1995;130:1224–7.
8. Mahdhaoui A, Bouraoui H, Amine MM, Mokni M, Besma T, Ernez Hajri S, Deridi G, Khelfa M, Bahri F, Yacoubi T, Sriha B, Ammar H. The transesophageal echocardiographic diagnosis of left atrial myxoma simulating a left atrial thrombus in the setting of mitral stenosis. Echocardiography. 2004;21:233–6.
9. Vieira MLC, Ianni BM, Mady C, Encinas J, Pommerantzeff PMA, Fernandes PP, Leal SB, Mathias Jr W, Andrade JL, Ramires JA. Left atrial myxoma. Three-dimensional echocardiographic assessment. Arq Bras Cardiol. 2004;82:284–6.
10. Borges AC, Witt C, Bartel T, Muller S, Konertz W, Baumann G. Preoparative two- and three-dimensional transesophageal echocardiographic assessment of heart tumors. Ann Thorac Surg. 1996;61:1163–7.
11. Mehmood F, Nanda NC, Vengala S, Winokur T, Dod HS, Ebenezer F, Patel V, Bodiwala K, Upendram S, Kirklin JK, McGiffin DC, Pacifico AD. Live three-dimensional transthoracic echocardiographic assessment of left atrial tumors. Echocardiography. 2005;22:137–43.
12. Turley AJ, Hunter S, Stewart M. A cardiac paraganglioma presenting with atypical chest pain. Eur J Cardiothorac Surg. 2005;28:352–4.
13. Reynen K. Cardiac myxoma. N Engl J Med. 1995;333:1610–7.
14. Salcedo EE, Cohen GL, White RD, Davison M. Cardiac tumors: diagnosis and management. Curr Probl Cardiol. 1992;17:73–137.
15. Pinede L, Duhaut P, Loire R. Clinical presentation of left atrial cardiac myxoma. A series of 112 consecutive cases. Medicine. 2001;80:159–72.
16. Glancy DL, Roberts WC. The heart in malignant melanoma. A study of 70 autopsy cases. Am J Cardiol. 1968;2:355–71.
17. Centofanti P, Di Rosa E, Deorsola L. Primary cardiac tumors: early and late results of surgical treatment in 91 patients. Ann Thorac Surg. 1999;68:1236–41.
18. Silverman NA. Primary cardiac tumors. Ann Surg. 1980;191:127–38.
19. Vander Salm TJ. Unusual primary tumors of the heart. Semin Thorac Cardiovasc Surg. 2000;12:89–100.
20. Voci P, Pizzuto F, Romeo F. Coronary flow: a new asset for the echo lab? Eur Heart J. 2004;25:1867–79.

Echocardiography of Cardiac Masses: From Two- to Three-Dimensional Imaging

8

Luigi P. Badano, Denisa Muraru, and Sabino Iliceto

Introduction

Tumors involving the heart can cause symptoms and signs due to obstruction of cardiac chambers and great vessels, pulmonary or systemic embolization, complete heart block and arrhythmias, or cardiac tamponade, although they are often also incidental findings. In the past, they were often discovered at autopsy. Nowadays, technologic advances in cardiovascular imaging have led to a substantial increase in antemortem diagnoses. Echocardiography is the imaging technique of choice to detect intracardiac masses in the clinical practice [1, 2]. This tool has the unique advantage of being able to provide a non-invasive dynamic assessment of cardiac masses, to evaluate their hemodynamic impact and the presence of associated abnormalities (Table 8.1). However, current echocardiographic techniques do not allow tissue characterization. In this chapter, we will focus on the echocardiographic characteristics of primary and secondary cardiac tumors.

Both transthoracic and transesophageal echocardiography have shown a good sensitivity to detect intracardiac tumors (93.3 and 96.8%, respectively, in one series of pathologically confirmed tumors) [3], but a lower detection rate for pericardial or paracardiac lesions. Although cardiac tumors can often be seen by two-dimensional transthoracic echocardiography, their location, size, and relationships with surrounding structures are better defined by transesophageal echocardiography.

Visualizing the suspected cardiac mass throughout the cardiac cycle in more than one view, with the appropriate transducer and scanner settings, are important rules for the proper characterization of the mass, avoiding the misinterpretation of artifacts. A thorough knowledge of normal anatomy, physiologic variants, and embryonic remnants, as well as familiarity with structural changes associated with various operative and interventional procedures are crucial and will decrease the likelihood of misdiagnosis. Finally, it is pivotal that clinical and personal information are available at the time of the study, to be used for interpreting echocardiographic findings in context.

Conventional (i.e., two-dimensional) echocardiography is a tomographic technique, and effective interpretation of images requires one to mentally integrate them into a three-dimensional (3D), stereoscopic reconstruction of the heart. For example, an intracardiac tumor may have quite variable site of attachment, shape, and size, requiring the echocardiographer to examine the tumor from a series of two-dimensional images and then to "mentally" reconstruct the tumor to define its size, shape, and attachment. To do this accurately, a clinician should understand the relationship of each two-dimensional tomographic image to one

L.P. Badano, M.D. (✉) • D. Muraru, M.D. • S. Iliceto, M.D.
Cardiology, Department of Cardiac, Thoracic and Vascular Sciences, University of Padua
Medical School, Via N. Giustiniani 2,
Padua 35128, Italy
e-mail: lpbadano@gmail.com

C. Basso et al. (eds.), *Cardiac Tumor Pathology*, Current Clinical Pathology,
DOI 10.1007/978-1-62703-143-1_8, © Springer Science+Business Media New York 2013

Table 8.1 Echocardiographic assessment of cardiac masses

Characterization of the mass	
Location	Intra- or extracardiac
Relationship with adjacent structures	
Site, mobility, and mode of implantation	
Route of access to the heart	Superior/inferior vena cava Pulmonary veins Uncertain
Shape and size (3D volume)	Largest diameters or maximal area
Hemodynamic/functional consequences	Obstruction and/or regurgitation by interfering with valve function Extracardiac compression Segmental wall motion abnormalities or restrictive disease due to direct infiltration of the myocardium Pericardial infiltration and/or effusion with variable degree of hemodynamic impairment
Vascularization	Contrast
Differential diagnosis	
Benign	
1. Embryonic remnants	Chiari network, Eustachian valve, etc.
2. Thrombi	Free-floating or attached (mural, device or catheter-related)
3. Benign cardiac tumors	
4. Vegetations	
Malignant	
1. Primary	
2. Metastatic	

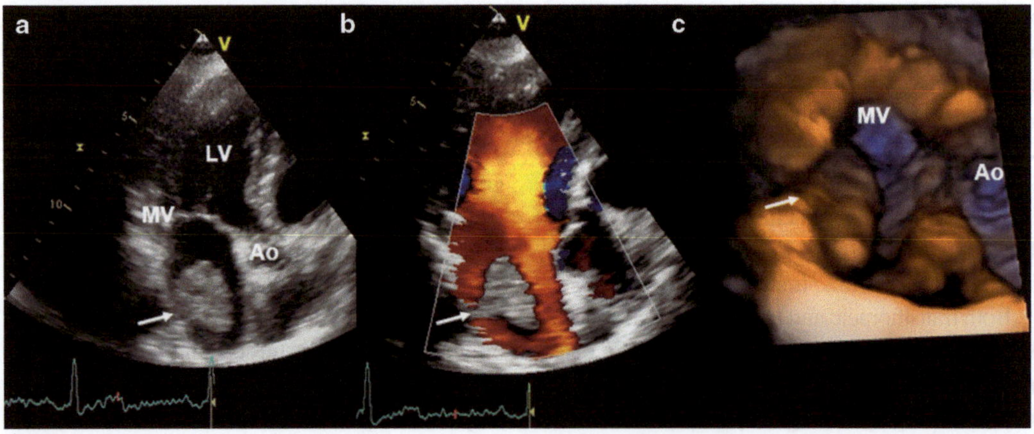

Fig. 8.1 Atypical left atrial myxoma. (**a**) At two-dimensional echocardiography, a large mass is seen attached by a short stalk (*white arrow*) to the left atrial free wall. Echodensity is not homogeneous; echolucencies within the mass represent hemorrhagic areas. A myxoma has been diagnosed at surgical inspection and then proven at histology. (**b**) Color flow two-dimensional echocardiography confirms the attachment of the mass to the left atrial free wall and shows no interference with mitral valve (MV) function. (**c**) Three-dimensional echocardiography showing the shape of the mass, its volume, and irregular surface. Mitral valve is seen in the background. *Ao* aortic valve, *LV* left ventricle, *MV* mitral valve

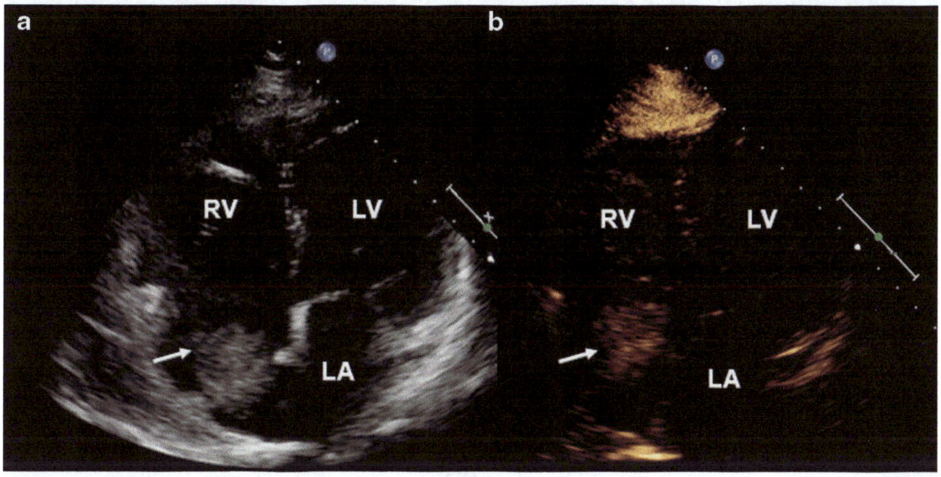

Fig. 8.2 Right atrial myxoma. (**a**) A large, not homogeneous and mobile mass (*arrow*) attached to the interatrial septum is visualized in the right atrium. (**b**). Partial enhancement of the mass tissue after intravenous injection of contrast agent suggesting a poorly vascularized mass (courtesy of Agata Barchitta, M.D., Ospedale CTO S Antonio, ULSS 16, Padova, Italy). *LA* left atrium, *LV* left ventricle, *RV* right ventricle

another. 3D echocardiography eliminates the need for cognitive reconstruction of image planes and use of geometric assumptions about the shape of structures for quantitation. This particularly applies to complex shapes such as intracardiac tumors (Fig. 8.1) [4–6]. Once a 3D data set is acquired, it can be cropped and sliced in many different ways. In addition, the possibility of rotating the data sets in the space allows the observer to obtain planes and views and to align structures in ways that were impossible to achieve with conventional two-dimensional echocardiography. Thus, additional information about mass location, shape, attaching interface, and relationships with adjacent structures can be derived from 3D data sets [7].

Contrast echocardiography is another echo modality which may be used to detect cardiac masses (i.e., in patients with inadequate acoustic window) and/or to differentiate among various types of cardiac masses [8, 9]. Three different echo contrast patterns can be seen in intracardiac masses, i.e., no enhancement at all by the contrast agent, suggesting the presence of thrombi since they are generally avascular; partial enhancement with decreased pixel intensity in comparison with the surrounding myocardium, suggesting a poorly vascularized mass such as myxoma (Fig. 8.2); and complete enhancement with higher intensity than adjacent myocardium, suggesting a highly vascularized tumor which is a characteristic of rapidly growing malignant tumors.

Myxoma

Myxomas can cause obstruction and/or regurgitation by interfering with valve function and frequently embolize, so that their immediate removal after diagnosis is mandatory.

Myxomas are usually solitary and are located most frequently (approximately 75% of the cases) in the left atrium (Fig. 8.1), with the remainder largely arising within the right atrium (Fig. 8.3a). Myxomas arising from the ventricles, mitral valve, as well as multiple myxomas (Fig. 8.3b) within the same cardiac chamber have also been exceptionally described. Therefore, a careful transesophageal echocardiographic study should be conducted preoperatively to be sure that all tumors have been detected and will be removed.

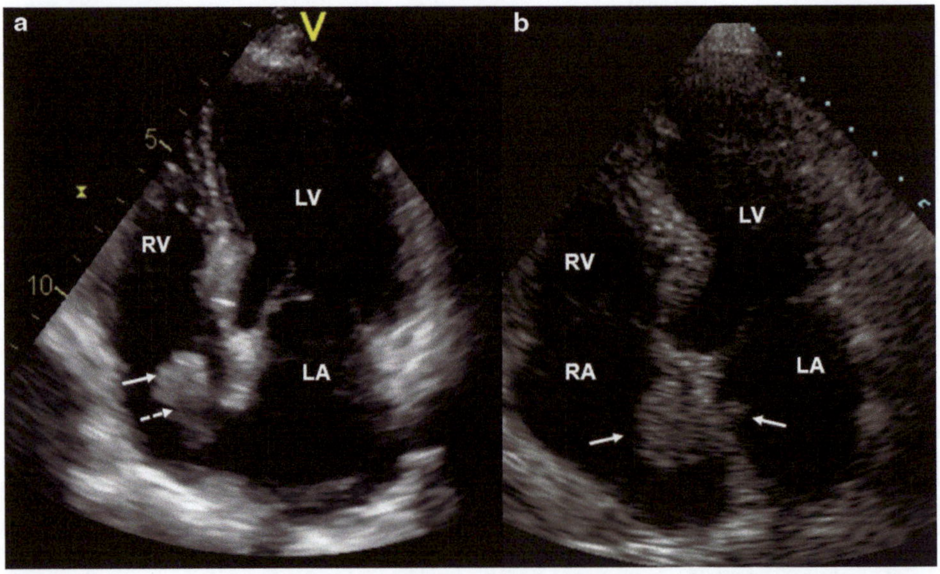

Fig. 8.3 (**a**) A large right atrial myxoma attached to interatrial septum. Areas of calcification (*arrow*) and echolucencies (*dashed arrow*) can be appreciated within this polypoid mass. (**b**) A large right atrial mass (*arrow*) attached to the interatrial septum, associated with a second smaller mass attached to the left side of interatrial septum (*arrow*), that were found to be myxomas at pathological examination. *LA* left atrium, *LV* left ventricle, *RA* right atrium, *RV* right ventricle

The typical atrial myxoma manifests as a single intracardiac homogeneous or finely speckled compact, rounded, or ovoid mass mass, isodense to the surrounding myocardium, attached to the interatrial septum near the fossa ovalis by a stalk-like pedicle. However, echocardiographic appearance can be also that of a polypoid, papillary, friable mass attached to the endocardium of any cardiac structure. Size can vary from less than 1 cm to an extent that virtually fills the whole atrium. The echogenity of myxomas may not be homogeneous, since they frequently contain cystic spaces, and areas of necrosis, hemorrhage, and calcification. Inhomogeneous appearance is useful to differentiate them from large thrombi. Mobility of myxoma depends on its size and the type of attachment; however, prolapsing of the tumor into the ventricles through the atrio-ventricular valves is a common characteristic of atrial myxomas. The attachment may be broad and hence they may also appear as immobile or hypomobile masses. The degree of functional obstruction to ventricular filling caused by the tumor can be qualitatively assessed by color Doppler flow imaging and measured by continuous-wave Doppler sampling of the ventricular inflow which will show, in case of significant obstruction, the typical tracing morphology of functional mitral (or tricuspid, in case of right atrial myxoma) stenosis.

Although transthoracic two-dimensional echocardiography has been found to be highly accurate in providing all relevant information for surgery [8], transesophageal echocardiography has a higher sensitivity in detecting myxomas in comparison with transthoracic echocardiography, especially in the setting of small myxomas, and should be performed in any case with the suspicion of intracardiac tumor or unknown source of embolism. Transesophageal echocardiography, particularly 3D modality, is also useful in very large myxomas nearly filling the atrial chamber, in close contact with large areas of atrial endocardium throughout the cardiac cycle, in which the stalk cannot be clearly visualized.

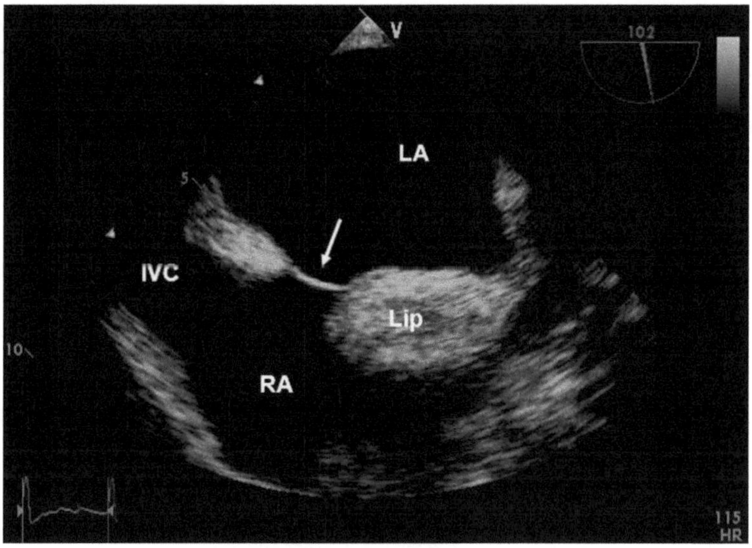

Fig. 8.4 Lipomatous hypertrophy of the interatrial septum. Transesophageal echocardiography shows the typical thickening of the interatrial septum (Lip) that spares the region of the fossa ovalis (*arrow*) giving the classic dumbbell appearance to the interatrial septum (courtesy of Pasquale Gianfagna, M.D., Cardiothoracic Department, Azienda Ospedaliero-Universitaria, Udine, Italy). *IVC* inferior vena cava, *LA* left atrium, *RA* right atrium

Postoperative echocardiography should be performed to document the complete excision of the tumor. Since recurrent myxomas have been reported, long-term follow-up is indicated, particularly in the familial form of the disease.

Cardiac Lipoma and Lipomatous Hypertrophy of Interatrial Septum

Lipomas are encapsulated, hyperdense, homogeneous tumors which can be found throughout the heart, typically in subepicardial or subendocardial location. Rarely, they can arise within the myocardium or from the valve leaflets. Occasionally, they may grow as broad-based, pedunculated masses into any of the cardiac chambers and may reach giant sizes and weigh up to 4.8 kg [10]. Usually, there is no calcification, necrosis, or intratumoral hemorrhage, as opposed to myxomas. Intrapericardial lipomas may cause compression of the heart and pericardial effusion.

Lipomatous hypertrophy of interatrial septum has often been included in reports of cardiac lipomas. Lipomatous hypertrophy of interatrial septum is defined as any deposit of fat in the atrial septum which exceeds 2 cm in transverse dimension (Fig. 8.4) [11]. It is associated with advanced age and obesity and caused by an increase in the number of adipocytes. Lipomatous hypertrophy of interatrial septum typically spares the fossa ovalis (giving rise to the characteristic "*dumbbell*" shape to the interatrial septum) and does not represent a true cardiac tumor [11]. In rare cases, an obstruction of inferior vena cava may occur.

Papillary Fibroelastoma

Papillary fibroelastomas are the most common tumors of the cardiac valves. Echocardiographically, they manifest as small (2–10 mm), usually single, mobile, pedunculated echo masses which can be filamentous, frond-like, or oval in shape, typically attached to the valve leaflets on either side of the heart. Due to their small size, papillary fibrobroelastomas could not be detected by transthoracic echocardiography.

Ninety percent of papillary fibroelastomas occur on valve surfaces, being more commonly found on the aortic valve (29%, where they can arise from both surface, Fig. 8.5) and on the mitral valve (25%, mainly arising from the atrial

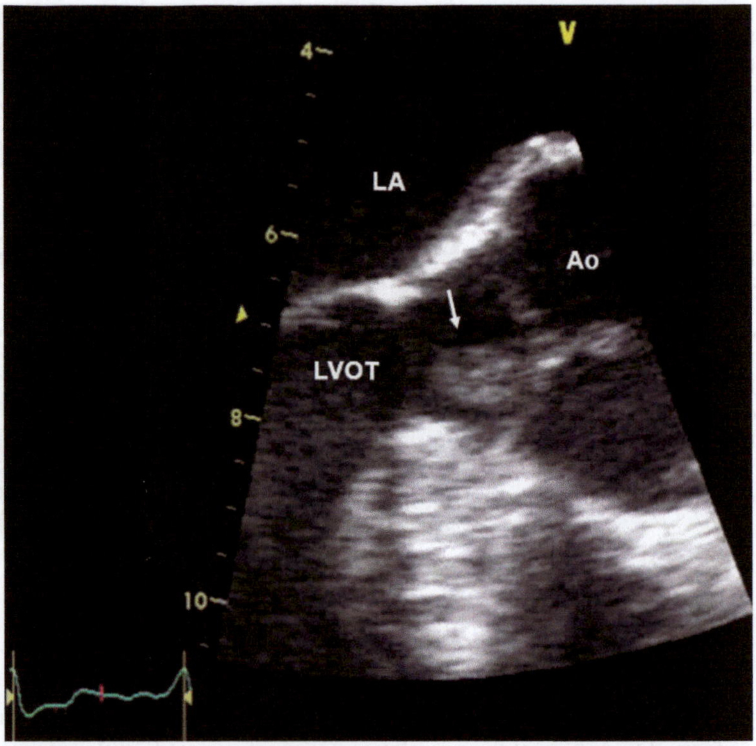

Fig. 8.5 Papillary fibroelastoma of the aortic valve. Transesophageal echocardiogram revealed a small, oval-shaped, highly mobile mass (*arrow*) attached to the body of the right coronary cusp of the aortic valve by a short stalk (courtesy of Pasquale Gianfagna, M.D., Cardiothoracic Department, Azienda Ospedaliero-Universitaria, Udine, Italy). *Ao* aorta, *LA* left atrium, *LVOT* left ventricular outflow tract

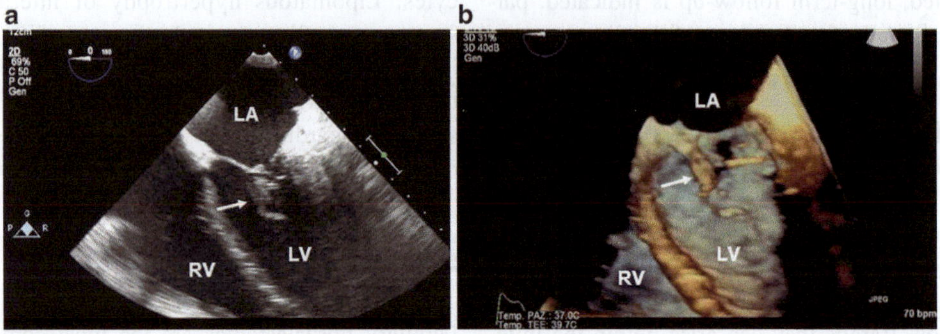

Fig. 8.6 Papillary fibroelastoma of the mitral valve. (**a**) Transesophageal echocardiogram showed a large, highly mobile mass on the ventricular side of the anterior mitral valve leaflet (*arrow*). (**b**) Three-dimensional echocardiography allowed the localization of this mass at the mid portion of the leaflet and a better appreciation of its morphology and size (courtesy of Pasquale Gianfagna, M.D., Cardiothoracic Department, Azienda Ospedaliero-Universitaria, Udine, Italy). *LA* left atrium, *LV* left ventricle, *RV* right ventricle

side, Fig. 8.6), than on the pulmonary (13%) or tricuspid valves (17%) [12]. Sixteen percent of papillary fibroelastomas have been reported to arise from nonvalvular surfaces (Fig. 8.7) and from the subvalvular apparatus of the mitral valve [13].

Papillary fibroelastomas often appear like infectious vegetations or Lambl's excrescences, which makes differential diagnosis difficult. Large mobile vegetations attached to the valves may mimic papillary fibroelastomas, but the clinical context suggestive of infective endocarditis helps

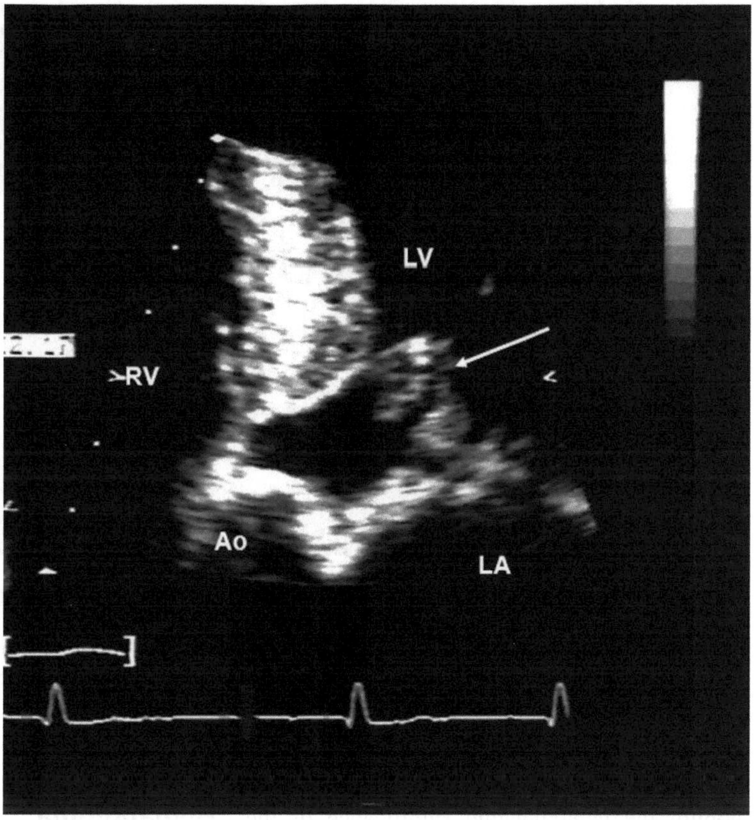

Fig. 8.7 Uncommon localization of papillary fibroelastoma on the endocardium of the interventricular septum. Transthoracic two-dimensional echocardiography, zoomed apical five-chamber view: a frond-like, highly mobile mass is attached to the left ventricular endocardium in the outflow tract (*arrow*). The mass was resected and found to be a fibroelastoma (courtesy of Pasquale Gianfagna, M.D., Cardiothoracic Department, Azienda Ospedaliero-Universitaria,Udine, Italy). *Ao* aortic valve, *LV* left ventricle, *LA* left atrium, *RV* right ventricle

in differentiating between them. Lambl's excrescences, which can be found as normal features in many adults, are filamentous, mobile, and avascular structures that generally arise at the closure line of the valves [14]. Papillary fibroelastomas are not as thin as Lambl's excrescences and, unlike the latter, they do not arise from the leaflet closure line, but from other regions on the valve surface. Fibroelastomas may also be confused with blood cysts, which are unusual, blood-containing, cystic structures that develop within atrio-ventricular valve leaflets. Blood cysts are sessile with a broader base, and thus less mobile than fibroelastomas.

Rhabdomyoma

Rhabdomyomas are the most common primary cardiac tumor in children and up to 50% of them are associated with tuberous sclerosis. These tumors are usually located in the myocardium of both ventricles and multiplicity is common (Fig. 8.8), but intracavitary growths can be found in more than 50% of patients. They may also originate within the atrium or in the atrio-ventricular junction. When occurring intramural, they appear as bright intramural masses with luminal extension. A circumscribed ventricular wall thickening of the left and/or right ventricle can be detected. When intracavitary, rhabdomyomas will more frequently appear as echodense structures, lobulated in shape and ventricular in origin. They may be associated with mechanical complications, such as outflow tract obstruction. Multifocal lesions are common.

Since regression of these tumors with complete resolution during infancy is expected in more than 80% of cases, surgery is indicated only in the setting of severe symptoms and signs and echocardiography is the technique of choice to

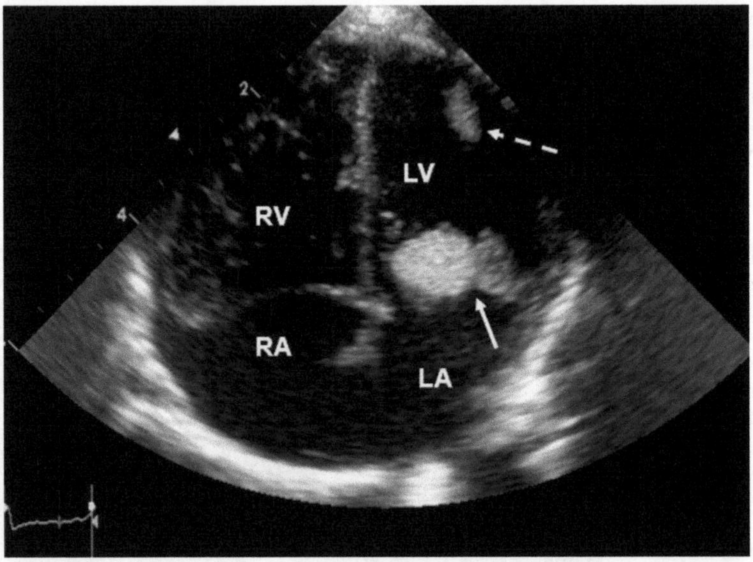

Fig. 8.8 Rhabdomyoma in a child with tuberous sclerosis. Transthoracic apical four-chamber view showing a large, lobulated, and echodense mass localized at the left atrio-ventricular junction (*arrow*). A smaller mass can be seen within the myocardium of the apical region of the left ventricular lateral wall (*dashed arrow*) (courtesy of Pasquale Gianfagna, M.D., Cardiothoracic Department, Azienda Ospedaliero-Universitaria, Udine, Italy). *LA* left atrium, *LV* left ventricle, *RA* right atrium, *RV* right ventricle

monitor the hemodynamic significance of the tumor and its evolution.

Fibroma

Echocardiographic appearance of cardiac fibroma is that of a single intramural (typically occurring in the interventricular septum, less frequently in the left ventricular free wall) hyperechogenic, noncontractile mass [15]. It may be confused with asymmetric hypertrophic cardiomyopathy or infiltrative myocardial disease, but usually its abnormal texture helps in reaching the correct diagnosis. The size of the mass may vary considerably, from 1 up to 10 cm. A pathognomonic echocardiographic feature of large fibromas is the presence of calcifications due to poor blood supply. Strain rate can be used to confirm the noncontractile nature of the mass [16]. In addition to its detection, echocardiography is useful to monitor the growth of the tumor and, postoperatively, to check for its recurrence.

Hemangioma

Hemangiomas can occur in any cardiac location and can arise from endocardium, myocardium, epicardium, or pericardium (Fig. 8.9a). Hemangiomas are typically intramyocardial, although most often involve the base of the heart. They appear as hyperreflective (but not calcific) masses varying in size (between 1 and 8 cm) and are usually associated with pericardial effusion. The vascularized nature of this tumor is difficult to be appreciated on conventional echocardiography. After contrast injection, the tumor is completely enhanced (Fig. 8.9b), showing a greater intensity than the surrounding myocardium [9, 17].

Teratoma

Intracardiac location of teratomas is very rare. They are usually located within the pericardial space, with a non-homogeneous echogenity and multicystic appearance and may present as a large hemopericardium causing hemodynamic compromise [18].

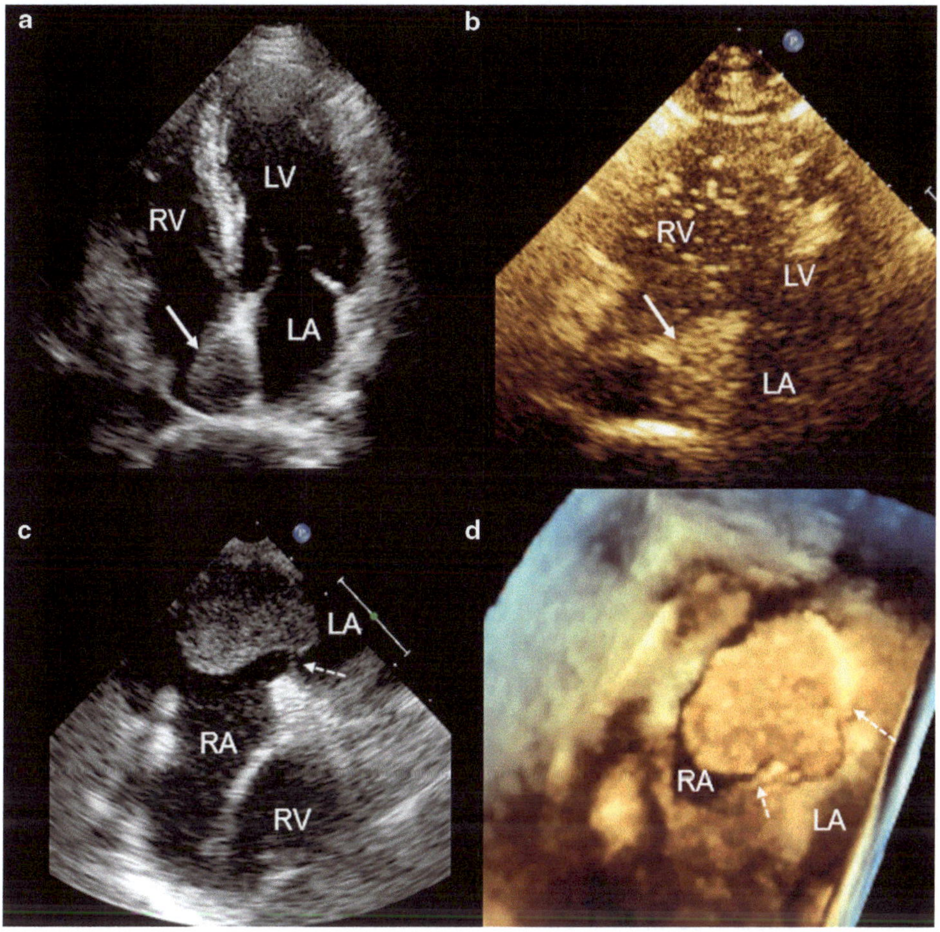

Fig. 8.9 A rare hemangioma of the interatrial septum. (**a**) Two-dimensional four-chamber apical view showing a large mass infiltrating the interatrial septum (*arrow*). (**b**) Complete enhancement of the mass tissue (*arrow*) with higher intensity than adjacent myocardium after intravenous injection of contrast agent, suggesting a highly vascularized tumor. (**c** and **d**) Transesophageal two- and three-dimensional image of the tumor highlighting the infiltration of the interatrial septum (*dashed arrow*). The three-dimensional data set allows a better appreciation of the shape of the mass, its volume, and its relationship with interatrial septum (*dashed arrow*) and right atrial walls (Courtesy of Agata Barchitta, M.D., Ospedale CTO S Antonio, ULSS 16, Padova, Italy). *LA* left atrium, *LV* left ventricle, *RA* right atrium, *RV* right ventricle

Sarcoma

Ninety-five percent of primary malignant tumors are sarcomas. Among these, angiosarcoma is the most frequent and, despite it can arise in any part of the heart, its most frequent location is the right atrium. The main echocardiographic characteristic, that helps to differentiate between benign myxomas and malignant angiosarcomas, is the evidence of infiltration of the cardiac wall and of the pericardium. Sarcomas may cause hemodynamic compromise as a result of obstruction anywhere in the right heart inflow or outflow tract. Angiosarcoma appears as a large, broad-based, mobile, inhomogeneous mass with hypodense necrotic and hemorrhagic zones

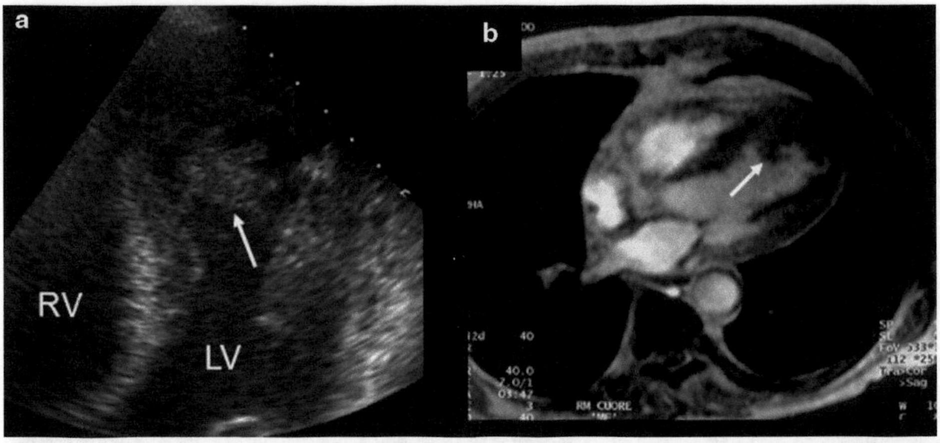

Fig. 8.10 Undifferentiated primary cardiac sarcoma of the left ventricle (localized at the apex and infiltrating left ventricular wall). The large size of the mass seen in this patient is not unusual for this tumor type, given its rapid and aggressive growth pattern. (**a**) Apical five-chamber view of the left ventricle showing an apical large polypoid mass (*arrow*) protruding into the left ventricular cavity. (**b**) Magnetic resonance imaging, four-chamber view, showing the mass infiltrating the left ventricular myocardium of the distal part of interventricular septum and apex (*arrow*). *LV* left ventricle, *RV* right ventricle

and a "cauliflower" shape. Infiltration of the pericardium, tricuspid valve, and vena cava can be frequently visualized. In the setting of a hemorrhagic pericardial effusion, a malignant tumor should be always considered [19].

Undifferentiated sarcoma (Fig. 8.10), malignant fibrous histiocytoma, leiomyosarcoma, rhabdomyosarcoma, osteosarcoma, fibrosarcoma, and liposarcoma are rare primary malignant cardiac tumors. Echocardiographic characteristics of the other cardiac sarcomas are similar to those listed for angiosarcomas, except they are not characteristically located within the right atrium, but elsewhere in the heart, predominantly within the left atrium. In the latter situation, they often originate from the roof of the left atrium or non-septal structures and this serves as a criterion of discrimination from myxomas. They appear as large, mobile, and inhomogeneous masses with zones of necrosis and hemorrhage and are indistinguishable from angiosarcoma. Only osteosarcomas which show typical calcifications within the mass can be differentiated from angiosarcomas.

Infusion of contrast can help in differentiating benign from malignant tumors. Highly vascular tumors like sarcomas become visually hyperenhanced and demonstrate quantitatively more perfusion than the adjacent myocardium [17].

Lymphoma

Primary cardiac lymphomas are defined as non-Hodgkin lymphomas involving only the heart/pericardium or as non-Hodgkin lymphomas with the bulk of the tumor located in the heart [20]. They are very rare in immunocompetent patients [21]. Their incidence is rising with the increasing prevalence of patients with AIDS or heart transplant. At echocardiographic examination, lymphomas commonly arise in the right atrium and appear as large, immobile, sometimes polypoid masses (Fig. 8.11) [22]. They frequently coexist with pericardial effusion.

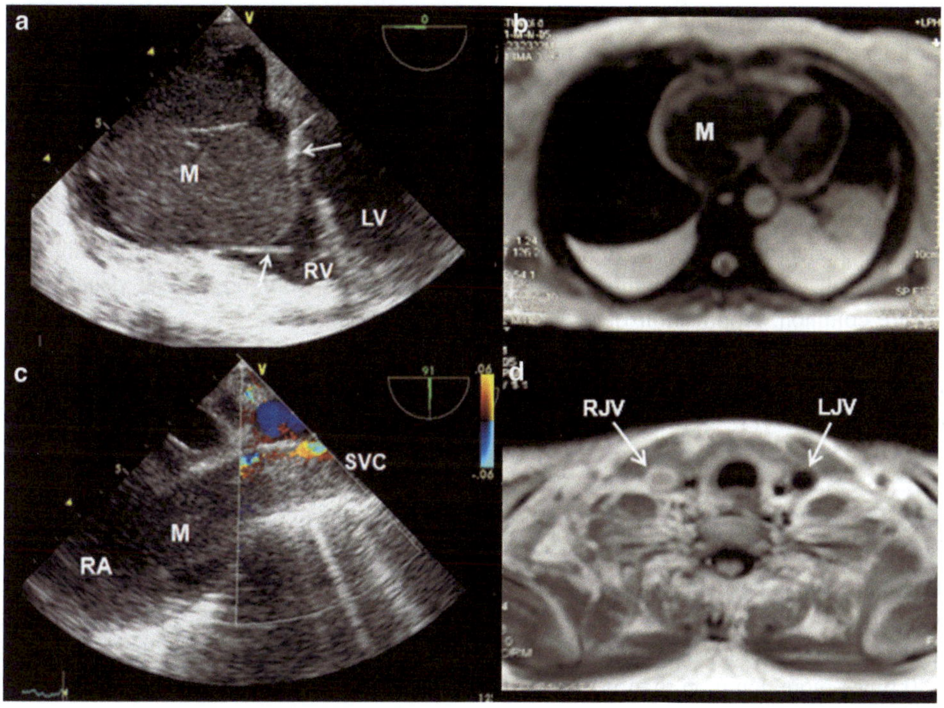

Fig. 8.11 Primary cardiac lymphoma in the right atrium. (**a**) At transesophageal echocardiography, a large mass fills almost completely the right atrium and prolapses through the tricuspid valve during right ventricular filling. (**b**) Magnetic resonance imaging. Four-chamber view showing the size of the tumoral mass (M) and its expansion within the right heart chambers. (**c**) Longitudinal view of the right atrium with superior vena cava at transesophageal echocardiography showing the extension of the tumor within the superior vena cava and the subsequently reduced blood flow through it. (**d**) CT scan showing the occlusion of the right jugular vein by the tumoral mass. *LV* left ventricle, *LJV* left jugular vein, *M* mass, *SVC* superior vena cava, *RA* right atrium, *RJV* right jugular vein, *RV* right ventricle

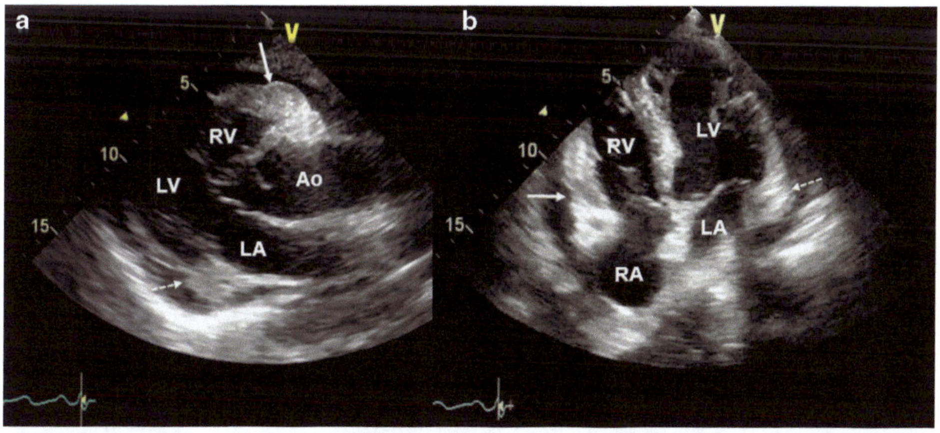

Fig. 8.12 Secondary cardiac lymphoma. At transthoracic echocardiography, the right ventricular free wall (*arrow*) appears thickened and hyperdense in both parasternal long-axis (**a**) and apical four-chamber (**b**) views. An additional intramyocardial, hyperdense, and oval-shaped mass can be appreciated at the posterior left atrio-ventricular junction (*dashed arrow*). Thickened pericardium and diffuse pericardial effusion are signs of pericardial involvement (courtesy of Pasquale Gianfagna, M.D., Cardiothoracic Department, Azienda Ospedaliero-Universitaria, Udine, Italy). *Ao* aorta, *LA* left atrium, *LV* left ventricle, *RA* right atrium, *RV* right ventricle

Secondary cardiac lymphomas show similar echocardiographic characteristics with primary cardiac lymphomas. Echocardiographic findings associated with cardiac metastases include the malignant pericardial effusion, sometimes associated to tumor masses with bizarre surface structures. The infiltrated cardiac walls appear as having a hyperdense pericardium and myocardium (Fig. 8.12). Wall motion abnormalities in these regions are common. Application of echo contrast agents can reveal the tumor perfusion and helps the distinction of the metastasis from the surrounding tissue.

Metastatic Cardiac Tumors

Cardiac metastases have been described in autopsy series in up to 20% of patients with malignancies of other organs (Fig. 8.13) and are up to 40 times more common than primary cardiac tumors [20, 23].

No malignant tumor preferentially metastasizes to the heart; however, melanomas (up to 64% of cases), leukemias, and lymphomas (up to 46%) are the tumors that most frequently manifest cardiac metastasis. Lung, breast, ovarian, and kidney cancer are also frequently involved [15, 20]. Although melanoma can manifest with the detection of intracardiac masses, the most common cardiac manifestation of melanoma is subclinical because it frequently invades the pericardial surface [15]. Indeed, pericardial effusion, with and without tamponade, is overall the most common echocardiographic finding in metastatic heart disease [24]. Solid material adherent to the visceral or parietal pericardium (either tumor or clotted blood) can be visualized within the effusion.

Both benign and malignant tumors can invade the heart through the inferior vena cava. The most common tumor that metastasizes to the heart through the inferior vena cava is the renal cell carcinoma (hypernephroma). Up to 43% of the patients with hypernephroma demonstrate inferior vena cava (Fig. 8.14) and/or right atrial involvement [25]. Among benign tumors, intravascular leiomyomatosis of pelvic or uterine origin can reach the right heart through the inferior vena cava.

Conclusions

Cardiac masses frequently pose a diagnostic challenge. Due to its wide availability and cost-effectiveness ratio, echocardiography is the first choice imaging modality for detection of cardiac tumors.

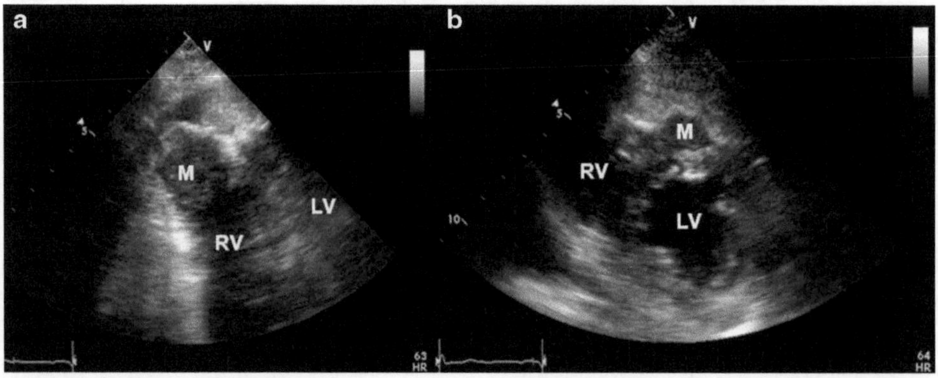

Fig. 8.13 Cardiac localization of metastases originating from a malignant tonsil tumor. Transthoracic echocardiography shows a hypodense, intramyocardial mass (M) localized at the apex of the right ventricle (**a**). In short-axis view (**b**), the mass can be easily differentiated from the surrounding myocardium (courtesy of Pasquale Gianfagna, M.D., Cardiothoracic Department, Azienda Ospedaliero-Universitaria, Udine, Italy). *LV* left ventricle, *RV* right ventricle

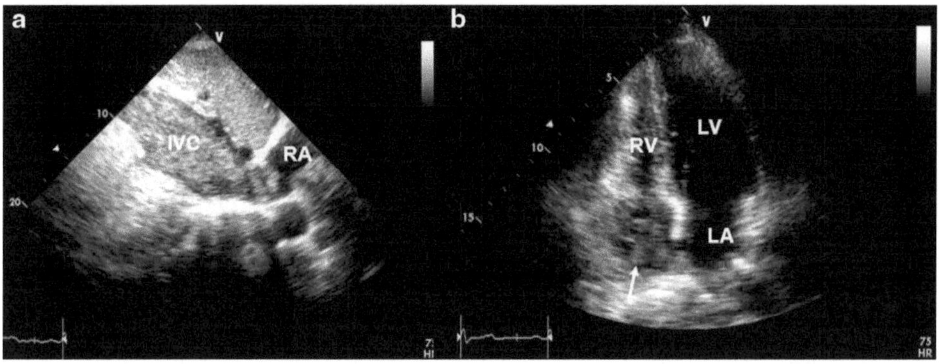

Fig. 8.14 Renal cell carcinoma (hypernephroma). A large hyperdense mass, filling almost completely the lumen of inferior vena cava and protruding into right atrium (*arrow*), can be appreciated at transthoracic echocardiography from both subcostal (**a**) and apical four-chamber view (**b**) (courtesy of Pasquale Gianfagna, M.D., Cardiothoracic Department, Azienda Ospedaliero-Universitaria, Udine, Italy). *IVC* inferior vena cava, *LA* left atrium, *LV* left ventricle, *RA* right atrium, *RV* right ventricle

Box 8.1 Practical Key Points for Echocardiographers

In the **left or right atrium**, the most common benign atrial masses are **myxomas**; *clinical context and contrast infusion provide important clues to distinguish from thrombi.*

In the **right atrium**, the most frequent malignant tumors are **angiosarcomas;** *other type of sarcomas usually originate from the left atrium.*

On **cardiac valves**, most common tumors are **papillary fibroelastomas**; *clinical history and hemocultures are key for differential diagnosis with vegetations.*

In the **ventricles** and in **children**, **rhabdomyomas** and **fibromas** are the most frequent; *rhabdomyomas are usually multiple and decrease in size and number with age.*

Malignant tumors are rapidly progressive and most commonly **secondary;** *pericardium, myocardium or veins with endocardial growth are typically involved, depending on their way of spread.*

Benign tumors may also be hemodynamically **"malignant"** by intramural growth, cavity obstruction or systemic embolization; *pericardial effusion, myocardial or valvular dysfunction may result from local invasion.*

The various echocardiographic techniques (transthoracic and transesophageal, contrast, and 3D ultrasound imaging) allow an accurate anatomic localization and a precise description of these masses, as well as an assessment of their hemodynamic impact. For cases that are not so straightforward, or for cases in which acoustic access is restricted, magnetic resonance imaging and computed tomography scanning are preferred over echocardiography to assess contiguous extracardiac involvement or the presence of metastatic disease. Integration of available clinical data with the knowledge of typical imaging characteristics and natural history of specific cardiac tumors is pivotal for an accurate non-invasive diagnosis.

References

1. Andrade MJ. Tumors and masses. In: Galiuto L, Badano LP, Fox K, Sicari R, Zamorano JL, editors. The EAE textbook of echocardiography. London: Oxford University Press; 2011. p. 355–69.
2. Auger D, Pressacco J, Marcotte F, Tremblay A, Dore A, Ducharme A. Cardiac masses: an integrative

approach using echocardiography and other imaging modalities. Heart. 2011;97:1101–9.
3. Meng Q, Lai H, Lima J, Tong W, Qian Y, Lai S. Echocardiographic and pathologic characteristics of primary cardiac tumors. Int J Cardiol. 2002;84: 69–75.
4. Muller S, Feuchtner G, Bonatti J, Müller L, Laufer G, Hiemetzberger R, Pachinger O, Barbieri V, Bartel T. Value of transesophageal 3D echocardiography as an adjunct to conventional 2D imaging in preoperative evaluating of cardiac masses. Echocardiography. 2008;25:624–31.
5. Mehmood F, Nanda NC, Vengala S, Winokur TS, Dod HS. Live three-dimensional transthoracic ecocardiographic assessment of left atrial tumors. Echocardiography. 2005;22:137–43.
6. Asch FM, Bieganski SP, Panza JA, Weissman NJ. Real-time 3-dimensional echocardiographic evaluation of intracardiac masses. Echocardiography. 2006;23:218–24.
7. Plana JC. Three-dimensional echocadiography to assess intra-cardiac masses. In: Badano LP, Lang RM, Zamorano JL, editors. Texbook of real-time three-dimensional echocardiography. London: Springer-Verlag; 2011. p. 111–9.
8. Mansencal N, Revault-d'Allones L, Pelage JP, Farcot JC, Lacombe P, Dubourg O. Usefulness of contrast echocardiography for assessment of intracardiac masses. Arch Cardiovasc Dis. 2009;102:177–83.
9. Bednarz JE, Spencer KT, Weinert L, Sugeng L, Mor-Avi V, Lang RM. Identification of cardiac masses and abnormal blood flow patterns with harmonic power Doppler contrast echocardiography. J Am Soc Echocardiogr. 1997;12:871–5.
10. Lang-Lazdunski L, Oroudji M, Pansard Y, Vissuzaine C, Hvas U. Successful resection of giant intrapericardial lipoma. Ann Thorac Surg. 1994;58:238–40.
11. O'Connor S, Recavarren R, Nichols LC, Parwani A. Lipomatous hypertrophy of the interatrial septum. Arch Pathol Lab Med. 2006;130:397–9.
12. Butany J, Nair V, Naseemuddin A, Nair GM, Catton GM, Yau T. Cardiac tumours: diagnosis and management. Lancet Oncol. 2005;6:219–28.
13. Gowda RM, Khan IA, Nair CK, Mehta NU, Vasavada BC, Sacchi TJ. Cardiac papillary fibroelastoma: a comprehensive analysis of 725 cases. Am Heart J. 2003;146:404–10.
14. Aziz F, Baciewicz FA. Lambl's excrescences. Tex Heart Inst. 2007;34:366–8.
15. Roberts WC. Primary and secondary neoplasms of the heart. Am J Cardiol. 1997;80:671–82.
16. De Cobelli F, Esposito A, Mellone R, Papa M, Varisco T, Besana R, del Maschio A. Late enhancement of a left ventricular cardiac fibroma assessed with gadolinium-enhanced cardiovascular magnetic resonance. Circulation. 2005;112:e242–3.
17. Kirkpatrick JN, Wong T, Bednarz JE, Spencer KT, Sugeng L, Ward RP, DeCara JM, Weinert L, Krausz T, Lang RM. Differential diagnosis of cardiac masses using contrast echocardiographic perfusion imaging. J Am Coll Cardiol. 2004;43:1412–9.
18. Tollens M, Grab D, Lang D, Hess J, Oberhoffer R. Pericardial teratomas (prenatal diagnosis and course). Fetal Diagn Ther. 2003;18:432–6.
19. Shanmugam G. Primary cardiac sarcoma. Eur J Cardiothor Surg. 2006;29:925–32.
20. Burke A, Virmany R. Tumours of the heart and great vessels. In: Burke A, Virmany R, editors. Atlas of tumour pathology. Washington, DC: Armed Forces Institute of Pathology; 1996.
21. Ceresoli GL, Ferrei AJM, Bucci E, Ripa C, Ponzoni M, Villa E. Primary cardiac lymphoma in immunocompetent patients: diagnostic and therapeutic management. Cancer. 1997;80:1497–506.
22. Zakja E, Badano LP, Sbrojavacca R, Malalan R, Gianfagna P, Fioretti PM. Unusual extension of an intracardiac primary lymphoma to the right jugular vein. J Cardiovasc Med (Hagerstown). 2007;8:652–5.
23. Peters PJ, Reinhardt S. The echocardiographic evaluation of intracardiac masses: a review. J Am Soc Echocardiogr. 2011;19:230–40.
24. Goldman JH, Foster E. Transesophageal echocardiographic (TEE) evaluation of intracardiac and pericardial masses. Cardiol Clin. 2000;18:860.
25. Almasi GH. Surgery for tumors with cavoatrial extension. Semin Thorac Cardiovasc Surg. 2000;12:111–8.

New Cardiac Imaging Techniques: Magnetic Resonance and Computed Tomography

9

Massimo Lombardi

Introduction

Primary tumors of the heart and of the pericardium are rare with an incidence at autopsy ranging from 0.0001 to 0.03%. Of these, the majority are benign and about 50% are myxomas. Nowadays, the diagnostic procedure implies an integrated use of cardiac imaging tools such as echocardiography, either transthoracic or trans-oesophageal, and two techniques with a large field of view such as magnetic resonance imaging (MRI) and multi-detector computerized tomography (MDCT). The last two have significant advantages and disadvantages which need to be considered for a better use of all the imaging modalities, with the purpose to obtain a final report as rich as possible of details (stadiation, topographic relations, hemodynamic effects, a probabilistic diagnosis of nature, etc.) to guide the following therapeutical approach which implies the surgical option [1].

Multi-detector Computerized Tomography

Among the advantages offered by MDCT the high spatial resolution is worthy of note mainly in the case of pulmonary, pleural, and mediastinal involvement, where MDCT reaches the highest accuracy among the different techniques and can be considered the reference method in the evaluation of lymph nodes. Furthermore, MDCT is extremely efficient in the detection of calcifications within the tumoral mass. Among cons, the relatively low temporal resolution might lead to low-quality images in the presence of tumoral masses with high mobility (Fig. 9.1). A MDCT study implies the administration of a large amount of ionizing radiations. When a benign tumor is suspected, with the possibility of even a complete healing (such as in the setting of a rhabdomyoma), the need of a regular and prolonged follow-up has to be considered in making the choice of the better and less risky imaging technique, particularly in a young patient.

Another limit of MDCT remains the scarce capability to evaluate the involvement of cardiac valves, although this can be easily overcome by the integrated use of echocardiography.

At present, it seems reasonable to consider among the advantages offered by MDCT its capability to evaluate the coronary anatomy when planning the surgical procedure, particularly in people aged more than 40 years [2] (Fig. 9.2).

Published papers consist mostly of single spectacular case reports [3, 4], but very few critical reviews do exist [5]. In general, MDCT can be considered a very efficient diagnostic tool capable of answering critical questions raised by the suspicion of a cardiac mass, besides the presence of the mass itself, such as its anatomical relations with the surrounding structures, the

M. Lombardi, M.D. (✉)
Cardiovascular MR Unit, Fondazione C.N.R./Regione Toscana "G. Monasterio", S. Cataldo Research Campus, Via Moruzzi. 1, 56010, Pisa, Italy
e-mail: massimo.lombardi@ftgm.it

C. Basso et al. (eds.), *Cardiac Tumor Pathology*, Current Clinical Pathology,
DOI 10.1007/978-1-62703-143-1_9, © Springer Science+Business Media New York 2013

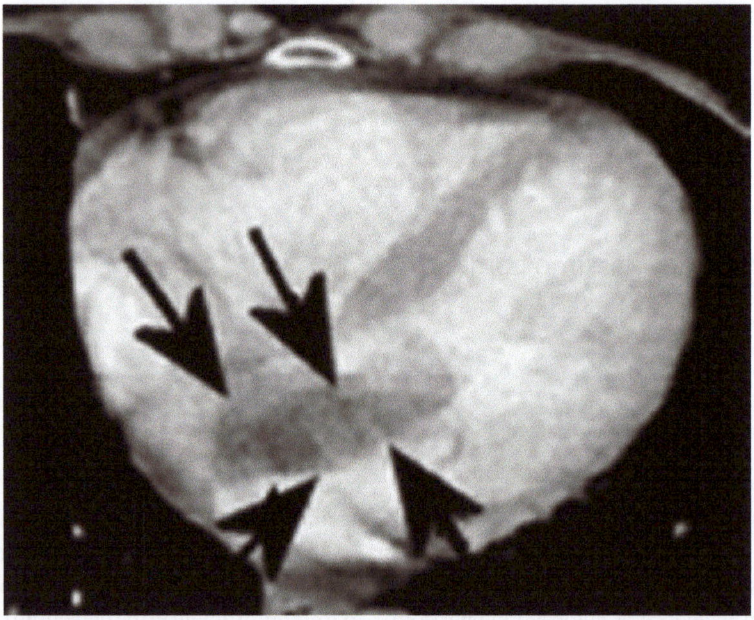

Fig. 9.1 Image obtained by MDCT scanner. Reprinted with permission of the Italian Society of Cardiology. A mass is visible inside the left atrium *(arrows)*. During the diastolic phase, the mass protrudes into the left ventricle through the mitral valve orifice

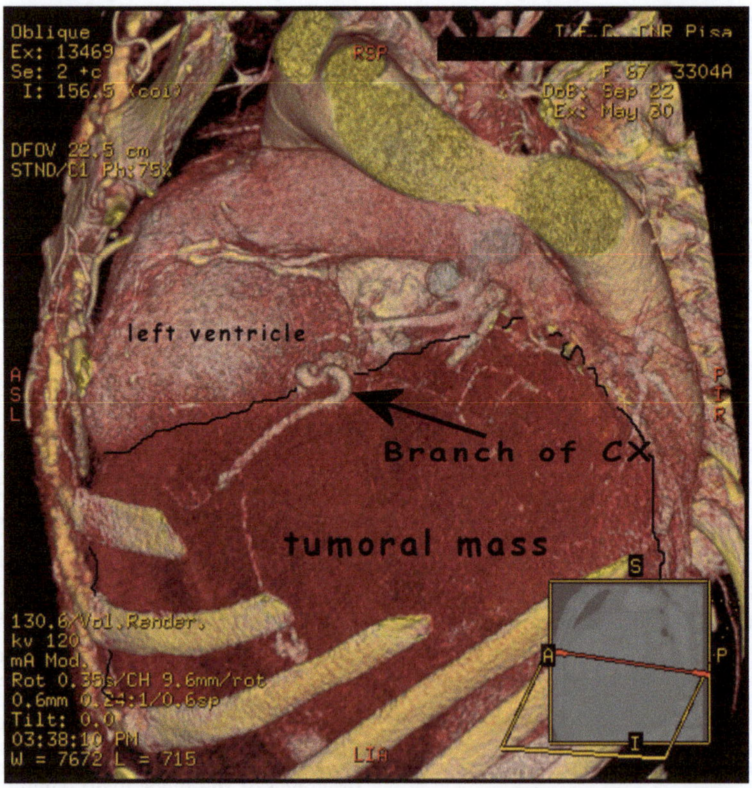

Fig. 9.2 Image obtained by MDCT scanner. A huge mass (22 cm anterior–posterior diameter) is clearly evident. The MDCT technique allows to identify the course of the branches of coronary arteries in relation with the mass

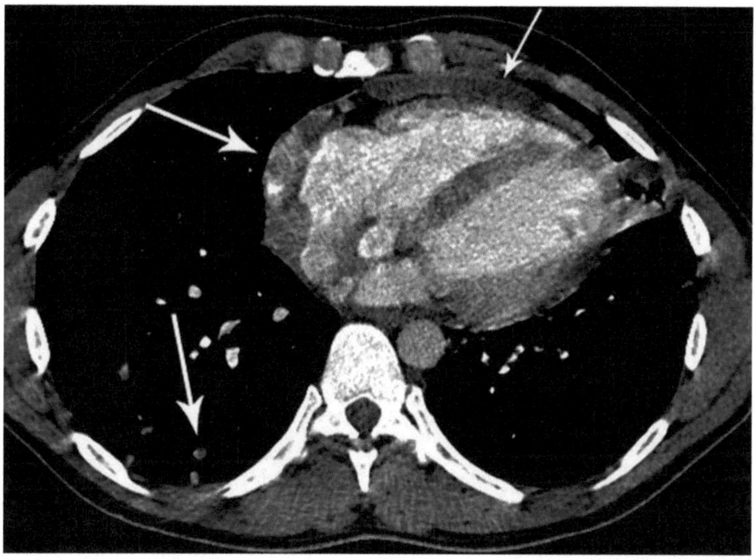

Fig. 9.3 Image obtained by MDCT scanner. Reprinted with permission of the Italian Society of Cardiology. At the level of the right atrium, a mass with irregular profile infiltrates both the pericardium and the myocardium *(arrows)*. The findings are compatible with the diagnosis of angiosarcoma. At the level of right lung, a small round shaped lesion consistent with metastasis is also detectable (courtesy of Dr. F. Cademartiri, Thorax Center, Rotterdam, The Netherlands)

infiltrative attitude (Fig. 9.3), the presence of calcifications within the mass, and the presence of hemorrhagic areas. To this purpose, the measurement in Hounsfield Units (HU) in the different regions of interest is mandatory. Unambiguous measurements can be performed only if high-quality images are obtained by a ECG-gated MDCT scanner of last generation [4, 5]. Finally, if the operator has enough experience, MDCT, like MRI, allows to differentiate between tumoral and thrombotic masses [5].

The wide availability of MDCT scanners and a diffuse experience of operators in the oncologic field are important advantages for the use of this technique when a cardiac mass is suspected. Furthermore, a MDCT examination is relatively easy to perform, requires a reduced scanning time, and is usually well tolerated by the patient even in the case of a critical clinical picture. Although the limit of a high heart rate (which is often associated with an intracardiac mass) is nowadays less relevant than in the past (high rotational speed, dual source technology, etc.), a heart rate more than 80 beats per minute considerably reduces the quality of images. Finally, since MDCT examination implies the administration of a large amount of iodine contrast agent, the renal function has to be always assessed.

Magnetic Resonance Imaging

The introduction of MRI for the evaluation of cardiovascular diseases has considerably modified the diagnostic strategy of imaging in cardiac and paracardiac masses. Such technique provides a complete multiplanar and noninvasive evaluation of the lesions involving the cardiac chambers, pericardium, and extracardiac structures, thus assuming a relevant role in providing diagnostic information useful for surgical planning. MRI is the most sophisticated imaging technique today available to characterize the tumoral mass in terms of morphology, dimensions, localization, extension, topographic relations, and infiltrative aspects of the surrounding structures.

Furthermore, one of the most interesting properties of MRI is the capability of differentiating among the various tissues, due to the relative differences in relaxivity which lead to high contrast among the tissues. With obvious limitations, a certain degree of tissue characterization is fea-

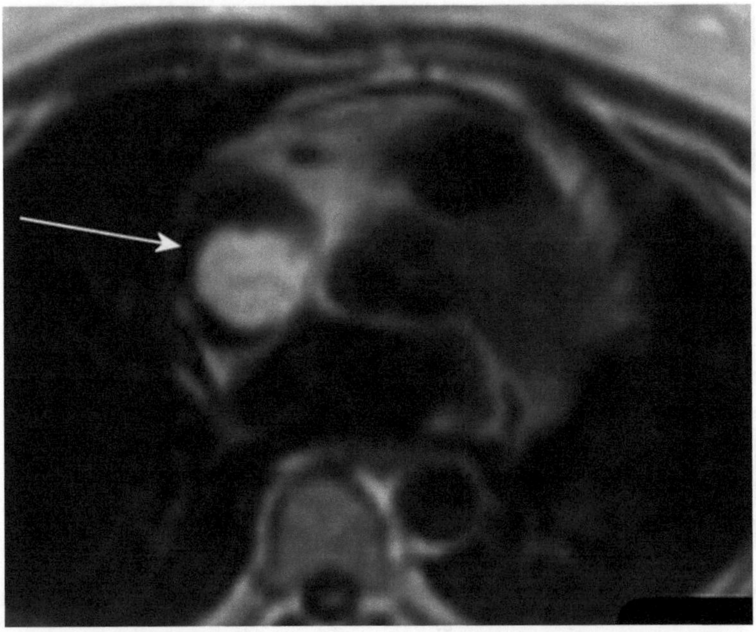

Fig. 9.4 Image obtained by MRI, SE T1 images. Reprinted with permission of the Italian Society of Cardiology. A lipoma (*arrow*) within the right atrial cavity is visible. The mass appears hyperintense in SE T1 images due to the adipose tissue

sible, such as the detection of lipomatous components, necrotic areas, hemorrhage, calcifications, myxoid tissue, vascularity, etc. Nevertheless, a precise tissue characterization in terms of histopathology is possible only in a few cases. Namely, it is almost definite when fat tissue is predominant, such as in the setting of a lipoma, where the capability of MRI to obtain images with fat suppression leads to a almost definitive diagnosis (Fig. 9.4). Similarly, myxoid tissue can be characterized very accurately (Fig. 9.5). However, in most of cases the diagnosis of nature of the mass is probabilistic, on the basis of certain findings which direct towards a kind of tumor rather than another.

A correct characterization of the cardiac and paracardiac masses requires integrated information that is obtainable with the different MRI sequences available. In other words, to properly characterize a cardiac or paracardiac mass, it is necessary to obtain weighted images in either T1, or T2, or IR (STIR), or T1/T2 , or T1 with spectral fat suppression, or in GRE T2* (for possible calcifications or hemorrhages inside the mass), and in T1 after contrast medium (0.1–0.2 mmol/kg) [6–8]. Often, a study of the dynamic of the contrast medium impregnation is performed utilizing "ad hoc perfusion" T1-weighted sequences. Obviously, the greater the vascularity of the mass, the faster and more intense the contrast medium impregnation would be. Dynamic sequences (cine SPGR, SSFP, etc.) are also useful to assess the function of the involved cardiac structures, and the effect on adjacent tissues and on the intracardiac blood flow dynamic (Fig. 9.6).

These are generally quite lengthy studies which at times may bring the operator/physician very close to the nature of diagnosis.

Properties of tissue composition affect the signal characteristics of myocardium with cardiac MRI. The myocardium is a water-based tissue that contains a large number of hydrogen protons and as such is ideally imaged with MRI. The surrounding epicardial fat, the fibrous pericardium and masses that affect the heart show different MRI signal characteristics, because they are composed of tissues that contain varying amounts of water or protons and therefore distort the signal characteristics of the normal myocardium. Thus, on the basis of tissue composition, MRI signal changes

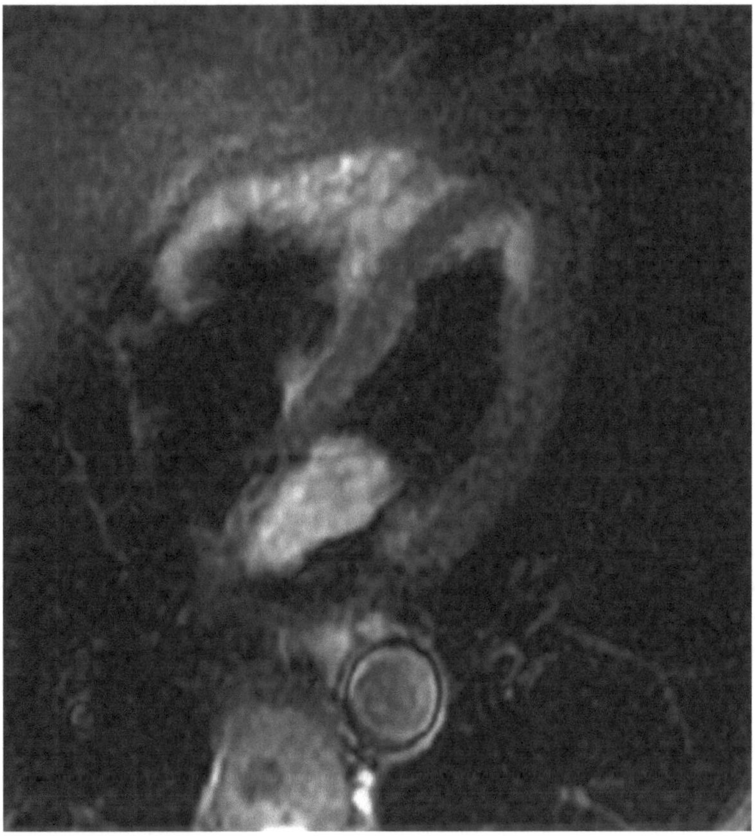

Fig. 9.5 Image obtained by MRI, Triple-IR sequence (STIR). Reprinted with permission of the Italian Society of Cardiology. A large myxoma is detectable within the left atrial cavity. The mass is protruding into the left ventricular cavity during the diastolic phase. The image has been obtained by a Triple-IR sequence (STIR) and the myxomatous tissue shows a marked hyperintense signal as compared to the surrounding structures. The signal hyperintensity in STIR images is always present in myxoid tissue, albeit this is not an exclusive characteristic

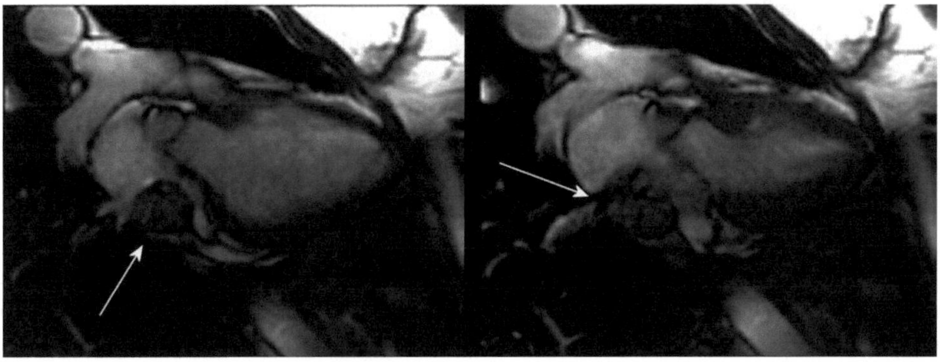

Fig. 9.6 Image obtained by MRI, SSFP sequence. Reprinted with permission of the Italian Society of Cardiology. Left atrial myxoma. *Left panel*: the tumoral mass is round shaped (*arrow*) and attached close to the ostium of a pulmonary vein. *Right panel*: during the cardiac cycle (systolic phase), the myxomatous mass obstacles the blood flow into the atrial cavity (temporal resolution 35 ms)

Table 9.1 Characteristics of the MRI signal from different tissues in the T1- and T2-weighted images

Tissue	T1	T2	Contrast agent
Liquid	Low(−−−)	High (+++)	Absent
Myxoid	Low (−−−)	High (+++)	Scarce
Collagen	Low (−−)	Low/high (−−/++)[a]	Scarce[a]
Adipose	High (+++)	High (++)	Absent
Necrosis	Low (−−)	High (+++)	Absent
Fibrous	Low (−−)	Low/high (−−/++)[a]	Scarce[a]
Calcium	Low (−−−)	Low (−−−)	Absent
Vascularized	Low (−−)	High (++)	Marked

[a]Signal and the contrast medium uptake depend on the vascularization and cellularity of the tissues

and, in some instances, the nature of normal or abnormal tissue can be inferred.

Table 9.1 reports the characteristics of signal of the various tissue components useful for a diagnostic orientation.

Benign Atrial Tumors

The benign lesions most frequently affecting the atrial chambers are the myxoma and the lipoma.

The *myxoma* originates from the endocardium as a polypoid, usually pedunculated mass (90%), or at times sessile with a large base of implantation; it shows mostly a smooth or, more rarely, a villous surface [9].

The most typical location is the atrial chamber (left atrium 75%, right atrium 18%, right ventricle 4%, left ventricle 3%).

Usually, the left atrial myxoma is attached to the interatrial septum at the level of the fossa ovalis; the stalk allows it to move freely inside the atrial chamber and sometimes to protrude into the left ventricle, during diastole, through the mitral valve orifice.

Clinically, it can be asymptomatic or mimic a mitral stenosis. When the site of origin is not typical, differential diagnosis with other masses is more difficult.

Typically, the myxoma produces an inhomogeneous signal due to the presence of fibrous, necrotic, hemorrhagic, and sometimes calcified areas within the mass (Fig. 9.7). In the context of the mass, hemorrhagic areas (81% of cases), thrombosis, or catabolites of hemoglobin (e.g., hemosiderin), are often detectable [10]. If the quantity of myxoid tissue is substantial, the lesion will have an elevated signal in the T2-weighted images (Fig. 9.5), while if the fibrous component prevails the mass will show a hypointense signal.

The presence of calcification is a common finding (56%), particularly frequent in the myxomas of the right atrium [11]. The calcium accounts for the areas of low signal in the context of the lesion, which is more evident in GRE T2* images. The drop of signal may be caused also by the effects of magnetic susceptibility, which are related to the presence of iron [12]. On the other hand, the hemorrhagic areas might exhibit a high signal in both T1 and T2 sequences [13].

It has been proven that the tumor enhancement after contrast medium administration depends on its tissue composition and that the zones which do not capture the contrast medium correspond to necrotic or cystic areas [14].

The differential diagnosis includes thrombotic masses and other less common lesions, such as cardiac sarcoma and papillary fibroelastoma (Fig. 9.8).

MRI without contrast agent generally does not help in differentiating myxoma from intracavitary thrombus, because both can present signal heterogeneity in SE images and low intensity in the GRE sequences [15]. However, a myxoma shows very intense signal in IR T2 images and a significant enhancement after contrast agent administration, while the thrombotic formation usually does not have such a behavior (Fig. 9.9) [16].

The *papillary fibroelastoma* is made up of fibrous tissue, elastic fibers, and a single layer of endocardial cells. The tumor is usually small sized, round shaped, and attached to the endocardium of the atrio-ventricular or semilunar valves [17] (Fig. 9.8). In the literature, there are no systematic descriptions on the behavior of the MRI signal for such lesion, and the diagnosis is generally based on echocardiography, due to the rapid movements of the mass during cardiac cycle and thus a not ideal visualization by MRI. However, it

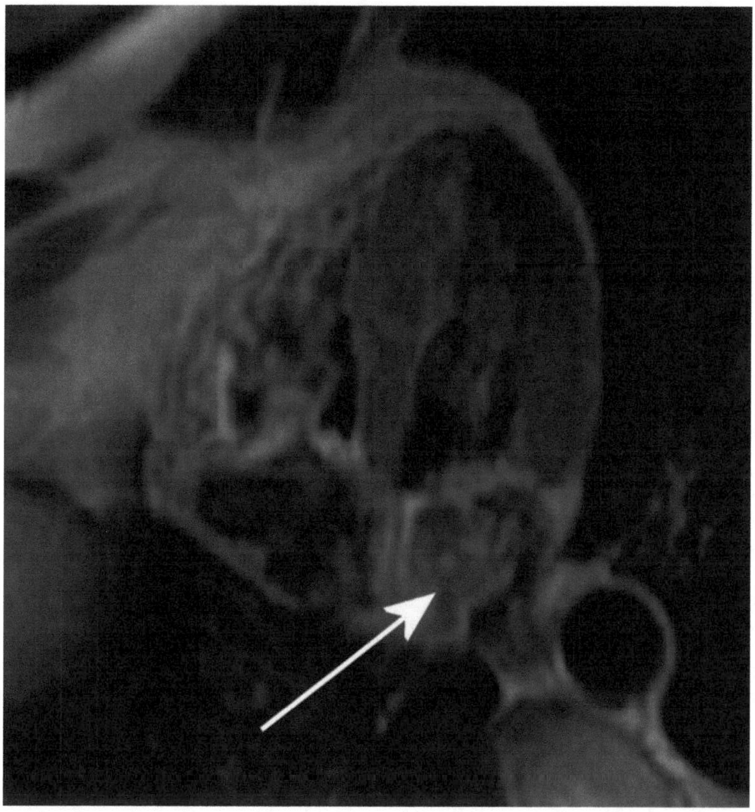

Fig. 9.7 Image obtained by MRI, SE T1 after the administration of Gd. Reprinted with permission of the Italian Society of Cardiology. Left atrial myxoma (same case of Fig. 9.5). Image in SE T1 after the administration of Gd-based contrast agent which is amplifying the dishomogeneity of signal intensity due to the composite structure of the tumoral mass *(arrow)* (myxoid, necrotic and calcified areas)

is worth noting that T2 images' signal intensity is usually lower in papillary fibroleastoma than in myxoma.

The *lipoma* is a relatively rare cardiac tumor. The properly called lipoma (Fig. 9.4) (encapsulated or surrounded by myocardium) should be clearly distinguished from the lipomatous hypertrophy of the interatrial septum. The latter entity consists of a non-capsulated adipose tissue deposition, which extends onto the epicardial fat. Half of the cardiac lipomas are subendocardial; the other half have a subepicardial and mesocardial location [18]. The left atrium and left ventricle are the most frequent locations.

Lipoma shows the characteristics of the MRI signal typical of the adipose tissue, i.e., elevated intensity of the signal in the T1- and T2-weighted images. In this case, the techniques of fat suppression easily confirm the adipose nature of the mass.

Benign Ventricular Tumors

Primary benign tumors of the ventricles are very rare in adults. The most frequent tumors of the left ventricle are the fibroma and the rhabdomyoma, which are more common in the pediatric population.

The *rhabdomyoma* is the most frequent tumor in children, and appears often as multiple nodules, either intramural or intracavitary. MRI signal characteristics are almost identical to those of the normal myocardium, as expected due to the origin of the tumor cells from cardiac myocytes.

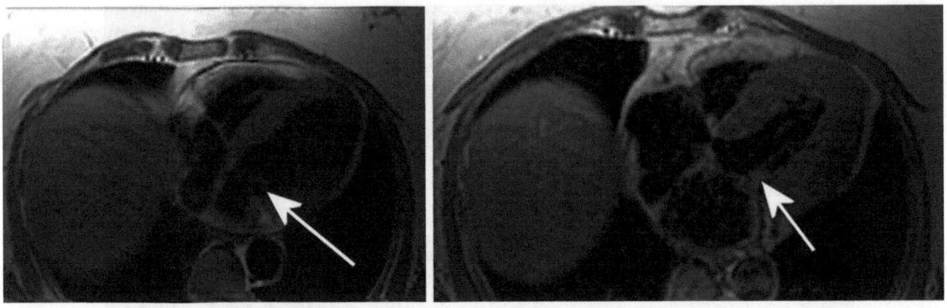

Fig. 9.8 Image obtained by MRI. Reprinted with permission of the Italian Society of Cardiology. Papillary fibroelastoma of the sub-valvular mitral apparatus. *Left panel*, image in SE T1: note the small, round shaped mass (*arrow*). *Right panel*, image in SE T1: same mass after the administration of Gd-based contrast agent

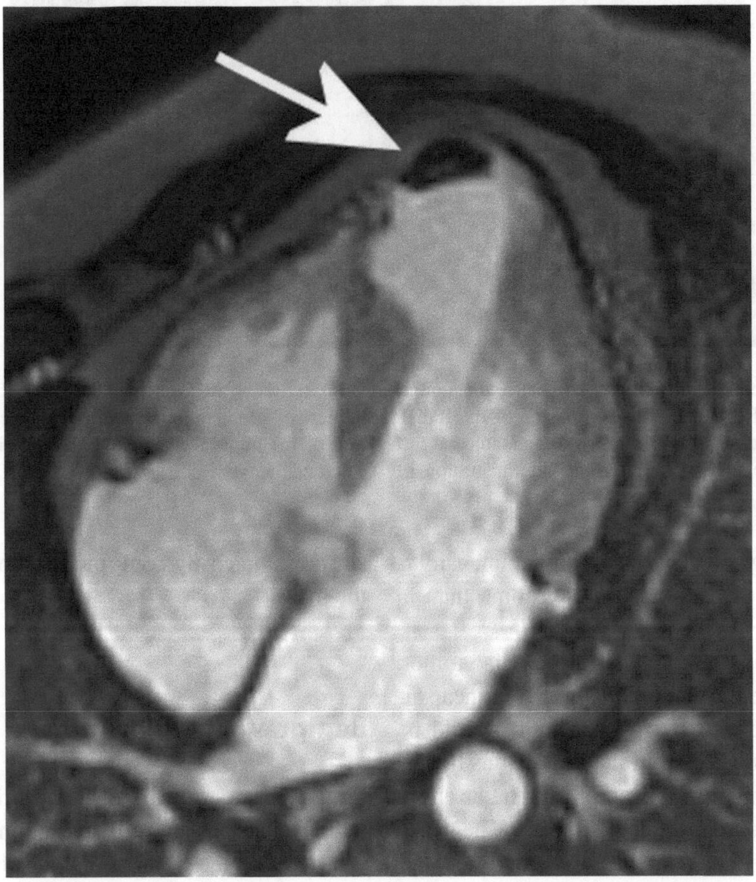

Fig. 9.9 Image obtained by MRI, after contrast agent administration using an IR-GRE sequence. Reprinted with permission of the Italian Society of Cardiology. Intraventricular apical thrombus (*arrow*)

The *fibroma* is the most frequent benign tumor of the left ventricle of the adult. It is usually intramural and it appears as an area of localized hypertrophy of the septum, of the apex, or of the free wall. Hypointense signal either in the T1 and in the T2 sequence is usually detected. After administration of contrast medium, it appears as formed by a hypointense

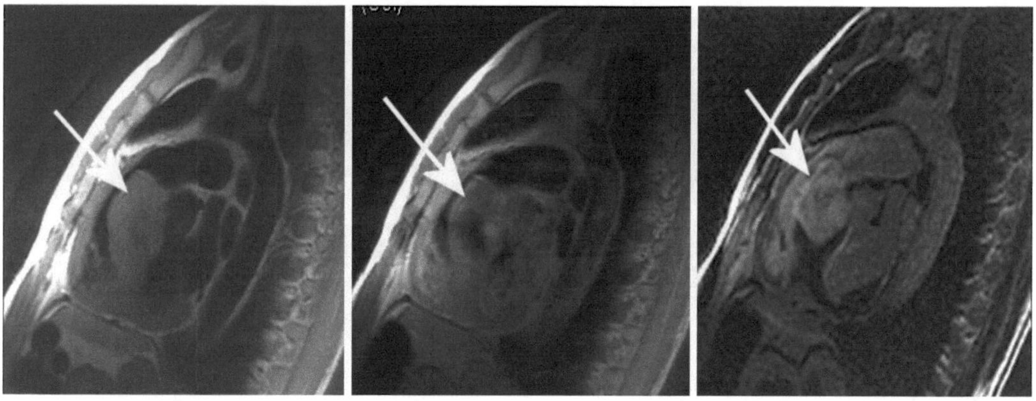

Fig. 9.10 Image obtained by MRI. Reprinted with permission of the Italian Society of Cardiology. Large fibroma of the interventricular septum (*arrows*). The fibromatous mass does not show any change in signal intensity in the different sequences utilized. After contrast agent administration, only a slight signal enhancement is detectable in the peripheral border of the mass. *Left panel*: image in SE T1. *Central panel*: image in SE T1 after the administration of paramagnetic contrast agent. *Right panel*: image obtained by GRE-IR sequence after the administration of paramagnetic contrast agent

core surrounded by an isointense "shell" [19] (Fig. 9.10).

In the right ventricle, myxomas, fibromas, and rhabdomyomas can be found.

Primary Malignant Cardiac Tumors

The malignant tumors of the heart are less frequent (10%) than the benign ones and more often localized in the right sections than in the left. Autopsy studies report an incidence of 0.001–0.28% [20]. Primary malignant tumors of the heart are extremely rare [20] and constitute a diagnostic dilemma as they are asymptomatic until they reach significant dimensions, and, even in these cases, the symptoms and signs are usually nonspecific. The advent of sophisticated imaging techniques has introduced the possibility of detecting such lesions in patients still not compromised and sometimes as casual findings, thus contributing to the characterization of the lesions and to the therapeutic decision.

The *angiosarcoma* is the most frequent (37%) among the primary malignant cardiac tumors [9]. It originates from endothelial cells, most frequently in the right atrium, with involvement of the pericardium, and frequently complicated by pericardial hemorrhage and tamponade. Despite the possible invasion of the pericardium, tumor cells in the pericardial fluid are rarely found.

Two variants of angiosarcoma are described, i.e., a well-defined mass protruding into the atrial cavity with preservation of the septum, or a diffusely infiltrating mass extending along the pericardium (Fig. 9.11). The presence of hemorrhage and necrotic areas is frequent and accounts for the typically heterogeneous signal of the tumor, which usually presents high intensity areas in the T1-weighted images, because of the presence of meta-hemoglobin due to hemorrhagic phenomena. In the setting of pericardial infiltration, a linear capture along the vascular structures is detectable.

Undifferentiated sarcomas are malignant soft tissue tumors that are negative to multiple immunohistochemical markers due to scarce or even absent differentiation. The majority of cases are reported in the left atrium (Fig. 9.12). The prognosis is generally poor. They usually appear as polypoid masses, isointense to the myocardium in MRI images, with wall thickening at the level of infiltration or with aspects similar to the angiosarcoma due to pericardial infiltration.

Rhabdomyosarcoma (4–7%) is a tumor which originates from the muscular striated fiber. The embryonal variant is the more common form and appears in infants, children, and young adults. Despite the low incidence, such neoplasm represents the most frequent form of malignant cardiac

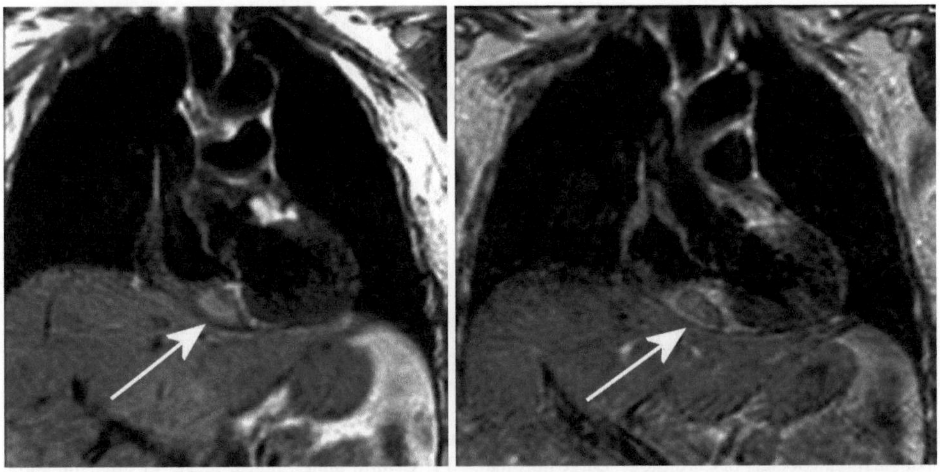

Fig. 9.11 Image obtained by MRI. Reprinted with permission of the Italian Society of Cardiology. Angiosarcoma. *Left panel*, T1-weighted images (coronal plane): the tumoral mass shows an hyperenhanced area due to metahemoglobin (post hemorrhage). *Right panel*, images after the administration of paramagnetic contrast agent: significant signal enhancement at the periphey of the mass

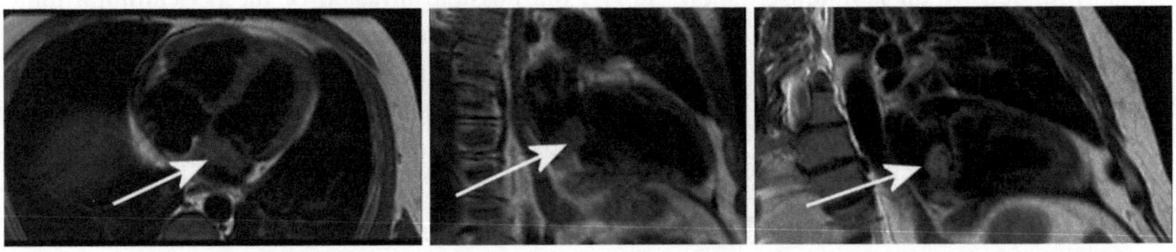

Fig. 9.12 Image obtained by MRI. Reprinted with permission of the Italian Society of Cardiology. Undifferentiated sarcoma of the left atrium (*arrow*). Histopathologic findings showed a mixture of myxoid tissue and histiocytes surrounded by necrotic and fibrotic areas (courtesy of Dr. Feola and Dr. Leonardi. Cardiologic Unit—Ospedale di Cuneo, Italy)

tumors in childhood. It can occur anywhere in the myocardium and it involves the ventricular chamber more frequently than other types of sarcoma (Fig. 9.13). These tumors are often multicentric, usually intramural, and can involve the pericardium. At difference from the angiosarcoma, the myocardium is always involved and the pericardium often presents nodular masses.

The characteristics of the MRI signal are variable (isointensity to the myocardium, hyperintensity in T2 in correspondence of cystic-like or necrotic areas).

Osteosarcomas (nowadays called undifferentiated pleomorphic sarcomas with areas of osseous differentiation) are a heterogeneous group of soft tissue sarcomas containing malignant cells that produce bone and fibrotic or chondroid tissue.

At difference from the metastatic osteosarcoma that often occurs in the right atrium, the primary cardiac osteosarcoma most often involves the left atrium and is aggressive with a very poor prognosis. The demonstration of bone component can be appreciated more easily through CT imaging.

Leiomyosarcoma usually originates from smooth muscle bundles of the subendocardial space, but they can also originate from the arteries and pulmonary veins and spread to the cardiac structures. It has a predisposition for the left atrial cavity, particularly at the level of the posterior wall. Affected patients are typically in their fourth decade. Also in this case the MRI features are not specific, i.e., lobulated masses, irregular in shape, often multiple with tendency to invade the pulmonary

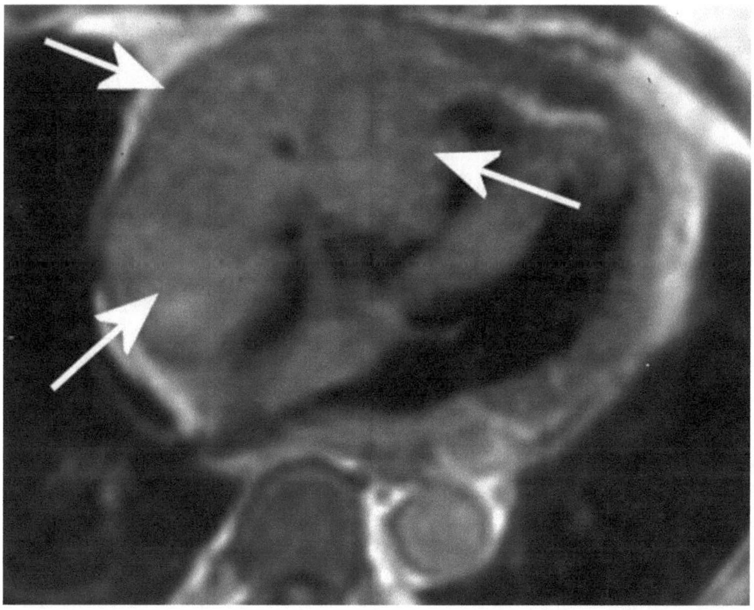

Fig. 9.13 Image obtained by MRI, SE T1-weighted image. Reprinted with permission of the Italian Society of Cardiology. Right atrial rhabdomyosarcoma. Large mass involving right chambers of the heart, with diffuse infiltration of cardiac walls, of the tricuspid valve and of the pericardium (*arrows*). The infiltrative growth and the dimensions are in keeping with an aggressive malignant tumor

veins or the mitral valve, showing an intermediate signal in T1 and a high one in T2.

Fibrosarcoma is a rare primary malignant cardiac tumor composed of fibroblasts and like other sarcomas preferentially involves the left atrium. It can also infiltrate the pericardial space, mimicking mesothelioma. It can appear heterogeneous in MRI images, but overall MRI features are not specific.

Liposarcoma is an extremely rare malignant primary cardiac tumor that contains lipoblasts. It has been usually described in the atria, although it has also been reported in the ventricles and in the pericardium, where it can develop either with a nodular aspect or diffuse involvement. At difference from the benign lipoma, the adipose component in primary liposarcoma is scarce or absent, thus explaining the limited value of MRI to achieve a precise histopathologic diagnosis.

Primary cardiac lymphoma is a extra-nodal lymphoma that involves exclusively the heart and the pericardium. Pericardial effusion is often present and drainage of the pericardial fluid, besides the palliative effect, has a diagnostic purpose, since lymphoma cells are detectable in the majority of cases. Thoracotomic cardiac mass biopsy is also frequently performed to achieve the diagnosis. Despite its rare occurrence, it is important to include primary cardiac lymphoma in the differential diagnosis of cardiac masses, since early chemotherapic treatment can give excellent results [21].

It mostly appears as multiple polypoid nodules, infiltrating the myocardium with undefined borders and protruding into the cardiac chambers (Fig. 9.14). The site most frequently affected is the right atrium; the pericardium is often involved with thickening by tumor infiltration. As compared with other primary malignant cardiac

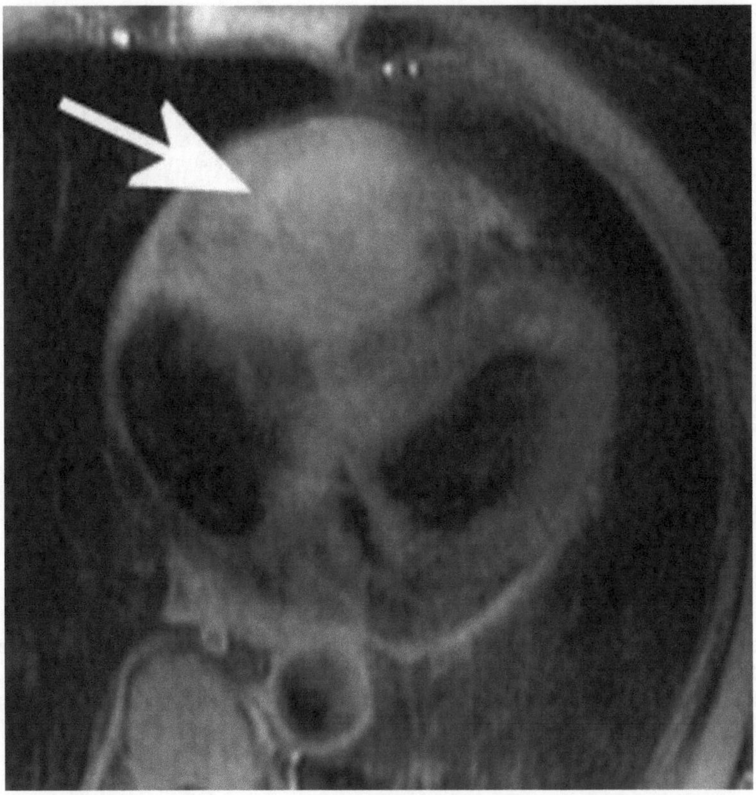

Fig. 9.14 Image obtained by MRI. Cardiac lymphoma. Diffuse involvement of the pericardium and of the myocardium of the right ventricle (*arrow*)

tumors, necrosis is less frequent. The MRI signal is mostly hypointense in T1 and hyperintense in T2, but it has also been reported as isointense to the myocardium; the enhancement pattern is also quite variable (homogeneous, dishomogeneous).

Diagnostic Accuracy

MDCT and MRI allow a sophisticated characterization of cardiac masses and not so rarely a diagnosis of the nature of the mass itself. The differential diagnosis between benign and malignant masses is usually obtained. However, from the data available a more prudent approach seems indicated. In a review by Hoffman et al. [22] of more than 200 cardiac masses, the MRI signal properties, the morphologic aspects (localization, dimensions, structural homogeneity, infiltrative attitude of surroundings tissues, pericardial and pleural effusion, displacement of extracardiac structures) and the uptake of contrast agent (see Table 9.2) were assessed in terms of diagnostic accuracy. None of the considered characteristics reached a sensitivity and a specificity of 100%. However, from the integrated use of all these findings a diagnosis of high probability is reachable.

More recently, a multicenter experience of 78 pediatric cardiac tumors evaluated by MRI demonstrated that reviewers, who were blinded to the histologic diagnoses, correctly diagnosed 97% of the cases, but included a differential diagnosis in 42% of cases [23]. Better image quality and more complete examination were associated with higher diagnostic accuracy. However, histologic diagnosis

Table 9.2 Diagnostic accuracy of morphologic characteristics and uptake of Gd-based contrast agent

Characteristic	Sensitivity	Specificity	PPV	NPV
Localization	0.86	0.58	0.58	0.86
Signal dishomogeneity	0.86	0.48	0.53	0.84
Infiltrative attitude	0.64	0.70	0.58	0.74
Dimension >5 cm	0.55	0.78	0.67	0.68
Pericardial effusion	0.50	0.88	0.73	0.73
Pleural effusion	0.50	0.91	0.79	0.73
Pleural and pericardial effusions	0.59	0.82	0.68	0.75
Increase of signal after Gd c.a.	0.88	0.34	0.42	0.83

Modified from Hoffman et al. [22]
PPV positive predictive value, *NPV* negative predictive value, c.a. contrast agent

remained the gold standard and in some cases malignancy could not be definitively excluded on the basis of cardiac MRI alone.

Cardiac Metastases and Pericardial Masses

MRI is very useful in evaluating the extracardiac extension of primary tumors of the heart, providing the information needed to plan the most appropriate surgical approach. Likewise, it allows to identify the presence of a cardiac involvement by extracardiac masses with excellent anatomical details. Therefore, when there is the suspicion of a secondary involvement of the heart, the physician generally asks for a MRI study. Moreover, metastases to the heart and the pericardium are much more common than primary cardiac tumors. The malignant tumors that more often secondarily affect the heart and pericardium are breast and lung carcinomas (Figs. 9.15 and 9.16), melanoma, lymphoma, and leukemia. Cardiac metastases appear as pulmonary or mediastinal masses that directly invade the heart, or like masses that protrude into the left atrium through the pulmonary veins or into the right atrium through the caval veins, or myocardial nodules. Sometimes, they can be suspected only for the presence of pericardial effusion. The high MRI contrast resolution allows to distinguish the tumor from the myocardium and between tumor, thrombus, and flow artifacts much more easily than other techniques, sometimes helping also in tissue characterization. For instance, metastases from melanoma show a signal hyperintensity in T1 images due to the paramagnetic effect of metals bound to melanin [24].

Among pericardial tumors, malignant primary mesothelioma, that can manifest as an isolated effusion or with pericardial thickening due to diffuse spreading or with bulky nodules, but without specific MRI signal characteristics (Fig. 9.17), is worthy of note. Pleural mesothelioma can also involve secondarily the pericardium.

Conclusions

Both MDCT and MRI have a very high value in the diagnostic workup of cardiac tumors. The MDCT has reached a diagnostic accuracy which was someway unexpected only a few years ago. It is the reference method to evaluate mediastinal lymph nodes, and to assess lung and pleural involvement. Due to the relatively easy and standardized scanning procedure, MDCT can be proposed as a robust method to detect cardiac and paracardiac masses, preferably in integration with echocardiography. MRI remains the most sophisticated tool in the clinical practice, although it is still available in a few specialized centers. However, the experience accumulated in the recent years has shown that it can be considered as the reference cardiac imaging tool because it is capable of answering many of the questions raised by the presence of a cardiac mass. Furthermore, the nonionizing nature of the technique induces to consider MRI as the ideal tool for follow-up, at difference from MDCT. Finally, the revision of the large amount of data available

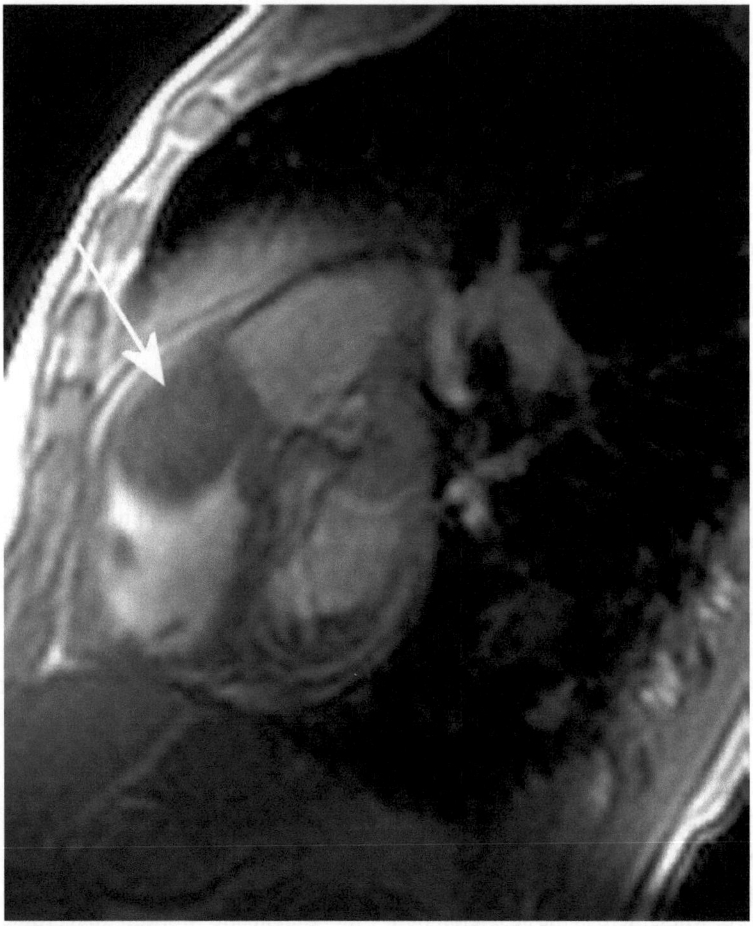

Fig. 9.15 Image obtained by MRI, in fast GRE and sagittal oblique plane. Metastasis of breast cancer at the level of right ventricular outflow tract *(arrow)*

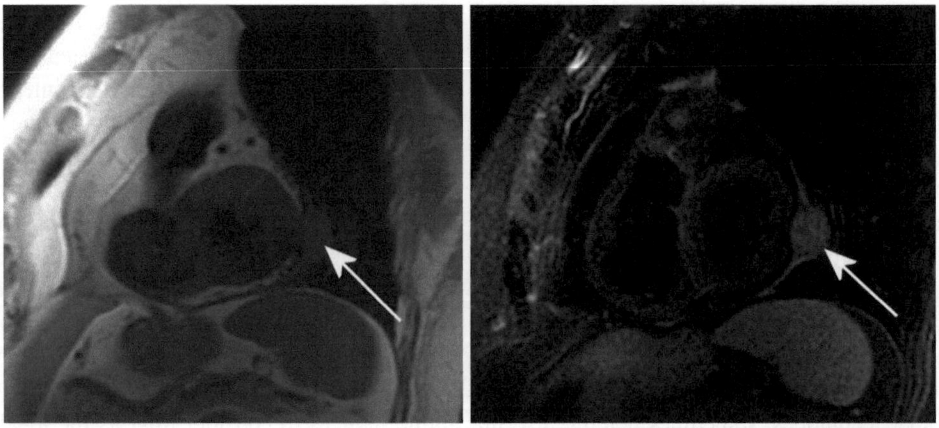

Fig. 9.16 Image obtained by MRI. Metastasis of lung cancer involving the pericardium (*arrows*). *Left panel*: image in SE T1. *Right panel*: image in triple-IR (STIR)

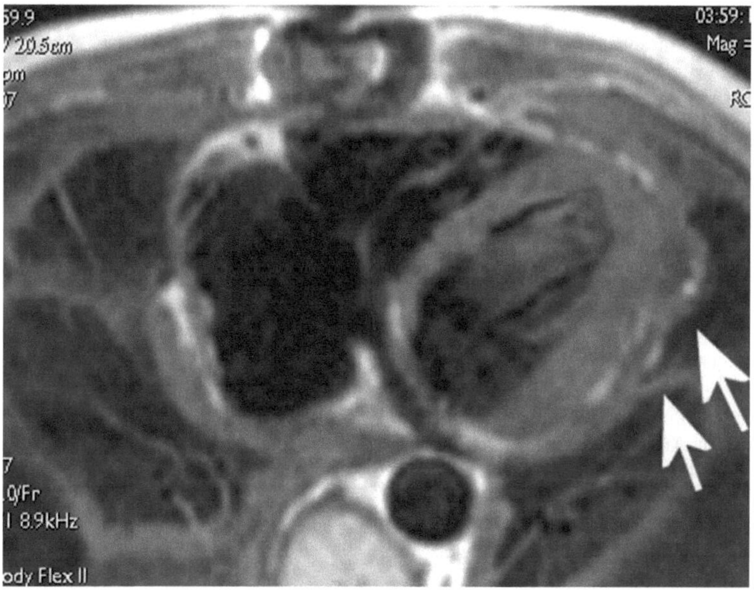

Fig. 9.17 Image obtained by MRI, SE T1-weighted image after the administration of paramagnetic contrast agent. Reprinted with permission of the Italian Society of Cardiology. Malignant mesothelioma of pericardium: note the presence of nodular thickening of the pericardium (*arrows*) with nonspecific signal characteristics

in scientific journals underline the need of an integrated use among the three imaging techniques (echocardiography, MDCT, and MRI) with the purpose to maximize the relative advantages [25].

References

1. Butany J, Nair V, Naseemuddin A, Nair GM, Catton C, Yau T. Cardiac tumours: diagnosis and management. Lancet Oncol. 2005;6:219–28.
2. Mollet NR, Cademartiri F, van Mieghem CAG, Runza G, McFadden EP, Baks T, Serruys PW, Krestin GP, de Feyer PJ. High-resolution spiral computer tomography coronary angiography in patients referred for diagnostic conventional coronary angiography. Circulation. 2005;112:2318–23.
3. Bootsveld A, Puetz J, Grube E. Incidental findings of papillary fibroelastoma on the aortic valve in 16 slice multi-detector row computed tomography. Heart. 2004;90:e35.
4. Wang HJ, Lin JL, Lin FY. Images in cardiovascular medicine. Cardiac hemangioma. Circulation. 2002; 106:2520.
5. Tatli S, Lipton MJ. CT for intracardiac thrombi and tumors. Int J Cardiovasc Imaging. 2005;21:115–31.
6. Lombardi M, Bartolozzi C. Risonanza Magnetica del cuore e dei vasi. Springer Verlag: Milano; 2004.
7. Higgins CB, De Roos A. Cardiovascular MRI and MRA. Philadelphia, PA: Lippincott Williams & Wilkins; 2003.
8. Manning W, Pennell DJ. Cardiovascular magnetic resonance. New York, NY: Churchill Livingstone; 2002.
9. Burke A, Virmani R. Tumors of the heart and great vessels. Atlas of tumor pathology, 3rd series, fasc 16. Washington, DC: Armed Forces Institute of Pathology; 1996.
10. Grebenc ML, Rosado-de-Christenson ML, Green CE, Burke AP, Galvin JR. Cardiac myxoma: imaging features in 83 patients. Radiographics. 2002;22:673–89.
11. Burke AP, Virmani R. Cardiac myxoma: a clinicopathologic study. Am J Clin Pathol. 1993;100:671–80.
12. Seelos KC, Caputo GR, Carrol CL, Hricak H, Higgins CB. Cine gradient refocused echo (GRE) imaging of intravascular masses: differentiation between tumor and nontumor thrombus. J Comput Assist Tomogr. 1992;16:169–75.
13. Masui T, Takahashi M, Miura K, Naito M, Tawarahara K. Cardiac myxoma: identification of intratumoral hemorrhage and calcification on MR images. Am J Roentgenol. 1995;164:850–2.
14. Matsuoka H, Hamada M, Honda T, Kawakami H, Abe M, Shigematsu Y, Sumimoto T, Hiwada K. Morphologic and histologic characterization of cardiac myxomas by magnetic resonance imaging. Angiology. 1996;47:693–8.

15. Gomes AS, Lois JF, Child JS, Brown K, Batra P. Cardiac tumors and thrombus: evaluation with MR imaging. Am J Roentgenol. 1987;149:895–9.
16. Funari M, Fujuta N, Peck WW, Higgins CB. Cardiac tumors: assessment with Gd-DTPA enhanced MR imaging. J Comput Assist Tomogr. 1991;15:953–8.
17. Edwards FH, Hale D, Cohen A, Thompson L, Pezzella AT, Virmani R. Primary cardiac valve tumors. Ann Thorac Surg. 1991;52:1127–31.
18. Puvaneswary M, Edwards JRM, Bastian BC, Khatri SK. Pericardial lipoma: ultrasound, computed tomography and magnetic resonance imaging findings. Aust Radiol. 2000;44:321–4.
19. Kiaffas MG, Powell AJ, Geva T. Magnetic resonance imaging evaluation of cardiac tumor characteristics in infants and children. Am J Cardiol. 2002;89:1229–33.
20. McAllister Jr HA. Primary tumors of the heart and pericardium. Curr Probl Cardiol. 1979;4:1–51.
21. Ceresoli FL, Ferreri AJ, Bucci E, Ripa C, Ponzoni M, Villa L. Primary cardiac lymphoma in immunocompetent patients: diagnostic and therapeutic management. Cancer. 1997;80:1497–506.
22. Hoffman U, Globits S, Schima W, Loewe C, Puig S, Oberhuber G, Frank H. Usefulness of magnetic resonance imaging of cardiac and paracardiac masses. Am J Cardiol. 2003;92:890–5.
23. Beroukhim RS, Prakash A, Buechel ER, Cava JR, Dorfman AL, Festa P, Hlavacek AM, Johnson TR, Keller MS, Krishnamurthy R, Misra N, Moniotte S, Parks WJ, Powell AJ, Soriano BD, Srichai MB, Yoo SJ, Zhou J, Geva T. Characterization of cardiac tumors in children by cardiovascular magnetic resonance imaging: a multicenter experience. J Am Coll Cardiol. 2011;58:1044–54.
24. Chiles C, Woodard P, Guiterriez R, Link KM. Metastatic involvement of the heart and pericardium: CT and MR imaging. Radiographics. 2001;21:439–49.
25. Krombach GA, Spuentrup E, Buecker A, Mahnken AH, Katoh M, Temur Y, Higgins CB, Günther RW. Heart tumors: magnetic resonance imaging and multislice spiral CT. Rofo. 2005;177:1205–18.

Surgical Management of Cardiac Neoplasms

10

Francesco Santini, Mariassunta Telesca, Giuseppe Faggian, and Alessandro Mazzucco

Introduction

Primary cardiac tumors are rare forms of heart disease reported in both adult and children and first described by Realdo Colombo in 1559 [1, 2]. Several occasional reports are available on this topic in the past medical literature. In 1809, Burns described an atrial tumor determining valvular obstruction [3]. A series of six atrial tumors, probably myxoma, was published by King in 1845 [4]. Barnes et al in 1934 made the first antemortem diagnosis of a cardiac sarcoma using electrocardiography and biopsy of a metastatic lymph node [5]. In 1936, Beck successfully resected a teratoma external to the right ventricle [6], and Mauer removed a left ventricular lipoma in 1951 [7].

However, prior to the advent of modern cardiac surgery the correct *antemortem* diagnosis of an intracardiac tumor was largely academic, since effective therapy was not possible. A new approach in the management of cardiac tumors was made possible by the introduction of cardiopulmonary bypass by Gibbon in 1953, and by the advent of echocardiography, which provided a noninvasive method for accurately diagnosing intracardiac mass [8–14].

F. Santini, M.D. (✉) • M. Telesca, M.D • G. Faggian, M.D • A. Mazzucco, M.D
Cardiac Surgery, University of Verona Medical School, Piazzale Stefani 1, 37126, Verona, Italy
e-mail: francesco.santini@univr.it

Indeed in the last decades, major advances in noninvasive cardiovascular diagnostic techniques—especially echocardiography, computed tomography, and magnetic resonance imaging (MRI)—have greatly facilitated the approach to cardiac neoplasm.

Clinical signs and symptoms of a cardiac tumor are often nonspecific and a high index of suspicion remains the most important element for diagnosis. Indeed, cardiac neoplasms can produce a broad array of systemic findings, including fever, cachexia, malaise, and arthralgias. Relevant signs and symptoms are considered:

1. progressive heart failure without apparent cause, not responsive to medical therapy
2. pericardial effusion, often hemorrhagic
3. persistent arrhythmias, Wolff-Parkinson-White syndrome, A–V blocks
4. embolic phenomena and symptoms mimicking systemic vasculitis or infective endocarditis
5. severe dizziness or syncope
6. signs of valvular or sub-valvular obstruction

When suspecting a more conventional valvular and/or myocardial disease, the presence of atypical signs may raise the suspicion of cardiac tumors. For example, left atrial myxomas may produce auscultatory findings similar to mitral stenosis, whose characteristics may change with patient position, and mimic the symptoms of a mitral disease. Furthermore, the well-described "tumor plop" is an early diagnostic sound sometimes confused with a third heart sound. The diagnostic tumor plop occurs just after the opening snap of the mitral valve and is believed

C. Basso et al. (eds.), *Cardiac Tumor Pathology*, Current Clinical Pathology,
DOI 10.1007/978-1-62703-143-1_10, © Springer Science+Business Media New York 2013

to be secondary to contact between the tumor and endocardial wall.

Cardiac tumors may display several findings on plain chest roentgenograms, usually nonspecific. These include alterations in cardiac contour, changes in overall cardiac size, specific chamber enlargement, alterations in pulmonary vascularity, pericardial effusions, and intracardiac calcification (rhabdomyomas, fibromas, hamartomas, teratomas, myxomas, angiomas). Visualization of intracardiac calcium in an infant or a child is unusual and should immediately raise the suspicion of an intracardiac tumor. Mediastinal widening, due to hilar and paramediastinal adenopathy, may indicate the spread of a malignant cardiac tumor.

Two-dimensional echocardiography, and more recently real-time three-dimensional echocardiography [15], provide adequate information regarding tumor size, attachment, and mobility, all important variables to plan operative resection of the cardiac mass. It may also facilitate the differentiation between left atrial thrombus and myxoma. Moreover, continuous-mode Doppler ultrasonography may be useful for evaluating the hemodynamic consequences of valvular obstruction and/or incompetence caused by cardiac tumors.

Transesophageal echocardiography provides an unimpeded view of the cardiac chambers and atrioventricular (AV) septa and appears to be superior to transthoracic echocardiography in many patients. Its potential advantages include improved resolution of the tumor and its attachment, and the ability to detect small masses not visualized by transthoracic echocardiography (<3 mm diameter). Transesophageal echocardiography has been routinely used to guide the percutaneous biopsy of right-sided cardiac masses, thus allowing successful sampling of the target tissue for preliminary histologic evaluation [16]. Transesophageal echocardiography should always be considered when the transthoracic study is suboptimal or confusing [17, 18].

Cardiac computed tomography (C-CT) can provide useful information in view of its high resolution and ability to accurately depict cardiac morphology without limitations because of acoustic windows. It can also provide some information regarding the nature of the tumor by measuring X-ray attenuation, and possible tumor expansion to adjacent tissues. Multidetector computed tomography (MDCT) is useful for the evaluation of calcification and fat content within a mass. Furthermore, the high spatial resolution of MDCT is beneficial to define small lesions, making this technique a useful tool for staging malignant tumors. CT appears also useful in the evaluation of the potential involvement of pericardial and extracardiac structures. C-CT however provides less information regarding characterization of tissues in comparison to cardiac MRI. Disadvantages of the method also include the use of radioactivity and of nephrotoxic contrast mediums [19–21].

Cardiac magnetic resonance imaging (C-MRI) allows for a more sophisticated assessment of the tumor relation to adjacent structures, thus improving the planning of a proper resection strategy. It also allows the detection of myocardial infiltration by the tumor and/or expansion of the mass to the pericardium or to adjacent structures [19–21]. C-MRI may also contribute to the characterization of the composition of the tumor by studying the signal in T1- and T2-weighted images, as well as the enhancement of the signal after gadolinium administration [22]. Recent technologic advances in cardiac MRI have resulted in the rapid acquisition of images of the heart with high spatial and temporal resolution and excellent myocardial tissue characterization [23]. Furthermore, administration of contrast medium may help to differentiate a cardiac tumor from a thrombus and/or from blood flow artifacts [19–23].

Cardiac catheterization and selective angiocardiography are usually not necessary since adequate preoperative information may be obtained by one or more of the above-mentioned less invasive imaging techniques. However, several circumstances exist in which the risk and expense of cardiac catheterization are outweighed by the supplemental information it may provide. These situations include cases in which (a) noninvasive evaluation has not been adequate; (b) a malignant cardiac tumor is considered likely (cardiac angiography may provide valuable information regarding the degree of myocardial, vascular, and/or pericardial invasion, as well as visualization of the vascular supply of the tumor, the source of its blood supply, and its relation to the coronary arteries); and (c) other cardiac lesions may coexist with a cardiac tumor (i.e., coronary artery disease) and possibly dictate a different surgical approach [24, 25].

The major angiographic findings in patients with cardiac tumors include (a) compression or displacement of cardiac chambers or large vessels, (b) deformity of cardiac chambers, (c) intracavitary filling defects, (d) marked variations in myocardial thickness, (e) pericardial effusion, and (f) local alterations in wall motion [24, 26].

The major risk of angiography is peripheral embolization due to dislodgement of a fragment of tumor or of an associated thrombus.

The diagnosis of cardiac tumors and the estimation of their grade cannot be made with the sole use of imaging methods and histological confirmation is always necessary. This can be achieved with minimally invasive techniques, such as cytological examination of pericardial or pleural fluid, or by means of echocardiographically aided percutaneous or transvenous cardiac biopsy. In cases where diagnosis cannot be established, biopsy via thoracoscopy or even thoracotomy may be needed [16, 27, 28].

Primary Benign Cardiac Tumors

Surgical Technique

The surgical management of cardiac tumors began in 1936 when Beck successfully resected a teratoma external to the right ventricle [6]. In 1951 Mauer resected a left ventricular lipoma [7] and Bhanson and Newman in 1952 removed a large right atrial myxoma using inflow caval occlusion [29]. In 1954 Crafoord for the first time removed successfully a left atrial myxoma using cardiopulmonary bypass [30], whereas Kay et al. first removed a left ventricular myxoma in 1959 [31]. By the early sixties, owing to the progressive safety of cardiopulmonary bypass and to the increased use of echocardiography, atrial myxomas started to be removed successfully on a more routine-based approach [8, 32].

Currently, operative excision is the treatment of choice for most benign cardiac tumors, very often resulting in a complete cure. Although many cardiac tumors appear histologically benign, they all are potentially lethal as a result of intracavitary or valvular obstruction, peripheral embolization, and/or disturbances of rhythm or conduction. Therefore, it is mandatory to carry out the operation promptly after the diagnosis is established [13, 14, 33–35].

Through a median sternotomy, intramural and intracavitary tumors must be excised under direct vision using the heart–lung machine (Fig. 10.1) with bicaval or femoral cannulation (Fig. 10.2). The potential dislodgment of tumor fragments constitutes one of the major risk of the operation and may result in peripheral emboli and/or the dispersion of micrometastases, which may seed peripherally. To reduce this risk, manipulation of the heart prior to cardiopulmonary bypass and aortic cross-clamp positioning should be minimized (*"no-touch technique"*), as in other circumstances when dealing with any intracardiac friable mass (i.e., thrombus).

During the preliminary maneuvers to set the cardiopulmonary bypass, a transesophageal echocardiography may result extremely useful to define in detail the anatomy of the intracardiac mass, its relationship with any valvular apparatus, to guide in an uneventful cannulation of the cardiac chambers, and to monitor the integrity of the tumor during the initial surgical manipulations.

After establishing cardiopulmonary bypass, under mild hypothermia, the heart is separated from the systemic circulation by an aortic cross-clamp followed by the infusion of blood or crystalloid cardioplegia administered antegradely into the aortic root, and/or retrogradely into the coronary sinus. Although some epicardial tumors may be removed without the aid of extracorporeal circulation, intramural and intracavitary tumors must be excised under direct vision. The surgical approach will depend on the location of the cardiac mass (right-, left-, combined atriotomy, aortotomy, etc.). In view of the potential multifocal location of

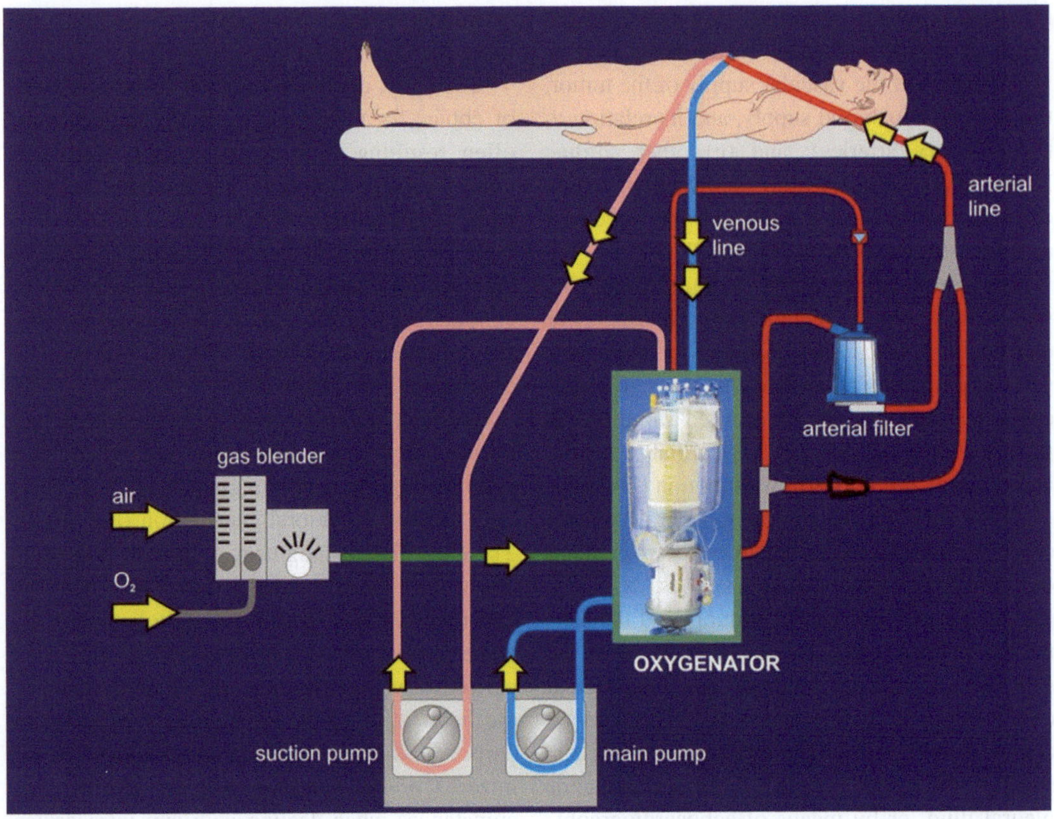

Fig. 10.1 Diagram of a cardiopulmonary bypass circuit. Venous blood is drained from the venae cavae/right atrium into the venous reservoir which is incorporated in the membrane oxygenator/heat exchanger unit. Arterialized blood exits the oxygenator and passes through a filter/bubble trap to the aortic cannula, which is usually placed in the ascending aorta. Suction systems and sources of gases are also represented

the cardiac tumors, all the cardiac chambers will need to be systematically explored. A good surgical exposure represents the fundamental principle to accomplish a complete, possibly *en bloc,* resection of the tumor. The ideal resection aims to include the tumor and a portion of the cardiac wall and/or interatrial septum, to which it is attached, spared by the disease. Variables with an impact on tumor resection are location, involvement of the myocardium and/or fibrous skeleton of the heart, and histology. To overcome the technical challenges of complete resection with accurate cardiac reconstruction, particularly of left-sided tumors with posterior extension, a technique of cardiac explantation, ex vivo tumor resection with cardiac reconstruction, and cardiac reimplantation—cardiac autotransplantation—has been successfully utilized [36–38].

Every care should be taken to remove the tumor without fragmentation. After tumor resection, the surgical field should be irrigated and carefully inspected for loose fragments. Whether blood removed from the surgical field during tumor manipulation should be discarded or returned to the pump circuit is controversial. Usually the cardiotomy suction is used during the operation, but the sole wall suction is utilized during the brief time that the tumor is actually excised in order to avoid tumor macroemboli entering the bloodstream via the perfusion circuit and the cardiotomy reservoir [8, 39, 40].

In the event of friable tumors located in the left (or right) cardiac chambers, the aorta (or the pulmonary artery) should be independently explored to exclude intraoperative migration of loose tumor fragments beyond the semilunar

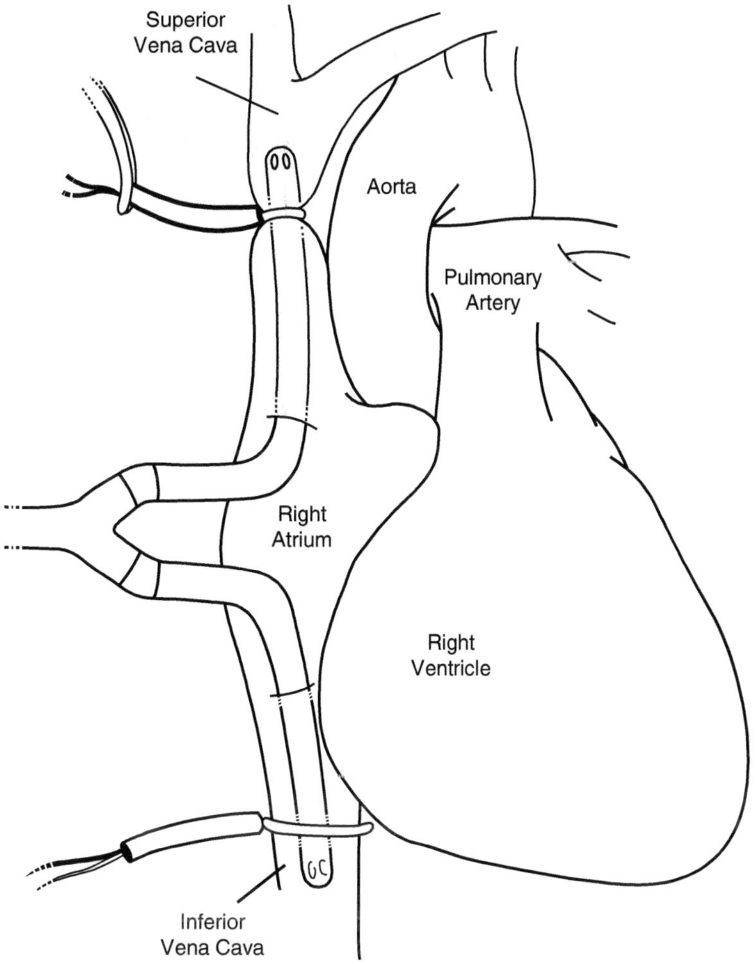

Fig. 10.2 Cannulation of the superior and inferior vena cava from incision in the right atrium. Caval snares are always used to allow safe opening of the right atrium

valves. The use of an intra-aortic filter (Edwards Embol-X System, Edwards Lifescience, Irvine CA) may help to reduce the event of systemic embolization in case of friable tumors located in the left cardiac chambers [41].

Ventricular tumors are usually approached through the AV valves if located in the ventricular inflow, or through the semilunar valves when located in the ventricular outflow tract.

In the event of tumors involving a cardiac valve, the surgical strategy should still aim to a complete resection of the mass, although trying to preserve the native valve by means of several well-described reparative techniques. When this is not possible, a valve prosthesis may be used.

The major surgical consideration in excision of ventricular tumors includes location, potential for a complete resection, preservation of adequate ventricular myocardium, maintenance of proper AV valve function, and preservation of the conduction system. It is not always possible to remove a ventricular tumor completely, and partial removal is only palliative. Children with extensive fibromas have been treated with cardiac transplantation. In selected cases of right ventricular tumors, a right heart bypass (cavopulmonary anastomosis) has also been utilized [11–14, 33, 42–48].

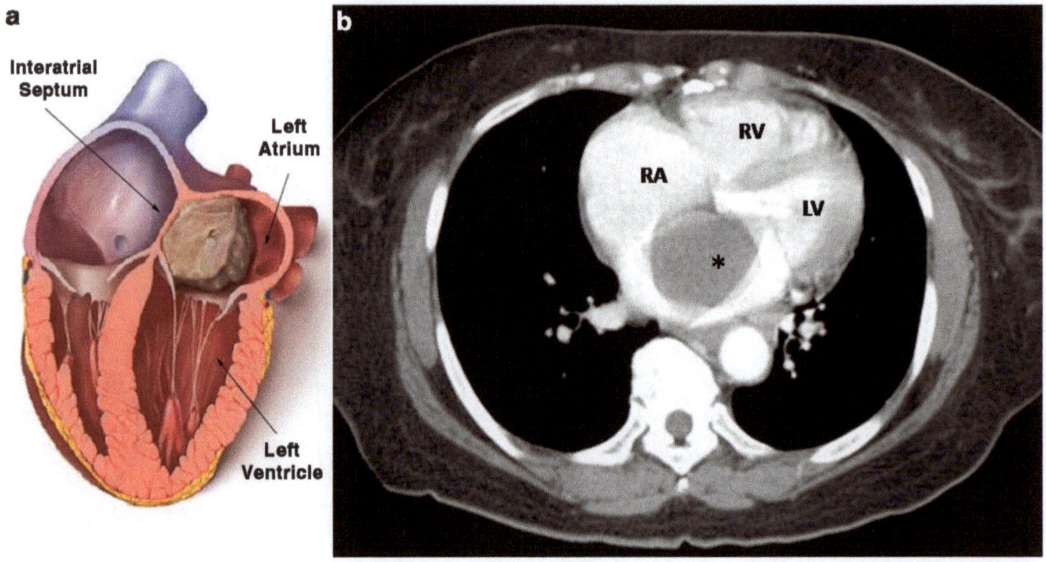

Fig. 10.3 (**a**) Diagram of a left atrial myxoma (75% of all cases) attached to the interatrial septum, above the mitral valve. (**b**) Cardiac-CT showing a left atrial mass (myxoma) (*asterisk*) attached to the interatrial septum. *RA* right atrium, *RV* right ventricle, *LV* left ventricle

Coming off cardiopulmonary bypass, transesophageal echocardiography may provide useful information on complete tumor excision, valve/prosthesis function in case of repair/replacement, absence of residual shunt in case of septal reconstruction, myocardial function, and de-airing.

Left Atrial Myxoma

Myxoma is the most common type of primary cardiac tumor, accounting for 1/3 to 1/2 of all cases. They may occur in any chamber of the heart but have a special predilection for the left atrium, from which approximately 75% originate. Left atrial myxomas generally arise from the interatrial septum at the border of the fossa ovalis (Fig. 10.3a, b), but can originate anywhere within the atrium, including the appendage. Surgical resection is the only effective therapeutic option for patients with cardiac myxoma and should not be delayed because death from obstruction to flow within the heart and/or embolization may occur in as many as 8% of patients awaiting operation [8]. Left atrial myxomas can be approached by an incision through the anterior wall of the left atrium, anterior to the right pulmonary veins, eventually extended behind both cavae to achieve greater exposure. Exposure and removal of large tumors attached to the interatrial septum however may be facilitated by a right atrial approach, which allows easy removal of tumor attached to the fossa ovalis with full-thickness and large excision at the site of attachment and easy patch closure of the atrial septum if necessary (Fig. 10.4a, b) [49]. As mentioned, the tumor should be removed without fragmentation. Nevertheless, after removal the surgical field should be irrigated and inspected for loose fragments. In case of atrial wall rather than septal attachment, large full-thickness excision of tumor insertion should be aimed whenever possible. A systematic inspection of the other cardiac chambers to exclude other tumor location potentially overlooked by the utilized imaging techniques is always recommended.

Histologic evaluation of the primary lesion is obviously mandatory to elaborate the most appropriate patient management and follow-up [11–14, 33, 35, 42, 49–51].

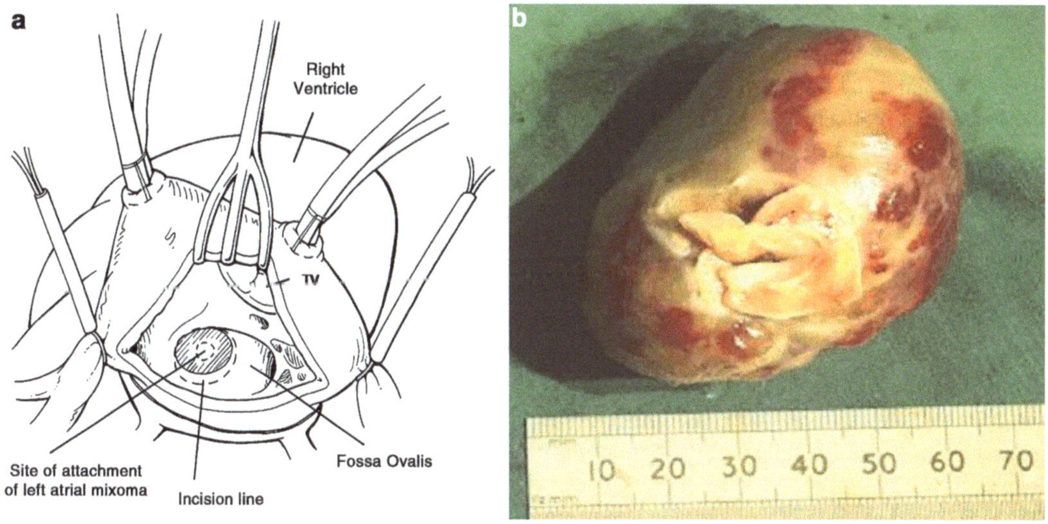

Fig. 10.4 (**a**) Right atriotomy and exposure of the left atrial myxoma through the fossa ovalis. Reprinted with permission of the Italian Society of Cardiology. *TV* tricuspid valve. (**b**) Left atrial myxoma with its base of attachment to the interatrial septum, excised with surrounding tissue

Right Atrial Myxoma

About 10 to 20% of all cardiac myxomas are found in the right atrium. Right atrial myxomas are more likely to have broad-based attachments; they also are more likely to be calcified and thus visible on chest radiographs. Right atrial myxomas can produce signs and symptoms of right-sided heart failure with venous hypertension, hepatomegaly, ascites, and dependent edema. The tumor may also simulate tricuspid valve stenosis by partially obstructing the valve orifice. If a patent foramen ovale is present, right to-left atrial shunting may occur with central cyanosis, and possible paradoxical embolization [8].

When approaching right atrial myxomas, intraoperative echocardiography may be extremely helpful to promote safe venous cannulation, avoiding mass trauma and/or poor venous return related to an impinging tumor. Both venae cavae may be cannulated directly and caval snares are always used to allow opening of the right atrium. However, when low- or high-lying tumor pedicles preclude safe transatrial cannulation, cannulation of the jugular or femoral vein can provide venous drainage of the upper or lower body [52]. The right atrium may be opened widely for resection of the tumor and reconstruction of the atrium using pericardium or polytetrafluoroethylene, keeping in mind that resection of large or critically placed right atrial myxomas may require careful preoperative planning and special perfusion strategies. The tricuspid valve and the right atrium, as well as the left atrium and ventricle, should always be inspected carefully for multicentric tumors in patients with right atrial myxoma, with or without familial occurrence [49–51].

Ventricular Myxomas

Ventricular myxomas (6–8%) occur more often in women and children and may be multicentric [12–15, 53]. Right ventricular tumors typically arise from the free wall, and left ventricular tumors tend to originate in the vicinity of the posterior papillary muscle.

Ventricular myxomas may be approached directly through the AV valve or by detaching portion of the AV valve, for mass exposure and resection, and reattachment after excision. Small tumors in either outflow tract can be removed through the outflow valve [8]. If necessary, the tumor is excised through a direct incision into the ventricle, but this is unusual. It is not necessary to remove the full thickness of the ventricular wall because no recurrences have been reported with partial-thickness excisions [49–51]. As mentioned for right atrial myxoma, in the presence of a ventricular myxoma inspection for other tumors is highly recommended because of the high incidence of multiple locations.

Overall 30-day mortality after removal of an atrial myxoma is below 5%, although excision of ventricular myxomas carries a higher risk (approximately 10%). Operative mortality may be increased by tumor unrelated variables such as advanced age, disability, and/or comorbidities. Long-term survival, freedom from complication, and quality of life are excellent in the nonfamilial form of myxoma [35, 48–51, 54, 55].

The recurrence of an intracardiac myxoma (described by 6 months and up to 11 years after the resection) may be related to an inadequate original resection, when at the same site of the original tumor, or to the presence of neoplastic fragments. Recurrence of nonfamilial sporadic myxoma is approximately 1–4% and possibly lower in patients with a normal DNA genotype [55, 56]. The rarer subgroup of patients with sporadic myxoma and abnormal DNA have a recurrence rate estimated at between 12 and 40%.

The recurrence rate is highest in patients with familial complex myxomas, all of whom exhibit DNA mutation [56]. Overall, recurrences are more common in younger patients. Most recurrent myxomas occur in the same or different cardiac chambers, and may be multiple particularly in familial complex myxomas. Extracardiac recurrence after myxoma excision, likely from embolization, local tumor growth, and invasion, has been observed in the brain, arteries, soft tissue, and bones [8].

In view of these considerations, patients who are treated initially for multicentric tumors, those whose tumors are removed from unusual locations in the heart or believed to have been incompletely resected and/or those with an abnormal DNA genotype, should be closely followed up [56, 57]. Furthermore, in those cases with delayed evidence of malignant characteristics within a resected mass mistakenly thought to be an *innocent* myxoma, complete patient rescreening is mandatory.

Lipoma

Lipomas are well encapsulated primary benign cardiac tumors, and consist of mature fat cells [9–12]. They are usually located in the subepicardium, in the left ventricle, in the right atrium, and in the interatrial septum (Fig. 10.5a, b). The non-encapsulated hypertrophy of the fat within the atrial septum, often in continuity with the epicardial fat, is known as *lipomatous hypertrophy.* Lipomatous hypertrophy is more common than cardiac lipoma, is more frequent in elderly, obese patients, and is usually an incidental finding during a variety of cardiac imaging or surgical procedures.

Often asymptomatic and incidentally discovered on routine chest roentgenogram, echocardiogram, or at surgery, lipomas may cause arrhythmias, conduction system disturbances, symptoms of heart failure, and sudden death, especially in cases where they reach a large size [58–60]. Large lipomas, particularly when associated with severe symptoms, should be resected. Smaller, asymptomatic tumors, incidentally discovered during cardiac operation undertaken for different indications, should be removed if excision is doable without adding risk to the primary procedure. In case of location in the atrial septum, patch reconstruction may be necessary. Cardiac lipomas are not known to recur.

Papillary Fibroelastoma

Papillary fibroelastomas are the most common tumors of the cardiac valves, accounting for 75% of all valvular tumors (Fig. 10.6a). They usually affect the elderly (age range 60 ± 16) [61], are generally small in size (<1 cm), and affect mainly the aortic or the mitral valve, even though tricuspid and pulmonary valves may also be affected. Occasionally, papillary fibroelastomas locate in the left ventricle, more often in the outflow tract, can be multifocal, and are associated with the hypertrophic obstructive cardiomyopathy [62–64]. Papillary fibroelastomas resemble a sea anemone with frond-like projections comprising dense elastin at the core of each frond, coated with collagen and lined by flat endocardial cells. Although frequently asymptomatic and often incidental findings at autopsy, papillary

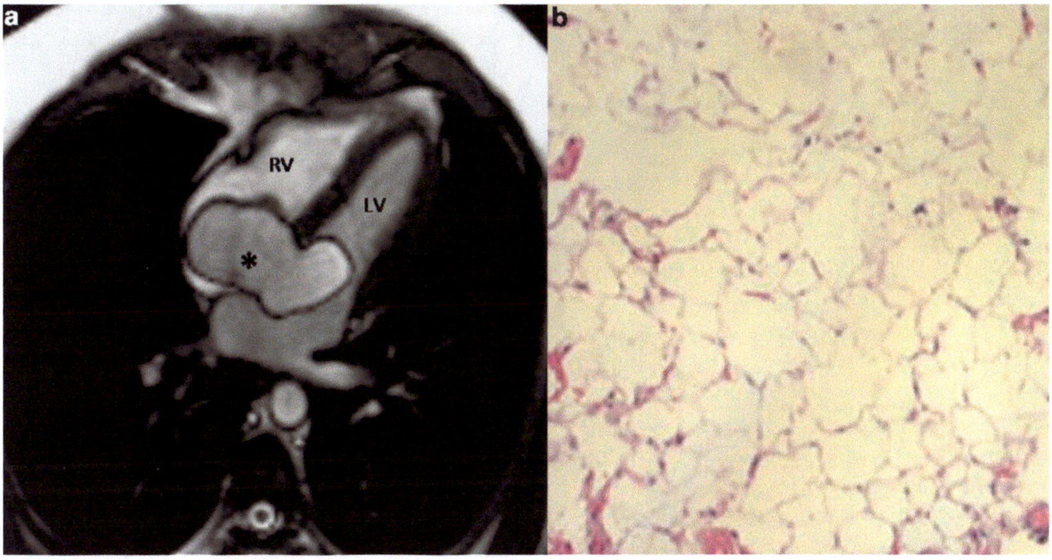

Fig. 10.5 (**a**) Cardiac-MRI of a huge lipomatous hypertrophy located in the interatrial septum (*asterisk*). *RV* right ventricle, *LV* left ventricle. (**b**) Microscopic views of the excised lipoma. Hematoxylin and eosin staining shows mature adipocytes (×100)

fibroelastomas are capable of producing obstruction of flow, particularly coronary ostial flow when located on the aortic valve (Fig. 10.6b). Most importantly, they may embolize to the coronary system or to the brain (or to the lung when right-sided), with potential life-threatening complications. Therefore, papillary fibroelastomas should be resected whenever diagnosed. In the event of a potential underlying coronary artery disease, invasive coronary angiography poses a significant risk of stroke in case of localization of the mass at the aortic valve level. In these patients, multislice-CT coronary angiography should be considered as a safer alternative [65]. Standard cardiopulmonary bypass with bicaval cannulation and conventional myocardial protection is utilized for tumor resection. Valve repair rather than replacement should follow the resection of these benign tumors whenever technically feasible, using conservative margins of resection with no observed recurrence after complete excision (Fig. 10.7a, b). In the rarer cases of a multifocal valve localization, valve replacement may be required. Worthy of note, the reported presence of dendritic cells and cytomegalovirus in the resected specimen suggests the possibility of a virus-induced tumor, therefore evoking the concept of a chronic form of viral endocarditis [66].

Fibroma

Fibromas are the second most common cardiac tumor of childhood, although they may also affect the adult population. These are solitary non-infiltrating intramural tumors, usually located in the left ventricle, mainly in the interventricular septum, and they are often mistaken for hypertrophic cardiomyopathy or apical thrombus (Fig. 10.8). Fibromas are non-encapsulated, firm, nodular, gray–white tumors potentially bulky, composed mainly of interlacing bundles of dense collagen and elastic fibers, and elongated fibroblasts. Deposits of calcium may be present. Symptoms may be related to chamber obstruction, impairment of contraction, and/or arrhythmias. Depending on size and location, fibromas may interfere with valve function, obstruct flow paths, or cause sudden death from conduction disturbances [8]. Surgical approach requires standard cardiopulmonary bypass with bicaval cannulation and conventional myocardial protection.

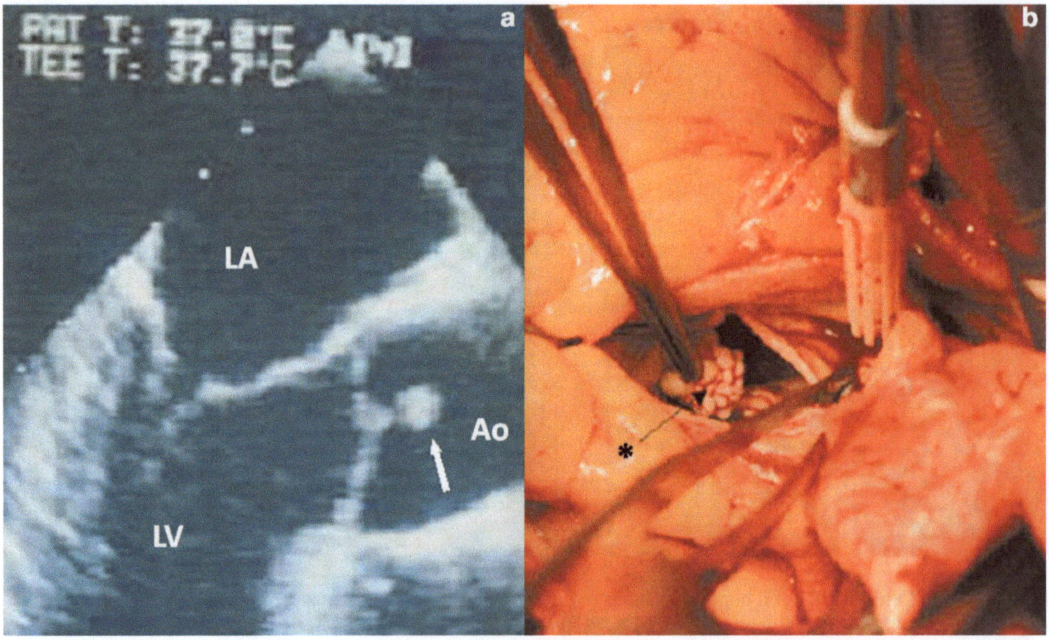

Fig. 10.6 (**a**) Transesophageal echocardiogram of a papillary fibroelastoma attached to the aortic valve (*arrow*). Reprinted with permission of the Italian Society of Cardiology. *LA* left atrium, *LV* left ventricle, Ao aorta. (**b**) Intraoperative view showing the papillary fibroelastoma attached to the right coronary aortic valve cusp (*asterisk*/*arrow*)

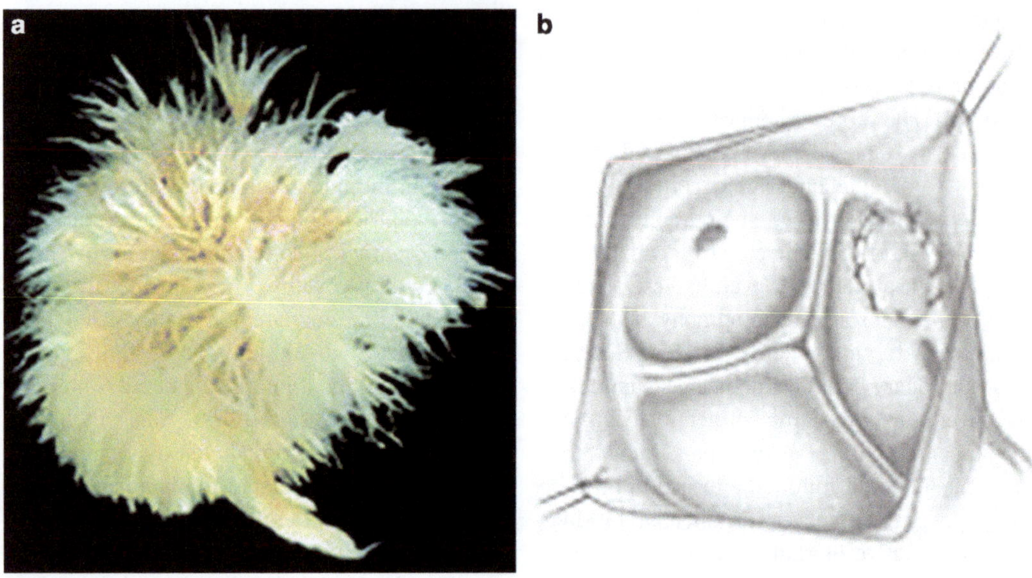

Fig. 10.7 (**a**) Papillary fibroelastoma after resection, with the typical sea anemone shape. (**b**) Diagram of an aortic valve patch reconstruction after repair. Reprinted with permission of the Italian Society of Cardiology.

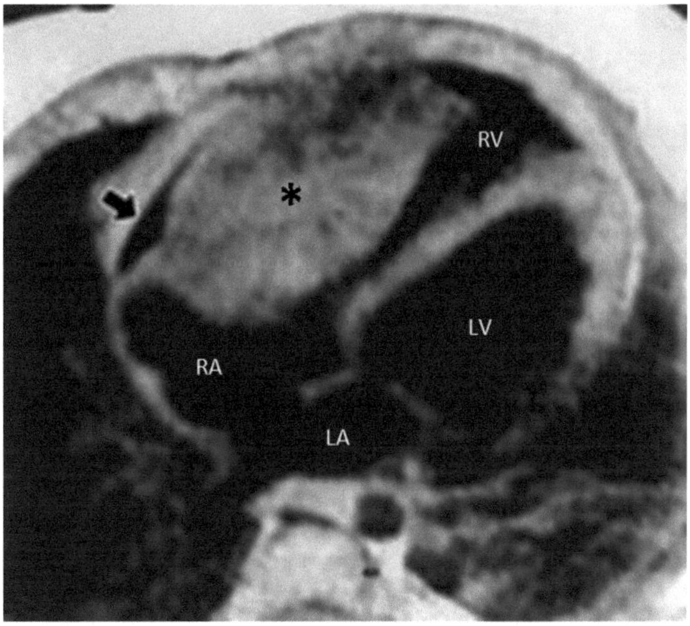

Fig. 10.8 Cardiac-MRI of a fibroma involving the right atrium and ventricle (*asterisk*), with associated pericardial effusion (*arrow*). Reprinted with permission of the Italian Society of Cardiology. *RA* right atrium, *RV* right ventricle, *LA* left atrium, *LV* left ventricle

Complete resection is usually successful when the tumor is localized, does not involve coronary arteries, AV valves, and/or the fibrous skeleton of the heart, and can be enucleated, usually through an epicardial approach, without entering the ventricle whenever possible. Video-assisted cardioscopy has been recently reported as a suitable and useful technique to assist removal of primary left ventricular fibroma with intracavitary extension [67]. Complete excision is usually curative. On the other hand, partial tumor removal is palliative although often followed by a prolonged survival [68]. Children with extensive fibromas, in good overall clinical conditions and with no specific contraindications, have been successfully treated with orthotopic cardiac transplantation [69]. In selected cases of extensive right ventricular tumors, a right heart bypass (cavo-pulmonary anastomosis) (Fig. 10.9a, b, c) has also been utilized [11–14, 33, 42–48] as a palliative solution or as a *bridge* to orthotopic cardiac transplantation [70].

Rhabdomyoma

Rhabdomyoma represents the most common cardiac tumor in children. Thought to be a myocardial hamartoma rather than a true neoplasm [71, 72], it usually presents during the first few days after birth. Occasionally sporadic, it is quite often associated with tuberous sclerosis (hereditary disorder characterized by hamartomas, seizures, developmental delay and behavioral problems, sebaceous adenomas) [53, 73, 74].

Rhabdomyomas are variable in size, usually multiple, and they affect the right and the left ventricle likewise. Firm, gray, nodular, and often intramural, they tend to project into the ventricular cavity, thus causing mechanical complications, such as obstruction of the ventricular outflow tract. On histology, they show large myocytes filled with glycogen and containing hyperchromatic nuclei. As for other intracardiac masses, clinical signs and symptoms depend on the size, location, and number of the tumors. Frequently enough, rhabdomyomas cause heart failure obstructing cardiac chambers and/or valvular orifice flow. Onset of symptoms may be represented by arrhythmias, particularly ventricular tachycardia, although sudden death may be the only effect of an undisclosed cardiac rhabdomyoma. Surgery may be advisable in symptomatic patients, without tuberous sclerosis, before 1 year of age. The tumor is removed easily in early infancy, and despite being non-encapsulated

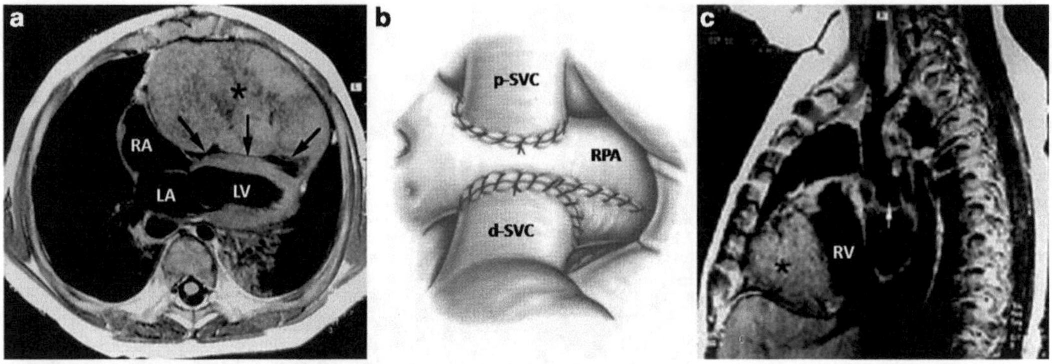

Fig. 10.9 Right heart bypass [cavo-pulmonary anastomosis (**b**, *diagram*)] in a case of extensive non-resectable right ventricular tumor (**a**, *asterisk*; *arrows* indicate residual right ventricular cavity). Reprinted with permission of the Italian Society of Cardiology. MRI control (**c**). *RA* right atrium, *RV* right ventricle, *LA* left atrium, *LV* left ventricle, p-*SVC* proximal superior vena cava, d-*SVC* distal superior vena cava, *RPA* right pulmonary artery

some can be completely resected. Partial resection may be conceivable to release the obstruction [75]. However, whenever planning a surgical strategy, it has to be considered that rhabdomyomas may regress spontaneously after birth, thus limiting indication to surgical resection to the actual symptomatic cases [73].

In case of multiple and extensive tumors, particularly in patients with tuberous sclerosis, surgery offers little benefit.

Other benign cardiac tumors (hemangioma, teratoma, paraganglioma, pheochromocytoma, cystic tumors of the AV node, etc.) are rarely observed. As mentioned, clinical signs and symptoms will be a result of intracavitary and/or valvular obstruction, peripheral embolization, and disturbances of rhythm or conduction, including sudden death. After the diagnosis, strict patient surveillance and multidisciplinary decision making relative to surgical indication are mandatory.

Primary Malignant Tumors

Malignant cardiac tumors continue to pose a therapeutic challenge to cardiac surgeons and oncologists because of the technical difficulty involved in extensive cardiac resections and the aggressive biological nature of the tumors.

Primary malignant tumors are relatively rare, accounting for upto 25% of all primary cardiac tumors in third level referral centers. They usually affect people aged 30–50 years, and are mainly represented by sarcomas (angiosarcoma, rhabdomyosarcoma, leiomyosarcoma, liposarcoma, osteosarcoma, fibrosarcoma, and malignant fibrous histiocytoma) and lymphomas [9–14]. Angiosarcomas are usually located in the right chambers of the heart (Fig. 10.10a, b), whereas other sarcomas affect the left atrium more frequently. Lymphomas with bi-atrial localization have also been reported (Fig. 10.11) [76]. Malignant tumors have usually a poor prognosis in view of the extensive infiltration of the myocardium, the frequent obstruction of intracardiac flow, and the occurrence of metastases [28]. Indeed, a metastatic spread has been demonstrated at autopsy in more than 75% of all patients who died of a primary cardiac sarcoma, mostly involving lungs, mediastinal lymph nodes, and spine. The nonspecific clinical signs and symptoms include congestive heart failure, dyspnea, atypical chest pain, malaise, anorexia, and weight loss. Arrhythmias, syncope, sudden death, pericardial effusion, and tamponade have also been reported [77]. Chest X-ray can offer indirect findings from the enlargement of cardiac chambers, the occurrence of calcification, or pericardial effusion. Two-dimensional echocar-

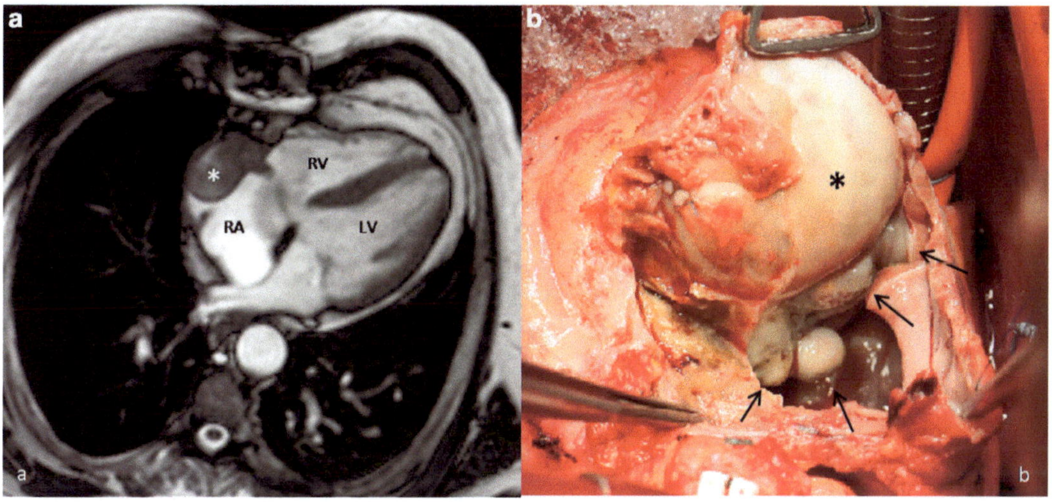

Fig. 10.10 (**a**) Cardiac-MRI of an angiosarcoma involving the right atrium and the right atrio-ventricular junction (*asterisk*). *RA* right atrium, *RV* right ventricle, *LV* left ventricle. (**b**) Intraoperative view of the tumor (*asterisk*), with multilobulated extensions (*arrows*)

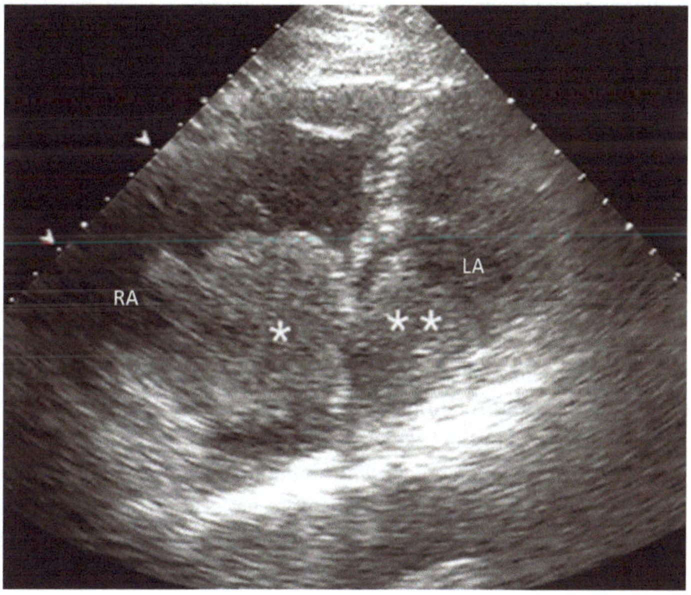

Fig. 10.11 Modified four-chamber echocardiographic view. Bi-atrial lymphoma filling almost entirely the right atrium (*asterisk*) and less extensively the left atrial chamber (*double asterisk*). *RA* right atrium, *LA* left atrium

diography provides adequate information regarding tumor location, size, attachment, and mobility all important variables to plan operative resection of the cardiac mass. If malignancy is suspected, chest CT and/or MRI may grossly guide on the histologic nature of the mass and provide detailed anatomy of the tumor, thus helping in staging and assessing its resectability. Cardiac catheterization may offer useful information about myocardial, vascular, and/or pericardial infiltration, and on the presence of tumor feeding vessels. Malignancy may be suggested and coronary involvement suspected by the evidence of a *tumor blush* (Fig. 10.12a, b), although this finding is not

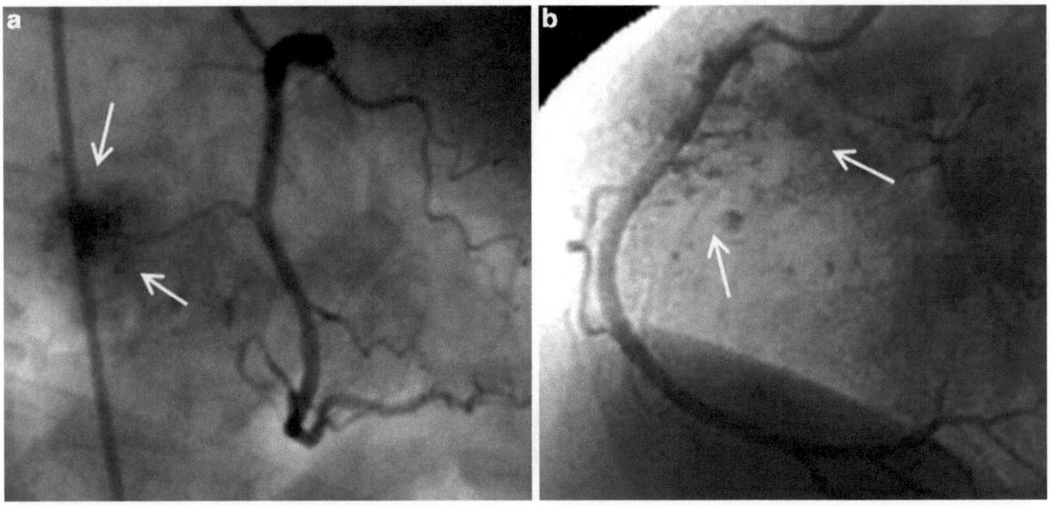

Fig. 10.12 Typical *tumor blush* (*arrows*) at coronary angiography in right atrial sarcomas

pathognomonic having been found also in myxomas [8]. Finally, transesophageal echocardiography guided transvenous endomyocardial biopsy is a very important tool to define tumor histology and to interpret metastatic lesions, thus helping to plan the most efficacious therapeutic strategy which usually involves a combination of surgery, chemotherapy, and radiation therapy [77–80].

The decision to resect a primary malignant tumor is based on several variables, including tumor location and size, histology, grade of myocardial infiltration, relationship with the cardiac valves and the fibrous skeleton of the heart, absence of metastatic spread, and potential for a radical excision of the mass. Other more general variables, such as age, overall clinical conditions, frailty, and comorbidities, will also need to be considered to finalize the surgical strategy [34, 36, 76–82].

Currently, chemotherapy, radiation therapy, or a combination of both are used as an adjuvant to decrease tumor size and facilitate surgical resection. In this perspective, a multidisciplinary decision-making approach relative to the overall therapeutic management is mandatory.

Based on the surgical approach and clinical behavior, cardiac sarcomas can be classified as right heart sarcomas, left heart sarcomas, and pulmonary artery sarcomas.

If complete resection is possible, respecting the anatomical and functional integrity of the heart, surgery provides better palliation and can improve survival vs. medical therapy alone [76–82].

As previously mentioned, a good surgical exposure represents the fundamental principle to accomplish a complete, possibly en bloc, resection of the tumor, encompassing the mass and about 1 cm portion of the surrounding cardiac tissue. Besides the routine use of cardiopulmonary bypass, deep hypothermia with circulatory arrest (<18 °C rectal temperature), providing a bloodless field unencumbered by cardiopulmonary bypass cannulas, can greatly improve exposure. Surgery may be technically demanding and the necessity of securing negative margins may entail further interventions such as coronary artery bypass, valve replacement, reconstructive procedures, pacemaker implantation, and pericardial repairs, thus resulting in an increased risk of postoperative complications.

To overcome the technical challenges of complete resection with accurate cardiac reconstruction, particularly of left-sided tumors with posterior extension, a technique of cardiac explantation, ex vivo tumor resection with cardiac reconstruction, and cardiac reimplantation—cardiac autotransplantation—has been utilized [36–38, 77, 78, 83]. Surgical outcomes with cardiac autotransplantation are excellent in patients who do not require concurrent pneumonectomy [77].

In selected cases of right ventricular tumors, a right heart bypass (cavo-pulmonary anastomosis) has also been utilized as a palliation to prolong survival [11–14, 33, 42–48].

The role of orthotopic cardiac transplantation in the management of locally advanced non-metastatic cardiac tumors appears to be limited. Indeed, it has been shown that about two-thirds of the so treated patients die of local recurrence or distant metastases within a year. Nevertheless, about 25% of the patients managed by orthotopic cardiac transplantation have a mean survival of more than 2 years without recurrent disease [44–46, 48, 78, 84]. The overall poor availability of donors however represent another important limitation to the role of orthotopic cardiac transplantation in this cohort of patients.

Despite a good local control often achievable with surgery, postoperative adjuvant therapy is recommended to all patients. Indeed, long-term survival is frequently poor due to metastatic tumor recurrence. This is particularly true in case of incomplete tumor resection [77, 78, 82, 85, 86].

Secondary Metastatic Cardiac Tumors

Metastatic cardiac tumors are far more frequent (approximately from 30- to 40-fold) than primary tumors of the heart. Although almost every type of malignant tumor has the potential to reach the heart, they usually arise from melanomas, lung, breast, and renal cancer, as well as lymphomas. Metastases may originate from blood dissemination via coronary arteries (melanoma, sarcoma, bronchogenic carcinoma) or lymphatic channels of cancer cells, direct extension via adjacent tissues (lung, breast, esophageal, and thymic tumors), or propagation via the superior or the subdiaphragmatic vena cava to the right atrium (liver, kidney tumors) (Fig. 10.13a, b). The pericardium is most often affected by direct extension of thoracic cancer, resulting in pericardial effusion which may contain masses comprising either cancer cells or blood clots and fibrin. The myocardium is the target of hematologous and/or retrograde lymphatic metastasis.

Cardiac metastases rarely are solitary and nearly always produce multiple microscopic nests and discrete nodules of tumor cells [8]. Clinical symptoms are quite rare and mainly related to pericardial effusion or cardiac tamponade. Arrhythmias, conduction block, and congestive heart failure have been occasionally reported [87–89].

Priority is given to the management of the primary focus of the disease and the cardiovascular complications that are manifested [28]. Surgical therapy is limited to relieve the recurrent pericardial effusions or, occasionally, cardiac tamponade (subxiphoid pericardiotomy, pericardial window) [90]. In most instances, these patients have widespread disease with limited life expectancies.

Abdominal and pelvic tumors (renal, hepatic, adrenal, uterine) on occasion may involve the inferior vena cava, with an intraluminal thrombotic extension to the right atrium. Renal cell cancer represents 1–3% of all visceral cancers and 85–90% of malignant kidney tumors and is most frequently responsible for this phenomenon (4–10% of all patients) (Fig. 10.13a, b) [91, 92]. Clinical symptoms are often few and nonspecific and related to the progressive obstruction of the inferior vena cava (ascites, peripheral edema) and/or to the presence of an abdominal mass.

CT-scan and/or MRI are used to study the primary focus of the disease, while two-dimensional echocardiography and in some instances perfusion lung scintigraphy are utilized to evaluate cardiopulmonary involvement. Radiation and chemotherapy are not effective in relieving the obstruction of blood flow. However, if the kidney can be fully removed, as well as the tail of tumor thrombus, survival can approach 75% at 5 years [91, 92]. Surgical intervention, in the absence of metastatic spread, besides to remove the primary focus of the disease, including the thrombus in the inferior vena cava, the adjacent lymphatic structures, and, eventually, the involved caval wall, aims to prevent potentially massive pulmonary

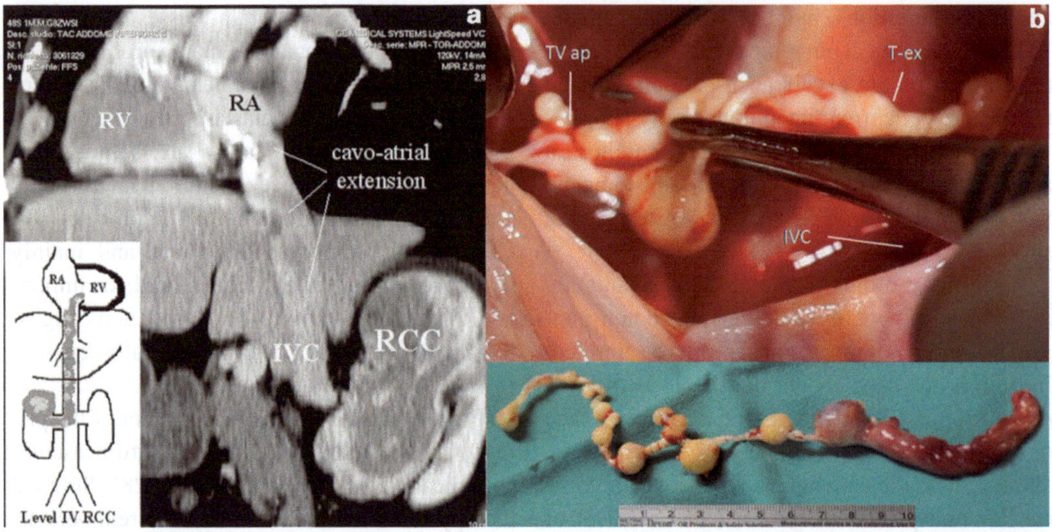

Fig. 10.13 (**a**) CT evidence of a right renal cell cancer (RCC) with neoplastic extension into the inferior vena cava (IVC) and right atrium (RA) [level IV cavoatrial tumor thrombus (*insert diagram*)]; *RV* right ventricle. (**b**) Intraoperative view. Tumor extension (T-ex) into the right atrium through the inferior vena cava (IVC), attached to the tricuspid valve apparatus (TV ap). Specimen after excision (*insert*)

embolism related to the fragmentation of the neoplastic tissue and/or thrombus. Renal cell tumors with atrial extension typically are approached with abdominal dissection to ensure full resectability of the renal tumor. Depending on the proximal extension of the tumor thrombus different surgical approaches have been recommended. In type III and IV disease, the exposure and isolation of the inferior vena cava are more extensive, requiring liver mobilization and sometimes an associated median sternotomy with or without the use of cardiopulmonary bypass and, in some circumstances, deep hypothermic circulatory arrest (DHCA) to improve exposure.

It is now accepted that neoplastic extension into the inferior vena cava is not a prognostically determining factor [92]. With no perinephric fat or lymph nodal involvement, it has been observed that the patients who undergo tumor excision with a radical nephrectomy and inferior vena cava thrombectomy have an overall and cancer-specific 5-year survival of 30–72%, with an operative mortality of 2.7–13% and an immediate palliation of symptoms of obstructive tumors [93–95].

References

1. Columbus MR. De Re Anatomica, Liber XV. Venice: N Bevilacque, 1559. p. 269.
2. Moes RJ, O'Malley CD. Realdo Colombo: on those things rarely found in anatomy. Bull Hist Med. 1960;34:508.
3. Burns A. Observations of some of the most frequent and important diseases of the heart. London: James Muirhead; 1809.
4. Goldberg HP, Glenn F, Dotter CT, Steinberg I. Myxoma of the left atrium: diagnosis made during life with operative and postmortem findings. Circulation. 1952;6:762.
5. Barnes AR, Beaver DC, Snell AMP. Primary sarcoma of the heart: report of a case with electrocardiographic and pathological studies. Am Heart J. 1934;9:480.
6. Beck CS. An intrapericardial teratoma and tumor of the heart: Both removed operatively. Ann Surg. 1942;116:161.
7. Mauer ER. Successful removal of tumor of the heart. J Thorac Surg. 1952;3:479.
8. Walkes JC, Smythe WR, Reardon MJ. Cardiac neoplasms. In: Cohn LH, editor. Cardiac surgery in the adult. 3rd ed. New York, NY: McGraw-Hill; 2008. p. 1479–509.
9. McAllister HA Jr, Fenoglio JJ Jr: Tumors of the cardiovascular system. In: Atlas of tumor pathology. Washington DC: Armed Forces Institute of Pathology, 1978 (fas. 15).

10. Smith C. Tumors of the heart. Arch Pathol Lab Med. 1986;110:371–4.
11. Butany J, Nair V, Naseemudin A, Nair GM, Catton C, Yau T. Cardiac tumors: diagnosis and management. Lancet Oncol. 2005;6:219–28.
12. Travis WD, Brambilla E, Muller-Hermelink H, Harris CC. Pathology and genetics of tumors of the lung, pleura, thymus and heart. Lyon: IARC Press; 2004.
13. Shapiro LM. Cardiac tumours: diagnosis and management. Heart. 2001;85:218–22.
14. Sarjeant JM, Butany J, Cusimano RJ. Cancer of the heart: epidemiology and management of primary tumors and metastases. Am J Cardiovasc Drugs. 2003;3:407–21.
15. Asch FM, Bieganski SP, Panza JA, Weissman NJ. Real-time 3-dimensional echocardiography evaluation of intracardiac masses. Echocardiography. 2006;23:118–24.
16. Abramowitz Y, Hiller N, Perlman G, Admon D, Beeri R, Chajek-Shaul T, Leibowitz D. The diagnosis of primary cardiac lymphoma by right heart catheterization and biopsy using fluoroscopic and transthoracic echocardiographic guidance. Int J Cardiol. 2007;118:39–40.
17. Engberding R, Daniel WG, Erbel R, Kasper W, Lestuzzi C, Curtius JM, Sutherland GR, Lambertz H, von Hehn A, Lesbre JP. Diagnosis of heart tumours by transoesophageal echocardiography: a multicentre study in 154 patients. European Cooperative Study Group. Eur Heart J. 1993;14:1223–8.
18. Tan CN, Fraser AG, Tan CN, Fraser AG. Transesophageal echocardiography and cardiovascular sources of embolism. Anesthesiology. 2007;107:333–46.
19. Restrepo CS, Largoza A, Lemos DF, Diethelm L, Koshy P, Castello P, Gomez R, Moncada R, Pandit M. CT and MR imaging findings of benign cardiac tumors. Curr Probl Diagn Radiol. 2005;34:12–21.
20. Araoz PA, Mulvagh SL, Tazelaar HD, Julsrud PR, Breen JF. CT and MR imaging of benign primary cardiac neoplasms with echocardiographic correlation. Radiographics. 2000;20:1303–19.
21. van Beek EJR, Stolpen AH, Khanna G, Thompson BH. CT and MRI of pericardiac and cardiac neoplastic disease. Cancer Imaging. 2007;7:19–26.
22. Sparrow PJ, Kurian JB, Jones TR, Sivananthan MU. MR imaging of cardiac tumors. Radiographics. 2005;25:1255–76.
23. O'Donnel DH, Abbara S, Chaithiraphan V, Yared K, Killeen RP, Cury RC, Dodd JD. Cardiac tumors: optimal cardiac MR sequences and spectrum of imaging appearances. AJR AmJ Roentgenol. 2009;193:377–87.
24. Fueredi GA, Knechtges TE, Czarnecki DJ. Coronary angiography in atrial myxoma: findings in nine cases. Am J Roentgenol. 1989;152:737–8.
25. Kumar SP, Kaul S, Saha PK, Miller MJ. Images in cardiology. Angiographic appearance of "tumour blush" produced by a large right atrial myxoma. Heart. 2006;92:751.
26. Singh RN, Burkholder JA, Magovern GJ. Coronary arteriography as an aid in left atrial myxoma diagnosis. Cardiovasc Intervent Radiol. 1984;7:40–3.
27. Jurkovich D, de Marchena E, Bilsker M, Fierro-Renoy C, Temple D, Garcia H. Primary cardiac lymphoma diagnosed by percutaneous intracardiac biopsy with combined fluoroscopic and transesophageal echocardiographic imaging. Cathet Cardiovasc Intervent. 2000;50:226–33.
28. Paraskevaidis I, Michalakeas C, Papadopoulos C, Anastasiou-Nana M. Cardiac tumors ISRN oncology 2011;2011:208929.
29. Bahnson HT, Newman EV. Diagnosis and surgical removal of intracavitary myxoma of the right atrium. Bull Johns Hopkins Hosp. 1953;93:150–63.
30. Crafoord C. Discussion on mitral stenosis and mitral insufficiency. In: Lam CR, editor. Proceeding of the international symposium on cardiovascular surgery, Henry Ford Hospital Philadelphia: WB Saunders, 1955. p. 202.
31. Kay JH, Anderson RM, Meihaus J, Lewis R, Magidson O, Bernstein S. Surgical removal of an intracavitary left ventricular myxoma. Circulation. 1959;20:88–96.
32. Malm JR, Bowman FO, Henry JB. left atrial myxoma associated with an ASD. J Thorac Cardiovasc Surg. 1963;45:490.
33. Stiller B, Hetzer R, Meyer R, Dittrich S, Pees C, Alexi-Meskishvili V, Lange PE. Primary cardiac tumors: when is surgery necessary? Eur J Cardiothorac Surg. 2001;20:1002–6.
34. Cusimano RJ. Surgical management of cardiac tumors. Semin Diagn Pathol. 2008;25:76–81.
35. ElBardissi AW, Dearani JA, Daly RC, Mullany CJ, Orszulak TA, Puga FJ, Schaff HV. Survival after resection of primary cardiac tumors: a 48-year experience. Circulation. 2008;118:S7–15.
36. Thomas CR, Johnson GW, Stoddard MF, Clifford S. Primary malignant cardiac tumors: update 1992. Med Pediatr Oncol. 1992;20:519–31.
37. Reardon MJ, DeFelice CA, Sheinbaum R, Baldwin JC. Cardiac autotransplant for surgical treatment of a malignant neoplasm. Ann Thorac Surg. 1999;67:1793–5.
38. Reardon MJ, Malaisrie SC, Walkes JC, Vaporciyan AA, Rice DC, Smythe WR, DeFelice CA, Wojciechowski ZJ. Cardiac autotransplantation for primary cardiac tumors. Ann Thorac Surg. 2006;82:645–50.
39. Attum AA, Johnson GS, Masri Z, Girardet R, Lansing AM. Malignant clinical behavior of cardiac myxomas and "myxoid imitators". Ann Thorac Surg. 1987;44:217–22.
40. Read RC, White HJ, Murphy ML, Williams D, Sun CN, Flanagan WH. The malignant potentiality of left atrial myxoma. J Thorac Cardiovasc Surg. 1974;68:857–68.
41. Schmitz C, Weinreich S, White J, Oengoeren I, Schneider R, Schneider D, Speth I, Pohl C, Welz A. Can particulate extraction from the ascending aorta reduce neurologic injury in cardiac surgery ? J Thorac Cardiovasc Surg. 2003;126:1829–38.
42. Bakaeen FG, Reardon MJ, Coselli JS, Miller CC, Howell JF, Latrie GM, Espada R, Ramchandani MK,

Noon GP, Weilbaecher DG, DeBakey ME. Surgical outcome in 85 patients with primary cardiac tumors. Am J Surg. 2003;186:641–7.
43. Aravot DJ, Banner NR, Madden B, Aranki S, Khaghani A, Fitzgerald M, Radley-Smith R, Yacoub MH. Primary cardiac tumors: is there a place for cardiac transplantation? Eur J Cardiothorac Surg. 1989;3:521–4.
44. Goldstein DJ, Oz MC, Rose EA, Fisher P, Michler RE. Experience with heart transplantation for cardiac tumors. J Heart Lung Transplant. 1995;14:382–6.
45. Gowdamarajan A, Michler RE. Therapy for primary cardiac tumors: is there a role for heart transplantation? Curr Opin Cardiol. 2000;15:121–5.
46. Dietl CA. Successful Fontan-type operation for nonresectable right ventricular tumor. Ann Thorac Surg. 1990;5:814–6.
47. Calderon M, Galvan J, Negri V, Verdin R. Right ventricular bypass for palliation of cardiac sarcoma. Tex Heart Inst J. 1996;23:178–9.
48. Hoffmeier A, Deiters S, Schmidt C, Tjan TD, Schmid C, Drees G, Fallenberg EM, Scheld HH. Radical resection of cardiac sarcoma. Thorac Cardiovasc Surg. 2004;52:77–81.
49. Bortolotti U, Maraglino G, Rubino M, Santini F, Mazzucco A, Milano A, Fasoli G, Livi U, Thiene G, Gallucci V. Surgical excision of intracardiac myxomas: a 20-year follow-up. Ann Thorac Surg. 1990;49:449–53.
50. Ipek G, Erentug V, Bozbuga N, Polat A, Guler M, Kirali K, Peker O, Balkanay M, Akinci E, Alp M, Yakut C. Surgical management of cardiac myxoma. J Card Surg. 2005;20:300–4.
51. Tasoglu I, Tutun U, Lafci G, Hijaazi A, Yener U, Ulus AY, Aksoyek A, Saritas A, Birincioglu L, Pac M, Katircioglu F. Primary cardiac myxomas: clinical experience and surgical results in 67 patients. J Card Surg. 2009;24:256–9.
52. Bakir I, Van Vaerenberg G, Deshpande R, Coddens J, Vanermen H. Right atrial tumor: a contraindication to minimally invasive surgery? Innovations. 2009;4:39–42.
53. Uzun O, Wilson DG, Vujanic GM, Parsons JM, De Giovanni JV. Cardiac tumours in children. Orphanet J Rare Dis. 2007;2:11–25.
54. Wu KH, Mo XM, Liu YL. Clinical analysis and surgical results of cardiac myxoma in pediatric patients. J Surg Oncol. 2009;99:48–50.
55. Actis Dato GM, De Benedictis M, Actis Dato A Jr, Ricci A, Sommariva L, De Paulis R. Long-term follow-up of cardiac myxomas (7–31 years). J Cardiovasc Surg. 1993;34:141–143.
56. Acebo E, Val-Bernal JF, Gómez-Román JJ, Revuelta JM. Clinicopathologic study and DNA analysis of 37 cardiac myxomas: a 28-year experience. Chest. 2003;123:1379–85.
57. Yokomuro H, Yoshihara K, Watanabe Y, Shiono N, Koyama N, Takanashi Y. The variations in the immunologic features and interleukin-6 levels for the surgical treatment of cardiac myxomas. Surg Today. 2007;37:750–3.
58. Gulmez O, Pehlivanoglu S, Turkoz R, Demiralay E, Gumus B. Lipoma of the right atrium. J Clin Ultrasound. 2009;37:185–8.
59. Breuer M, Wippermann J, Franke U, Wahlers T. Lipomatous hypertrophy of the interatrial septum and upper right atrial inflow obstruction. Eur J Cardiothorac Surg. 2002;22:1023–5.
60. Verberkmoes NJ, Kats S, Tan-Go I, Schönberger JP. Resection of a lipomatous hypertrophic interatrial septum involving the right ventricle. Interact Cardiovasc Thorac Surg. 2007;6:654–7.
61. Gowda RM, Khan IA, Nair CK, Mehta NJ, Vasavada BC, Sacchi TJ. Cardiac papillary fibroelastoma: a comprehensive analysis of 725 cases. Am Heart J. 2003;146:404–10.
62. Yoda M, Tanabe H, Kanou H, Sawada H, Suma H. Multiple papillary fibroelastomas in rare locations of aortic valve and left ventricular outflow tract: a case report. J Heart Valve Dis. 2009;18:575–7.
63. Kobayashi Y, Saito S, Yamazaki K, Kurosawa H. Multiple papillary fibroelastoma in left ventricle associated with obstructive hypertrophic cardiomyopathy. Interact Cardiovasc Thorac Surg. 2009;9:921–2.
64. Kumar TK, Kuehl K, Reyes C, Talwar S, Moulick A, Jonas RA. Multiple papillary fibroelastomas of the heart. Ann Thorac Surg. 2009;88:e66–7.
65. de Visser RN, van Mieghem C, van Pelt NC, Weustink AC, Kerker JP, Galema TW. Papillary fibroelastoma of the aortic valve and coronary artery disease visualized by 64-slice CT. Nat Clin Pract Cardiovasc Med. 2008;5:350–3.
66. Grandmougin D, Fayad G, Moukassa D, et al. Cardiac valve papillary fibroelastomas: clinical, histological and immunohistochemical studies and a physiopathogenic hypothesis. J Heart Valve Dis. 2000;9:832.
67. Araji OA, Gutierrez-Martin MA, Miranda N, Barquero JM. Video-assisted cardioscopy for removal of primary left ventricular fibroma. Interact Cardiovasc Thorac Surg. 2010 Feb;10:344–5.
68. Agarwala BN, Starr JP, Walker E, Bacha EA. Surgical issues in giant right ventricular fibroma. Ann Thorac Surg. 2004;78:328–30.
69. Valente M, Cocco P, Thiene G, Casula R, Poletti A, Milanesi O, Fasoli G, Livi U. Cardiac fibroma and heart transplantation. J Thorac Cardiovasc Surg. 1993;106:1208–12.
70. Waller BR, Bradley SM, Crumbley 3rd AJ, Wiles HB, McQuinn TC, Bennett AT. Cardiac fibroma in an infant: single ventricle palliation as a bridge to heart transplantation. Ann Thorac Surg. 2003;75:1306–8.
71. Garson Jr A, Smith Jr RT, Moak JP, Kearney DL, Hawkins EP, Titus JL. Incessant ventricular tachycardia in infants: myocardial hamartomas and surgical cure. J Am Coll Cardiol. 1987;10:619–26.
72. Nicks R. Hamartoma of the right ventricle. J Thorac Cardiovasc Surg. 1964;47:762.
73. Geva T, Santini F, Pear W, Driscoll SG, Van Praagh R. Cardiac rhabdomyoma. Rare cause of fetal death. Chest. 1991;99:139–41.

74. Degueldre SC, Chockalingam P, Mivelaz Y, Di Bernardo S, Pfammatter JP, Barrea C, Sekarski N, Jeannet PY, Fouron JC, Vial Y, Meijboom EJ. Considerations for prenatal counselling of patients with cardiac rhabdomyomas based on their cardiac and neurologic outcomes. Cardiol Young. 2010;20:18–24.
75. Padalino MA, Basso C, Milanesi O, Vida VL, Moreolo GS, Thiene G, Stellin G. Surgically treated primary cardiac tumors in early infancy and childhood. J Thorac Cardiovasc Surg. 2005;129:1358–63.
76. Santini F, Innocente F, Gilioli E, Rossi A, Ferrara A, Brunelli M, Faggian G, Mazzucco A. Primary bi-atrial Burkitt lymphoma with severe inflow impairment in an immunocompetent patient. Cardiovasc Pathol. 2009;18:123–5.
77. Blackmon SH, Patel A, Reardon MJ. Management of primary cardiac sarcomas. Expert Rev Cardiovasc Ther. 2008;6:1217–22.
78. Putnam JB, Sweeney MS, Colon R, Lanza LA, Frazier OH, Cooley DA. Primary cardiac sarcomas. Ann Thorac Surg. 1991;51:906–10.
79. Neragi-Miandoab S, Kim J, Vlahakes GJ. Malignant tumours of the heart: a review of tumour type, diagnosis and therapy. Clin Oncol. 2007;19:748–56.
80. Gupta A. Primary cardiac sarcomas. Expert Rev Cardiovasc Ther. 2008;6:1295–7.
81. Park BJ, Bacchetta M, Bains MS, Downey RJ, Flores R, Rusch VW, Girardi LN. Surgical management of thoracic malignancies invading the heart or great vessels. Ann Thorac Surg. 2004;78:1024–30.
82. Bakaeen FG, Jaroszewski DE, Rice DC, Walsh GL, Vaporciyan AA, Swisher SS, Benjamin R, Blackmon S, Reardon MJ. Outcomes after surgical resection of cardiac sarcoma in the multimodality treatment era. J Thorac Cardiovasc Surg. 2009;137:1454–60.
83. Blackmon SH, Patel AR, Bruckner BA, Beyer EA, Rice DC, Vaporciyan AA, Wojciechowski Z, Correa AM, Reardon MJ. Cardiac autotransplantation for malignant or complex primary left-heart tumors. Tex Heart Inst J. 2008;35:296–300.
84. Crespo MG, Pulpon LA, Pradas G, Serrano S, Segovia J, Vegazo I, Salas C, Espana P, Silva L, Burgos R. Heart transplantation for cardiac angiosarcoma: should its indication be questioned? J Heart Lung Transplant. 1993;12:527–30.
85. Poole GV, Meredith JW, Breyer RH, Mills SA. Surgical implications in malignant cardiac disease. Ann Thorac Surg. 1983;36:484–9.
86. Janigan DT, Husain A, Robinson NA. Cardiac angiosarcomas: a review and case report. Cancer. 1986;57:852–91.
87. Hanfling SM. Metastatic cancer to the heart: review of the literature and report of 127 cases. Circulation. 1960;2:474–83.
88. Weinberg BA, Conces Jr DJ, Waller BF. Cardiac man ifestation of noncardiac tumors, part I: direct effects. Clin Cardiol. 1989;12:289–96.
89. Chiles C, Woodard PK, Gutierrez FR, Link KM. Metastatic involvement of the heart and pericardium: CT and MR imaging. Radiographics. 2001;21: 439–49.
90. Lestuzzi C, Bearz A, Lafaras C, Gralec R, Cervesato E, Tomkowski W, DeBiasio M, Viel E, Bishiniotis T, Platogiannis DN, Buonadonna A, Tartuferi L, Piazza R, Tumolo S, Berretta M, Santini F, Imazio M. Neoplastic pericardial disease in lung cancer: impact on outcomes of different treatment strategies. A multicenter study. Lung Cancer. 2011;72:340–7.
91. Prager RL, Dean R, Turner B. Surgical approach to intracardial renal cell carcinoma. Ann Thorac Surg. 1982;33:74–7.
92. Chiappini B, Savini C, Marinelli G, Suarez SM, Di Eusanio M, Fiorani V, Pierangeli A. Cavoatrial tumor thrombus: single-stage surgical approach with profound hypothermia and circulatory arrest, including a review of the literature. J Thorac Cardiovasc Surg. 2002;124:684–8.
93. Posacioglu H, Ayik MF, Zeytunlu M, Amanvermez D, Engin C, Apaydin AZ. Management of renal cell carcinoma with intracardiac extension. J Card Surg. 2008;23:754–8.
94. Kalkat MS, Abedin A, Rooney S, Doherty A, Faroqui M, Wallace M, Graham TR. Renal tumours with cavoatrial extension: surgical management and outcome. Interact Cardiovasc Thorac Surg. 2008;7:981–5.
95. Yazici S, Inci K, Bilen CY, Gudeloglu A, Akdogan B, Ertoy D, Kaynaroglu V, Demircin M, Ozen H. Renal cell carcinoma with inferior vena cava thrombus: The Hacettepe experience. Urol Oncol. 2010;28:603–9.

Cardiac Metastases

11

Furio Silvestri, Gianfranco Sinagra,
and Rossana Bussani

Introduction

Primary and secondary tumors of the heart are one of the least addressed and understood subjects in oncology and there have been a few systematic studies relating to this subject [1–3].

Although primary heart tumors are extremely rare, with a rate of incidence between 0.001 and 0.28% in various autopsy studies [2], the heart can be the target of metastases from any extracardiac malignant neoplasm able to spread to distant sites. Apart from this, the issue of cardiac metastases has a significant clinical impact as cardiac metastases can cause alterations in cardiac function. Any sign of cardiac dysfunction in a patient affected by cancer should alert clinicians to the possibility of metastases [4]. One might also generally add that when a patient with no clinical history develops a cardiac dysfunction with no apparent cause, clinicians should take into consideration the possibility of a cardiac metastasis amongst the various hypotheses.

The rates of cardiac metastasis reported in the literature are highly variable (Table 11.1) and, at least in our experience, have no specific time-related trends [5–15]. The relatively low rate of cardiac metastases has been ascribed to the contractile strength of the heart, the specific metabolism of the myocardium, the velocity of the coronary blood flow, and the lymphatic network that drains from the heart [3].

Although there are no known specifically cardiotropic malignant neoplasms, some nevertheless involve the heart with a higher frequency than others, such as melanoma and mediastinal primary tumors. The likelihood of tumoral diffusion to the heart depends therefore on several factors i.e., the specific biological potential of the main tumor, its location (and its proximity to the heart), and the contractile and drainage capacity of the myocardium.

Therefore, it is logical to assume that in most cases neoplasms that have a generalised secondary diffusion involve the heart.

Clinical Manifestations

As previously mentioned, cardiac metastasis can be the first or even the only sign of a clinically undiagnosed malignant neoplasm. Generally, if a focal myocardial metastasis does not give a clear symptomatic clinical picture, more extensive involvement of the pericardium or other cardiac areas can determine dramatic clinical situations causing clinical emergencies. Symptoms differ according to the areas involved. Meta-tumoral pericardial effusions and cardiac masses can be easily detected by transthoracic and transesophageal

F. Silvestri, M.D. • R. Bussani, M.D. (✉)
Department of Pathologic Anatomy, University of Trieste Medical School, Cattinara Hospital, Trieste, Italy
e-mail: bussani@univ.trieste.it

G. Sinagra, M.D.
Cardiovascular Department, University of Trieste Medical School, Cattinara Hospital, Trieste, Italy

C. Basso et al. (eds.), *Cardiac Tumor Pathology*, Current Clinical Pathology,
DOI 10.1007/978-1-62703-143-1_11, © Springer Science+Business Media New York 2013

Table 11.1 Overview of the literature

Author	Neoplasms *N.*	Cardiac metastases *N.* (%)
Walther [5]	2,027	46 (2.3)
Willis [6]	342	17 (4.9)
Hanfling [7]	694	127 (18.3)
Berge & Sievers [8]	2,595	122 (4.7)
Kline [9]	716	61 (8.5)
Karwinski & Svendsen [10]	2,564	130 (5.1)
Mukai et al. [11].	6,240	953 (15.0)
Manojlovic [12]	477	39 (8.2)
MacGee [13]	1,311	57 (4.3)
Silvestri et al. [14]	1,928	162 (8.4)
Bussani et al. [15]	7,289	662 (9.1)

ultrasound imaging, computerised tomography scan, high-resolution CT, and magnetic resonance [16]. The cytological analysis of the pericardial effusion also may allow us to detect and characterize the neoplastic cells.

- Pericardial metastases
  A pericardial effusion, often with a haemorrhagic pattern, is frequently the first sign of a metastatic cardiac involvement [17]. The effusion, often of conspicuous proportions, can cause an increase of the central venous pressure, a paradoxical pulse, low QRS voltages, and right atrioventricular diastolic collapse. Should pulseless electrical activity occur, a pericardiocentesis must be performed immediately.
- Myocardial metastases
  In the case of secondary cardiac intramural localisations, the clinical picture is obviously proportional to the degree of myocardial infiltration or, in any case, related to the site of parietal infiltration. Typical manifestations are the following: more or less significant arrhythmias such as atrial flutter or fibrillation, premature beats or ventricular arrhythmias, conduction disturbances, and complete atrioventricular block, especially when the conduction system has been infiltrated. Whenever there is a widespread ventricular involvement, the clinical pattern may include congestive heart failure. One can add to this the possible damage to the myocardium from the antineoplastic drugs, as well as the direct toxic effect to the myocardium from infiltration of the tumor. Although not frequent, a myocardial infarction can occur and can be due to several factors, such as a neoplasm-induced embolus in the coronary tree, a perivascular tumoral invasion, or an extrinsic compression by a severe meta-tumoral pericardial effusion.
- Metastases to the endocardium or intracavitary lesions.
  Some tumors can spread along the inferior vena cava reaching the right atrium and producing an intracavitary lesion, leading sometimes to obstruction. The most typical of these tumors are the carcinoma of the kidney and the hepatocellular carcinoma. These types of lesions can sometimes become so invasive that they obliterate completely the chamber and block the movement of the tricuspid valve, resulting in a clinical pattern similar to pericardial constriction or restrictive myocardial disease. In addition, it is also possible that the metastatic mass can become eroded and shed small neoplastic emboli in the pulmonary arterial system.

Another risk is the formation of neoplastic thrombi within the pectinate muscles of the right atrium or the trabeculae of the right ventricle, the latter generally with no clinical manifestations.

Neoplastic thrombi are also possible in the left atrium, following tumoral embolism through the pulmonary veins, generally in patients with lung carcinoma. Large thrombi can block the mitral valve.

Metastatic Pathways to the heart

Cardiac metastases can affect, also in combination, the pericardium, the epicardium, the myocardium, the endocardium, and the cardiac chambers, or sometimes rapidly develop intracavitary neoplastic thrombi. Tumors can spread to the heart through four possible pathways, i.e., by direct extension, through the bloodstream, through the lymphatic system, and by intracavitary diffusion through either the inferior vena cava or the pulmonary veins.

Pericardial Involvement

The main metastatic pathways are the direct invasion from intrathoracic neoplasms, a retrograde lymphatic spread through tracheal or bronchomediastinal lymphatic channels, or secondary spread of metastases from the myocardium and epicardium.

Epicardial or Myocardial Metastatic Involvement

The metastatic routes are a retrograde lymphatic spread through tracheal or bronchomediastinal channels, as extensions secondary to an already metastasised pericardium or through the bloodstream.

Endocardial Involvement

The spread routes are a direct haematogenous dissemination to the cardiac chambers followed by intracavitary lodging, or the extension of the metastases from the myocardium.

There is a subtle interactive relationship between the haematic and lymphatic network of the heart. The heart has a three-tiered lymphatic network: the subepicardial, the myocardial, and the subendocardial nets. Drainage of the lymphatics forms a major trunk that drains the whole heart and rests against the anterior side of the pulmonary artery. Multiple lymphatic channels drain the lymph from the heart to the mediastinum. There is also a common cardiac and pulmonary lymphatic duct draining directly into the mediastinum [18].

The subepicardial lymphatic plexus is formed by a net of capillaries and drainage ducts [19]. During diastole, the blood pressure in the ventricles drives the lymphatic drainage from the endocardial net to the myocardial one. During systole, cardiac contractions drive lymph from the myocardial lymphatics to the subepicardial ones. The pressure of the dilated heart against the pericardium at the end of diastole drains lymph from the subepicardial net into the main lymphatic trunk that emerges from the heart.

Obstruction to the lymphatic flow causes multiple alterations that make the lymphatic drainage more complex, if not impossible, increasing tissue damage. For example, a direct relationship between coronary perfusion and lymphatic flow has been described [20]. Experimental studies have shown that no contrast medium is absorbed by the lymphatics in the absence of coronary perfusion, while, as the coronary flow restores, the absorption and lymphatic drainage are re-established and become visible once again.

If intramural lymphatics are obstructed by neoplastic emboli, lymph will stagnate in the myocardial areas upstream of the obstruction, and the lymphatic drainage from the endocardium to the epicardium will be partially or totally inhibited. This causes tissue damage, due to both lymph stasis and inadequate drainage thus favouing increased proliferation of neoplastic cells in the undrained regions. As a result of increased pressure, the lymphatic vessel wall may also break, leading to interstitial tumor spread.

Myocardial contraction has two effects, one hindering the metastatic process, and the other promoting it. Cardiac contraction, as a matter of fact, on one hand hinders the spreading of intramural neoplastic metastases by facilitating the lymphohaematic drainage and therefore displacing any cardiac neoplastic emboli; on the other hand, it helps the diffusion of tumoral cells along the epicardial surface.

The key event leading to the diffusion of metastases is, therefore, the blockage of the common lymphatic node by neoplastic cells coming from metastasised lymph nodes of the mediastinum. This causes the slowing down of the lymph flow in the myocardium and the retrograde migration and proliferation of neoplastic cells towards the epicardium [21].

Once the neoplastic cells have reached and colonised the epicardium, neoplastic emboli can penetrate the intramural lymphatics as the lymphatic vessels follow closely the arterial ones. The damage to the myocardium caused by the stasis of the lymph flow as well as by the toxic effect of both the tumor and chemotherapy can further reduce myocardial contractility that in its turn further

Table 11.2 Malignant tumors and cardiac metastases at autopsy, Department of Pathologic Anatomy, University of Trieste, Italy (1994→2008)

	Autopsy, *N*.	Neoplasms		Cardiac metastases	
		N	%	*N*	%
Males	12,559	5,777	46.0	535	9.0
Females	13,072	4,186	32.0	370	9.0
Total	25,631	9,963	39.0	905	9.0

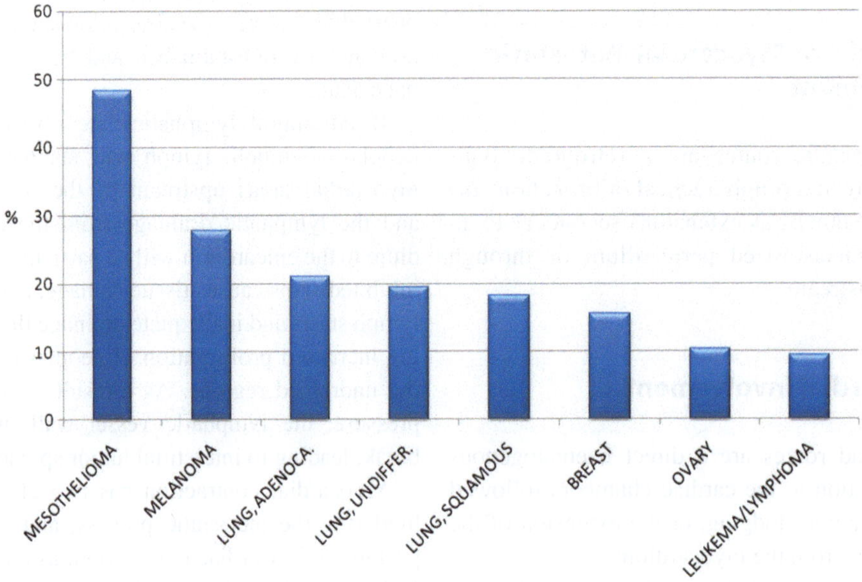

Fig. 11.1 Frequency of cardiac metastases from different type of primary malignant neoplasms

impairs the drainage of the lymph and facilitates the penetration and proliferation of the tumor in the myocardium.

Epidemiology of Cardiac Metastases

Few papers have been published in the literature on cardiac metastases, possibly because of the international trend to perform fewer postmortem examinations [14].

In our Department of Pathologic Anatomy, University of Trieste, Italy, in spite of a reduced global autopsy rate in the last years, the postmortem examinations of in-hospital deceased remains consistently above 60%.

In our Department, 25,631 postmortem studies were performed (12,559 men and 13,072 women) in the time frame between 1994 and 2008. In 9,963 cases, one or more malignant neoplasms were found (39% of total autopsy studies). Cardiac metastases were found in 905 cases (9% of all malignant tumors) (Table 11.2). While there was a gender difference in the rate of malignant tumors, 46% in men and 32% in women, there was no difference as far as cardiac metastases were concerned.

The incidence of primary tumors was decreasing with age (52% in patients aged ≤64 years vs. 26.7% in patients >85) as well as the incidence of cardiac metastases (16.7% in the younger cases and 4% in the over 85). This pattern was evident for every tumor detected and is probably due to the less aggressive biological characteristics of tumors in the elderly.

The tumors with the highest rate of heart metastases were the following (Fig. 11.1):

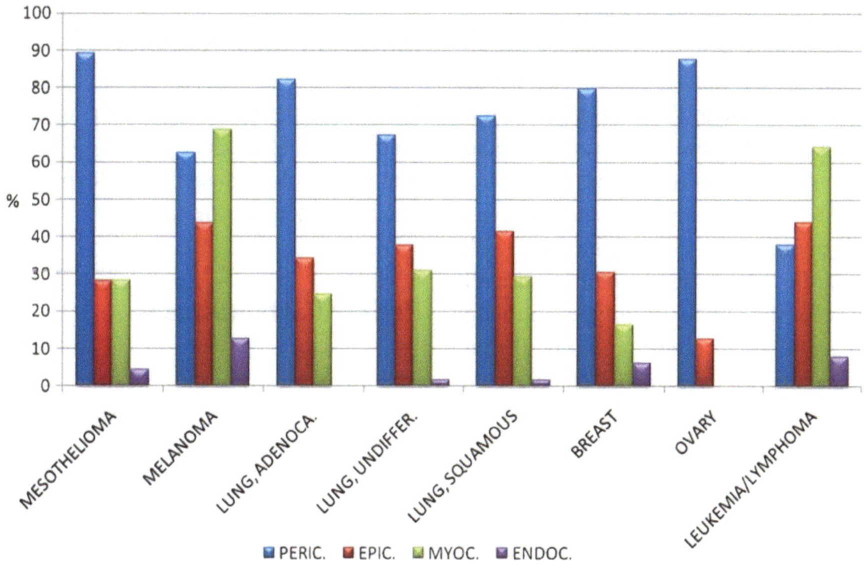

Fig. 11.2 Location of cardiac metastases by type of primary malignant neoplasm

pleural mesothelioma (48.4%), melanoma (27.8%), lung adenocarcinoma (21.0%), undifferentiated carcinoma of the lung (19.5%), lung squamous cell carcinoma (18.2%), and breast carcinoma (15.5%). High rates of cardiac metastases have also been observed in ovarian carcinomas (10.3%), lymphomyeloproliferative neoplasms (9.4%), bronchioalveolar (9.8%), gastric (8.0%), renal (7.3%), and pancreatic (6.4%) carcinomas.

When taking into consideration only tumors with multiple distant metastases, the incidence of cardiac involvement significantly increases reaching a global rate of 14.2%. The tumors that show a higher cardiac metastatic rate are melanoma, bronchioalveolar carcinoma, and renal carcinoma.

With the exception of mesothelioma (57.3% men vs. 30% women), there was no gender difference.

In our series, the heart was the only target of metastasis in 14 out of 905 cases. They were respectively five cases of lung squamous cell carcinoma, three cases of breast carcinoma, two lymphoma, one carcinoma of the oesophagus, two pleural mesothelioma, and one carcinoma of the kidney. About two-thirds of all cardiac metastases involved the pericardium [69.4%], one-third the epicardium [34.2%] or the myocardium [31.8%], and only 5% the endocardium. The tumors with the highest pericardial involvement were (Fig. 11.2) mesothelioma, lung adenocarcinoma, ovary, stomach, and prostate carcinoma. The epicardium was more frequently involved by melanoma, lung squamous cell carcinoma, and bronchioalveolar carcinoma. The myocardium was more often the target of melanoma and lymphomyeloproliferative processes, whereas the endocardium was particularly involved by melanoma, kidney and hepatic carcinoma.

While there was no significant age difference between the patients presenting heart metastases from mesothelioma or lung or breast carcinoma and those with metastases in other sites, this was not the case for leukemic or lymphomatous processes, prostatic or ovarian neoplasms, cancers of the stomach or pancreas, where the age of the patients with heart metastases was significantly lower of that of patients who presented carcinomas spreading to different sites.

As far as lung carcinomas, the rates of metastasis differed according to the specific histotype.

Adenocarcinoma spreads to the heart in 26% of cases, squamous cell carcinoma in 23.4%, undifferentiated carcinoma in 21.2%, and bronchioalveolar carcinoma in 17.4%. For all the lung cancer histotypes, however, the most affected area was the pericardium (82.2% of adenocarcinomas, 72.4% of squamous cell carcinoma, and 67.2% of undifferentiated carcinomas). The remaining cardiac structures show proportionally similar rates for the various histotypes, although we should highlight a certain preferential trend for the epicardium from squamous cell carcinoma (41.4%), while no cases of adenocarcinoma spreading to the endocardium were found.

Morphological Aspects

Heart metastases can present a wide variety of morphological aspects according to the type of tumor, its site, its spreading capacity, and the manner of permeating the heart.

Pericardial Metastases

The neoplastic infiltration can be focal, diffuse, or massive, with or without metaneoplastic fibrin-blood effusion (Fig. 11.3).

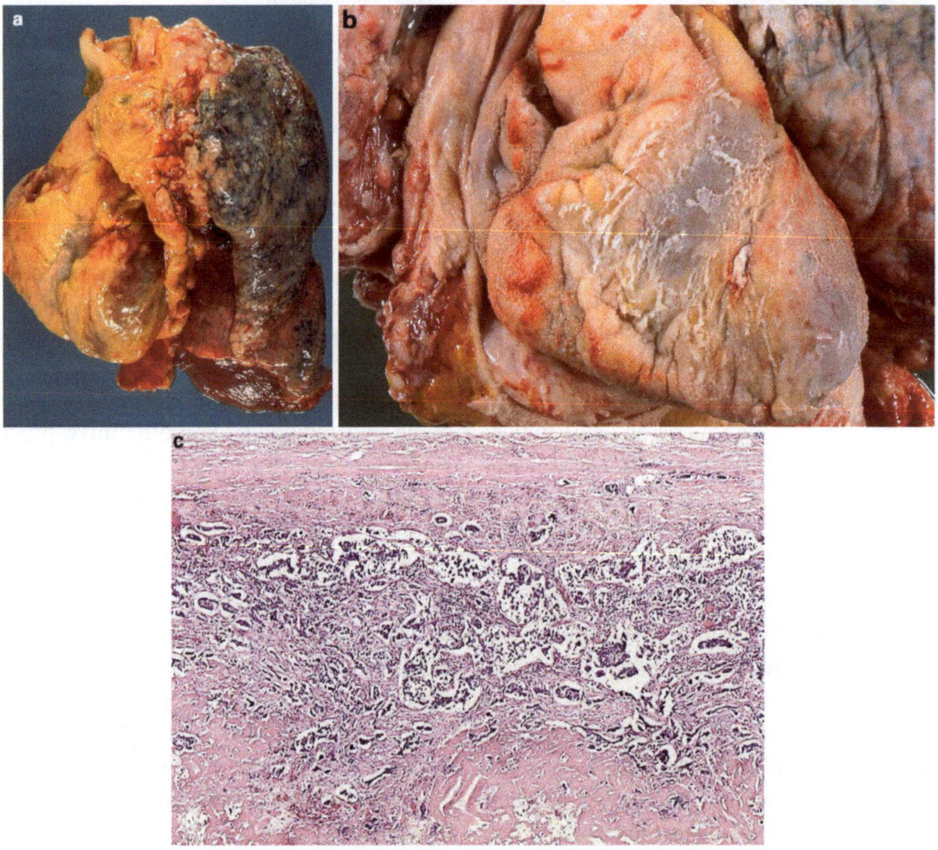

Fig. 11.3 Pericardial metastases usually present clinically as pericardial effusion especially in diffuse and haemorrhagic forms. (**a**) Neoplastic infiltration of the pericardium by direct invasion by an undifferentiated thyroid carcinoma. (**b**) Massive tumoral infiltration of the pericardium by a lung adenocarcinoma. (**c**) Histology of extensive lymphatic colonisation by carcinomatous cells (same case)

Epicardial Metastases

The neoplastic infiltration can present a micro- or macronodular or diffuse aspect (Fig. 11.4). Also in this case, the infiltration can originate from the flaking of cancerous cells from pericardial-infiltrated areas followed by secondary epicardial colonisation (usually a nodular infiltration), as well as from the lymphatic blockage (Fig. 11.5).

Spread to the epicardium may occur not only through the lymphatic pathway (multifocal or diffuse) but also through the bloodstream (in this

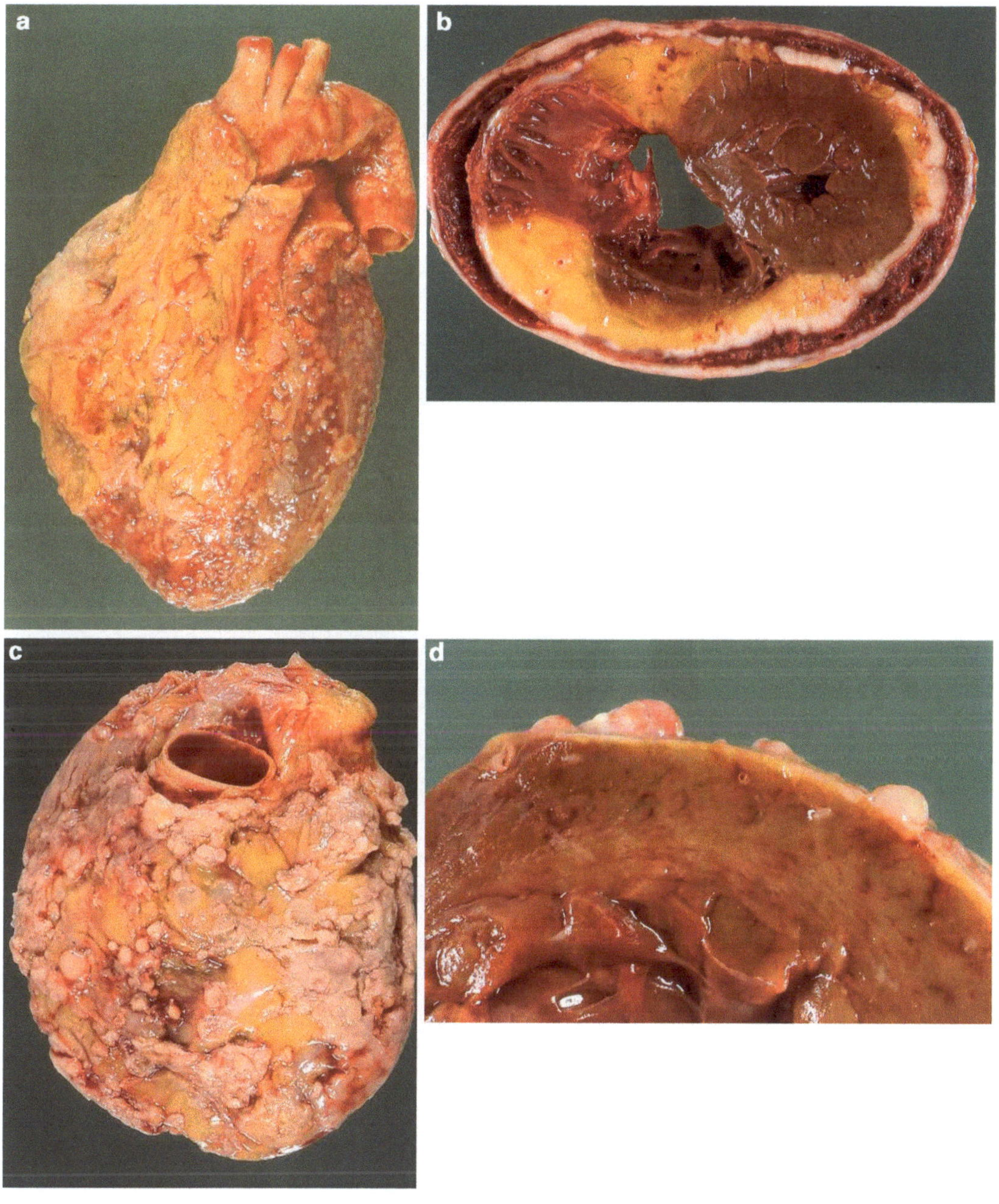

Fig. 11.4 Epicardial metastases. The neoplastic infiltration can present a micronodular (**a, b**) or a macronodular aspect (**c, d**). Frequently the metastatic involvement presents a haemorrhagic pattern (**e, f**)

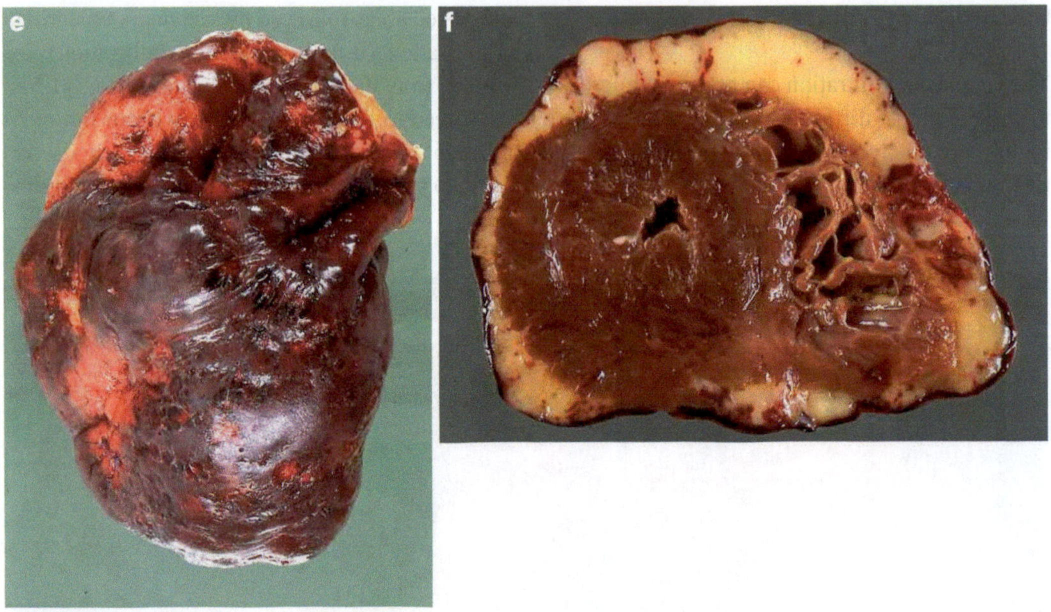

Fig. 11.4 (continued)

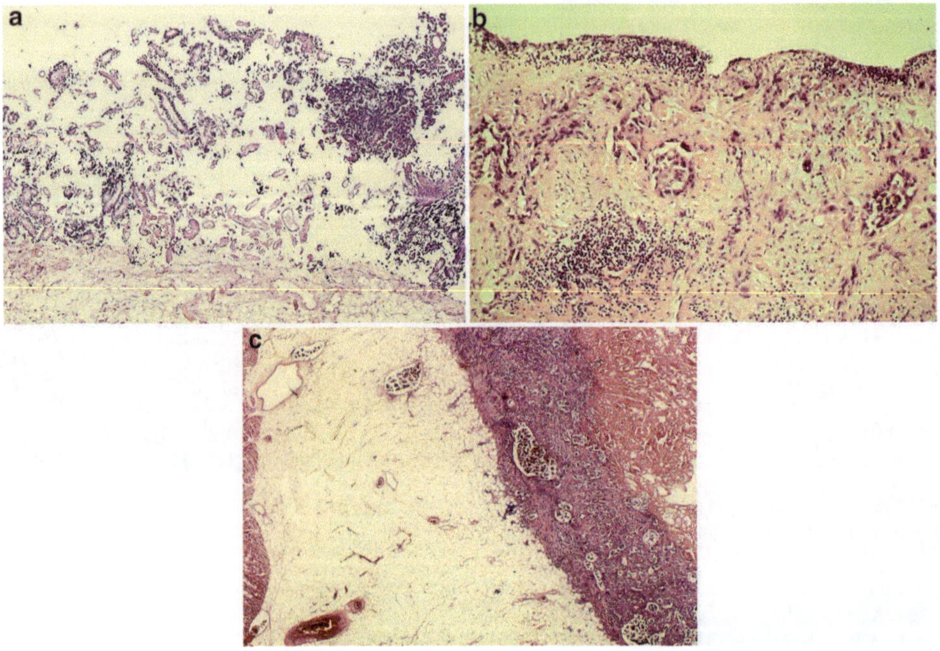

Fig. 11.5 (**a**) Flaking of neoplastic cells from pericardium to epicardium. (**b**) Lymphatics permeated with carcinomatous cells. (**c**) Haemorrhagic pattern of epicardial metastatic involvement

case the pattern tends to be micro-focal, and is often due to the neoplastic spread from intramural colonised areas of the myocardium).

When a diffuse carcinomatous spread occurs, a tight yellow-whitish mesh of lymphatics permeated with neoplastic cells can be seen on the epicardium.

Another interesting pattern is that of the "wave front extension". When there is an endolymphatic epicardial involvement and the heart develops dysfunction for various reasons (coronary artery, valvular, either due to the chemotherapy, or to the same lymphatic stagnation), the contractility of the myocardium is further greatly reduced. As a consequence, both the lymphatic drainage and the arterial and venous blood flow are decreased, and the lymphatic structure is dilated allowing a wide homogeneous tumoral wave front progression from the epicardium to the myocardium.

The pericardial effusion seen in neoplastic peri-epicarditis is often characterized by a full-fledged haemorrhage. This is very likely due to both the damage of the thin capillary wall caused by the release of inflammatory-related noxious substances as well as by hyperdilation of the vascular lumen due to congestion.

Myocardial Metastases

In our experience there has been no preferential involvement of a ventricular chamber from intramural invasion. There are, however, conflicting observations in the literature regarding ventricular involvement. According to some authors, the right ventricle is particularly affected [3, 11, 22]. They attribute this to the low pressure in the chamber and to the decreased systolic function of the ventricle, which facilitates the lodging of metastases. In other studies, the left ventricle seems to be the most affected [23–25], while other authors suggest that there is no preferential metastatic involvement [26, 27]. In our series, both ventricular chambers and the interventricular septum were affected as a result of a diffuse and non-preferential haematogenous spread.

Metastatic cells can target the myocardium following two routes, i.e., they can either proliferate and spread along the lymphatic channels that run along the vessels from the epicardium into the same myocardium, or through the bloodstream. Blood embolisation may result in lesions of remarkable size, which can sometime compress the surrounding myocardium and cause secondary hypoperfusion. Should occlusive endocoronaric neoplastic emboli occur, overt intramural metaneoplastic infarctions may result. Intramural metastases of the myocardium progressively increase in size and can spread to both the epicardial and endocardial components (Fig. 11.6). Neoplastic infiltration of the coronary sinus is extremely rare: in this setting, the carcinomatous cells infiltrating the fatty tissue of the basal heart region invade the atrium and involve the coronary sinus, which has been occluded by a neoplastic thrombosis.

The neoplastic invasion secondary to lymphoma almost always replaces the myocardium, with broad areas globally infiltrated by a homogeneous white-greyish tissue, with the typical "fish meat" pattern [28].

In spite of the massive loss of contractile mass, cardiac symptoms can be absent or aspecific [29]. In the few existing reports [30], the myocardium seems mostly involved by non-Hodgkin's lymphomas (78.3% vs. 66.7% of Hodgkin's lymphomas), whereas the pericardium is mostly affected in Hodgkin's lymphomas. Echocardiography may reveal a thickened myocardium, an anomalous myocardial structure, and abnormal wall contractility.

Endocardial Metastases

In the endocardium, the metastatic lesions are mainly located in the right atrium (Fig. 11.7c) or ventricle. Left atrial or ventricular lesions are relatively uncommon. The anchorage of neoplastic cells to the right chambers endocardium is favoured by lower intracavitary pressure, by the slower blood flow, and by the lower contractile strength, which are all typical of this regions. Furthermore, the neoplastic cells usually come

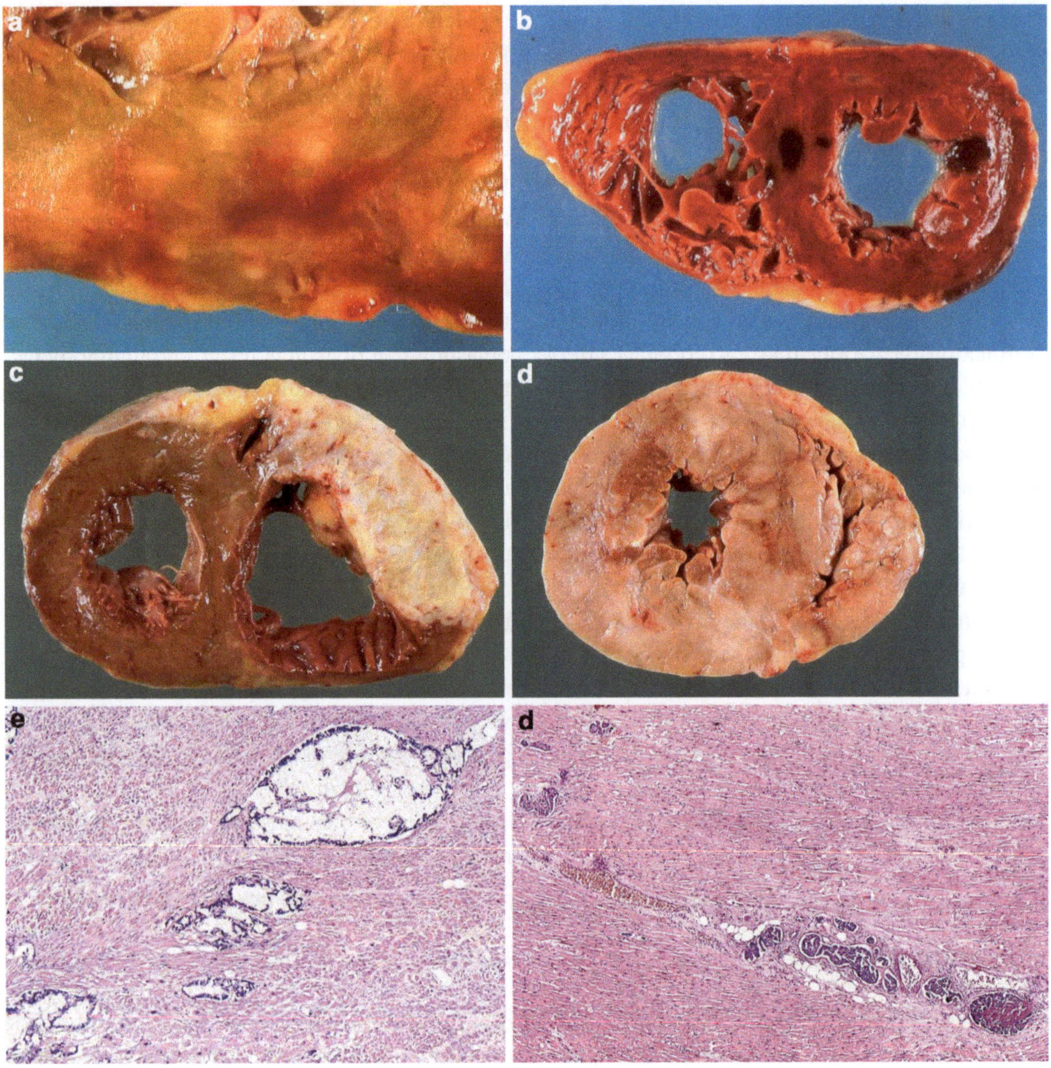

Fig. 11.6 Myocardial metastases. Multiple types and extension of intramural metastatic lesions are shown. (**a**) Small metastases from a squamous esophageal carcinoma. (**b**) Septal and ventricular metastases from a cutaneous melanoma. (**c**) Extensive transmural infiltration by an undifferentiated carcinoma of the lung. (**d**) Biventricular lymphomatous invasion. (**e**) Metastatic cells spreading along the lymphatic vessels, sometimes located near haematic vessels (**f**)

from the inferior vena cava (tumors of the kidney, liver, and uterus) or superior one (thyroid tumors), thus entering the right atrium first. Macroscopically, small, multiple thrombotic/neoplastic intertrabecular formations are often found in the right ventricle. At other times, large neoplastic thrombi can be found in the right atrium or right ventricle, where they can often cause haemodynamic obstruction and sometimes superficial erosion and fragmentation resulting in pulmonary microembolism (Fig. 11.7a).

Heart valves are an unusual target for metastases [31, 32] which is probably due to two factors, i.e., the absence of vessels in the normal valvular stroma and the continuous cusp motion. When valvular involvement occurs, the most likely pattern is that of a neoplastic thrombotic endocarditis: thrombotic material mixed with neoplastic

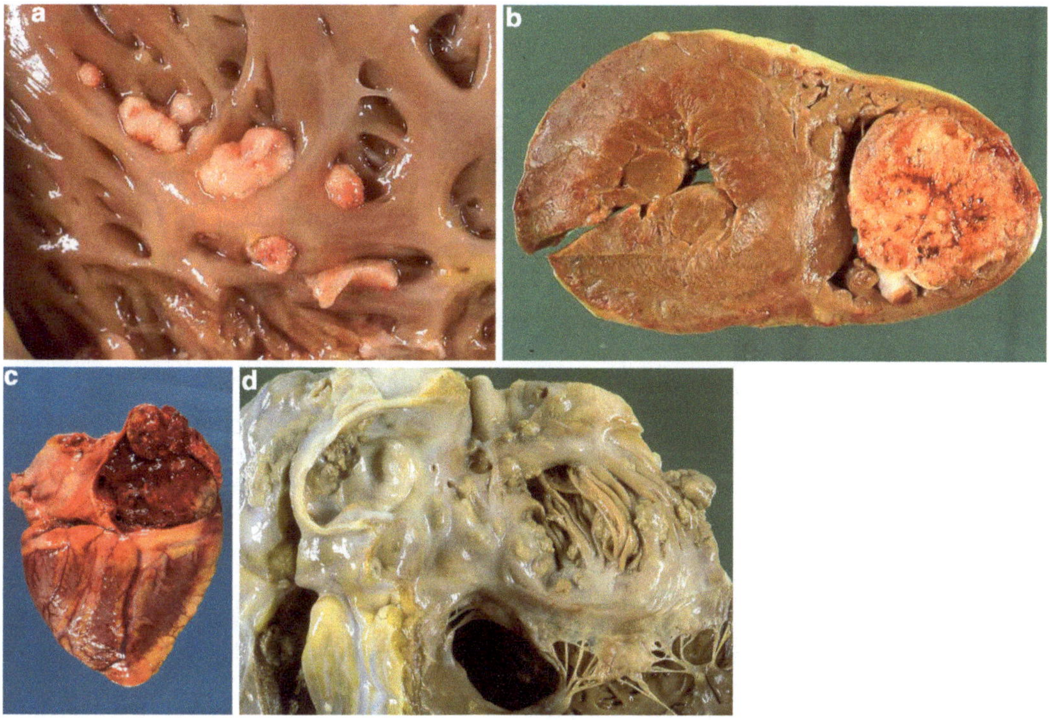

Fig. 11.7 Endocardial metastases. (**a**) Multiple small metastatic lesions in the endocardium of the right ventricle from a squamous pharyngeal carcinoma. (**b**) Extensive metastasis from a renal carcinoma occupying the entire ventricular chamber. (**c**) Massive neoplastic thrombosis of the right atrium in a patient with hepatocellular carcinoma. (**d**) Multiple, large metastatic nodules from a cutaneous melanoma in the right atrium; the lesions involve the sino-atrial node region too

elements superimpose upon an endocardium already damaged by hemodynamic and flogistic factors. This is facilitated by a state of hypercoagulation typical of many tumors [33, 34]. In our experience of thousands of postmortem examinations, we found only one case of neoplastic thrombotic endocarditis of the tricuspid valve in a patient affected by a poorly differentiated follicular carcinoma of the thyroid [35].

The Clinical Diagnosis of Pericardial Metastases

As a metastatic pericardial effusion is often the first clinical sign of a malignant tumor in patients with no history of cancer, the cytodiagnostic analysis of the same effusion can be the first step towards the determination of the origin of the neoplastic cells. Another option is the histopathological assessment of pericardial biopsy specimens after thoracotomy [1].

Patients with a metastatic carcinoma of unknown primary location represent a relatively common clinical problem which requires very important management and therapeutic decisions in order to solve it [36].

One of the most frequent examples is that of pericardial metastases from an adenocarcinoma. This tumor quite often has no histopathological characteristic pointing to the anatomical location of the primary tumor. Even though the most likely chance is that of a metastasis from a lung carcinoma [37, 38], immunohistochemical markers should nevertheless be used to get the best possible indications of the origin of the tumor.

The first goal is to understand whether the tumor is a lung adenocarcinoma, a reactive mesothelial proliferation, or an epithelial mesothelioma.

From a histochemical point of view, mucicarmine and periodic acid-Schiff stain with diastase digestion are useful to characterise the cytoplasmic mucin vacuoles, which are usually present, in variable proportions, in adenocarcinomas, while they are completely absent in mesothelioma cells. In mesotheliomas, cytoplasmic hyaluronic acid is revealed by colloidal iron or Alcian Blue. The most likely immunohistochemical algorithm for lung adenocarcinoma is the following: peripheral or membrane keratin positivity and TTF1 ("Thyroid Transcription Factor 1"), BerEP4, leu-M1, and CK7 positivity. Mesotheliomas, on the contrary, are always positive to keratins, but only to the cytoplasmic component, and to vimentin and calretin.

Unfortunately, as yet, there is no mesothelioma-positive and adenocarcinoma-negative immunohistochemical marker. The immunohistochemical diagnosis of mesothelioma can only be reached by exclusion.

The next step is to trace any other primary locations of adenocarcinomatous spread to the heart. According to some authors, a specific panel of markers (BCA225, CEA, CA125, CA19-9) could be fairly predictive for such neoplasms [39] as colon, breast, lung, and ovarian carcinomas. However, the sensitivity of these immunophenotypes is quite low, as they are expressed in varying rates by 32–39% of metastatic cells.

Other markers can also be useful. For instance, lung carcinomas are CK7 positive and CK20 negative, whereas colon adenocarcinomas are CK7 negative. On the other hand, it is easy to confirm the thyroid or prostatic origin of a pericardial metastasis as TTF1 and thyroglobulin can be used for thyroid carcinomas and prostatic-specific antigen for the prostatic carcinomas.

Cell clusters originating from a metastasised squamous cell lung carcinoma are usually CK5 positive and CK7, CK20 and TTF1 negative, whereas undifferentiated lung carcinomas are negative also for CK5 but positive for NSE (neuron-specific enolase), cromogranine and calcitonin.

No specific markers exist for breast carcinoma either [40]. Besides morphological data, CK7 positivity and CK20 negativity, oestrogen and progestogen receptors can be used, and in the past few years the so-called "gross cystic disease fluid protein-15", which seems to correlate significantly with this tumor.

A number of specific immunohistochemical panels can now permit the exact classification in the case of pericardial metastases secondary to various neoplasms, such as lymphoma (CD3, CD20, CD10, CD15, CD30, etc.), melanoma (S100, HMB45), myeloma (light-chain immunoglobulins), testicular neoplasms (CD30, hCG, CEA, alfa-feto protein) and those of the urothelial area (CK5-6, CK7, CK 20).

Immunohistochemical markers are also a fundamental tool in the diagnosis of cardiac spread from sarcomas (keratin negative and positivity to specific mesenchymal line markers).

References

1. Virmani R. Tumors metastatic to the heart and pericardium. In: Virmani R, Burke A, editors. Atlas of tumor pathology. Tumors of the heart and great vessels. 3rd Series, Fascicle 16. Washington, DC: AFIP; 1995. p. 195–209.
2. McAllister Jr HA. Tumours of the heart and pericardium. In: Silver MD, editor. Cardiovascular pathology, vol. 2. 2nd ed. New York, NY: Churchill Livingstone Inc; 1991. p. 1297–333.
3. Prichard RW. Tumors of the heart: review of the subject and report of one hundred thirty-seven cases. Arch Pathol. 1951;51:98–128.
4. Wenger NK. Pericardial disease in the elderly. Cardiovasc Clin. 1992;22:97–103.
5. Walther HE. Krebsmetastasen. Basel: Benno Schwabe; 1948. p. 37–42.
6. Willis RA. The spread of tumours in the human body, vol. 3. 2nd ed. London: Butterworths; 1952. p. 42.
7. Hanfling SM. Metastatic cancer to the heart. Review of the literature and report of 127 cases. Circulation. 1960;22:474–83.
8. Berge T, Sievers J. Myocardial metastases. A pathological and electrocardiographic study. Br Heart J. 1968;30:383–90.
9. Kline IK. Cardiac lymphatic involvement by metastatic tumor. Cancer. 1972;29:799–808.
10. Karwinski B, Svendsen E. Trends in cardiac metastasis. APMIS. 1989;97:1018–24.
11. Mukai K, Shinkai T, Tominaga K, Shimosato Y. The incidence of secondary tumors of the heart and

pericardium: a 10-year study. Jpn J Clin Oncol. 1988;18:195–201.
12. Manojlovic S. Metastatic carcinomas involving the heart. Review of post-mortem examination. Zentralbl Allg Pathol Anat. 1990;136:657–61.
13. MacGee W. Metastatic and invasive tumours involving the heart in a geriatric population: a necropsy study. Virchows Arch A Pathol Anat Histopathol. 1991;419:183–9.
14. Silvestri F, Bussani R, Pavletic N, Mannone T. Metastases of the heart and pericardium. G Ital Cardiol. 1997;27:1252–5.
15. Bussani R, De-Giorgio F, Abbate A, Silvestri F. Cardiac metastases. J Clin Pathol. 2007;60:27–34.
16. Butany J, Naseemuddin A, Nair GM, Catton C, Yau T. Cardiac tumours: diagnosis and management. Lancet Oncol. 2005;6:219–28.
17. Vaitkus PT, Hermann HC, LeWinter MM. Treatment of malignant pericardial effusion. JAMA. 1994;272:59–64.
18. Cui Y, Urschel JD, Petrelli NJ. The effect of cardiopulmonary lymphatic obstruction in heart and lung function. Thorac Cardiov Surg. 2001;49:35–40.
19. Patek PR. The morphology of the lymphatics of the mammalian heart. Am Heart J Anat. 1939;64: 203–49.
20. Jellinek H, Gabor G, Solti F, Veress B. The problem of the coronary changes due to disturbance of vascular wall permeability. Angiology. 1967;18:179–87.
21. Riquet M, Grand B, Arame A, Pricopi CF, Foucault C, Dujon A, Le Pimpec Barthes F. Lung cancer invading the pericardium: quantum of lymph nodes. Ann Thorac Surg. 2010;90:1773–7.
22. Yater WM. Tumors of the heart and pericardium: pathology, symptomatology and report of 9 cases. Arch Int Med. 1931;48:627–66.
23. Scott RW, Garvin CF. Tumors of the heart and pericardium. Am Heart J. 1939;17:431–6.
24. Burnett RC, Shimkin MB. Secondary neoplasms of the heart. Arch Int Med. 1954;33:205–18.
25. Kayser K, Mattfeldt T, Mobius HJ. Herz metastasierung beim primaren Bronchuskarzinom. Eine retrospektive Autopsiestudie. Pathologe. 1986;7:143–8.
26. Willis RA. The spread of tumors in the human body. London: J&A Churchill Ltd.; 1933. p. 259–68.
27. Pratt CB, Dugger DL, Johnson WW, Ainger LE. Metastatic involvement of the heart in childhood rhabdomyosarcoma. Cancer. 1973;31:1492–7.
28. Roberts WC, Glancy DL, De Vita Jr VT. Hodgkin's disease, lymphosarcoma, reticulum cell sarcoma and mycosis fungoides. A study of 196 autopsy cases. Am J Cardiol. 1968;22:85–107.
29. Meng Q, Lai H, Lima J, Tong W, Qian Y, Lai S. Echocardiographic and pathological characteristics of cardiac metastasis in patients with lymphoma. Oncol Rep. 2002;9:85–8.
30. Moore JA, De Ran BP, Minor R, Arthur J, Fraker TD. Transesophageal echocardiographic evaluation of intracardiac lymphoma. Am Heart J. 1992;124:514–6.
31. Hallahan DE, Vogelzang NJ, Borow KM, Bostwick DG, Simon MA. Cardiac metastases from soft-tissue sarcomas. J Clin Oncol. 1986;4:1662–9.
32. Deck AJ, True LD, Higano CS. Tricuspid valve metastasis from testicular carcinoma: a case report and review of the literature. Urology. 2000;56:330.
33. Nand S, Messmore H. Hemostasis in malignancy. Am J Hematol. 1990;35:45–55.
34. Patterson WP, Ringenberg QS. The pathophysiology of thrombosis in cancer. Semin Oncol. 1990;17:140–6.
35. Bussani R, Silvestri F. Neoplastic thrombotic endocarditis of the tricuspid valve in a patient with carcinoma of the thyroid. Report of a case. Pathol Res Pract. 1999;195:121–4.
36. Dennis JL, Hvidsten TR, Wit EC, Komorowski J, Bell AK, Downie I, Mooney J, Verbeke C, Bellamy C, Keith N, Oien KA. Markers of adenocarcinoma characteristic of the site of origin: development of a diagnostic algorithm. Clin Cancer Res. 2005;11:3766–72.
37. Tamura A, Matsubara O, Yoshimura NH, Kasuga T, Akagawa A, Aoki N. Cardiac metastasis of lung cancer. A study of metastatic pathways and clinical manifestations. Cancer. 1992;70:437–42.
38. Loire R, Hellal H. Neoplastic pericarditis. Study by thoracotomy and biopsy in 80 cases. Presse Med. 1993;22:244–8.
39. Brown RW, Campagna LB, Dunn K, Cagle PT. Immunohistochemical identification of tumor markers in metastatic adenocarcinoma. A diagnostic adjunct in the determination of primary site. Am J Clin Pathol. 1997;107:12–9.
40. Wick MR, Lillemoe TJ, Copland GT, Swanson PE, Manivel JC, Kiang DT. Gross cystic disease fluid protein-15 as a marker for breast cancer: immunohistochemical analysis of 690 human neoplasms and comparison with alpha-lactalbumin. Hum Pathol. 1989;94:18–26.

12 Systemic Therapy, Radiotherapy, and Cardiotoxicity

Chiara Lestuzzi, Gianmaria Miolo, and Antonino De Paoli

Introduction

Malignant cardiac tumors are usually sarcomas or Non-Hodgkin Lymphomas (NHL). The treatment of NHL is based on chemotherapy (CT), and surgery is commonly used as a rescue therapy to treat severe hemodynamic impairment by a large mass. CT is often effective over a short period of time in NHL (Figs. 12.1 and 12.2) and is the first choice treatment approach. The cyclophosphamide, doxorubicin, vincristine, and prednisone (CHOP) regimen has been the mainstay of therapy for several decades, and the addition, in recent years, of Rituximab (R, a monoclonal antibody) has increased its efficacy without affecting toxicity; therefore, R-CHOP is the most commonly used first-line therapy even in elderly patients, usually as many as 6–8 cycles are given [1, 2]. In non-responders or relapsing patients, high-dose therapy followed by autologous stem cell transplantation may be considered. Several standard high-dose regimens may be used: ifosphamide, carboplatin, etoposide (ICE), the same plus Taxol (TICE), etoposide, methyl prednisolone, high-dose cytarabine, cisplatin (ESHAP), dexamethasone, cisplatin, cytarabine (DHAP), and dexamethasone, cisplatin, gemcitabine (GDP) [1].

Although more frequent than primary lymphomas, cardiac sarcomas are very rare and most of the published experiences consist of case reports or small patient series. Also large institutions usually see roughly one patient/year or less (a few major referral centers may see up to 3–5 patients/year), which makes it impossible to plan randomized studies to assess the best treatment approach [3–7]. Cardiac sarcomas are a small subgroup of the more frequent (albeit rather rare) sarcomas of other sites (they represent roughly 1/100 of all sarcomas), and in most cases they pertain to the soft tissue sarcomas (STS) group. Therefore, the basic therapeutic approach should be based on extrapolation of data from the most frequent tumor sites, including STS of the extremities and trunk [4, 7–9].

Nevertheless, this approach may also be affected by some of the peculiar characteristics of cardiac compared to noncardiac sarcomas. Cardiac sarcomas tend to be high grade, angio- or leiomyosarcoma in histological subtype, and they usually have a propensity to occur at a younger age [8–10]. In addition, cardiac sarcomas are often metastatic at presentation and complete

C. Lestuzzi, M.D. (✉)
Department of Cardiology, Centro di Riferimento Oncologico (CRO), IRCCS, National Cancer Institute, Via F. Gallini 2, Aviano (PN) 33081, Italy
e-mail: clestuzzi@cro.it

G. Miolo, M.D.
Department of Medical Oncology, Centro di Riferimento Oncologico (CRO), IRCCS, National Cancer Institute, Via F. Gallini 2, Aviano (PN) 33081, Italy

A. De Paoli, M.D.
Department of Radiation Oncology, Centro di Riferimento Oncologico (CRO), IRCCS, National Cancer Institute, Via F. Gallini 2, Aviano (PN) 33081, Italy

C. Basso et al. (eds.), *Cardiac Tumor Pathology*, Current Clinical Pathology,
DOI 10.1007/978-1-62703-143-1_12, © Springer Science+Business Media New York 2013

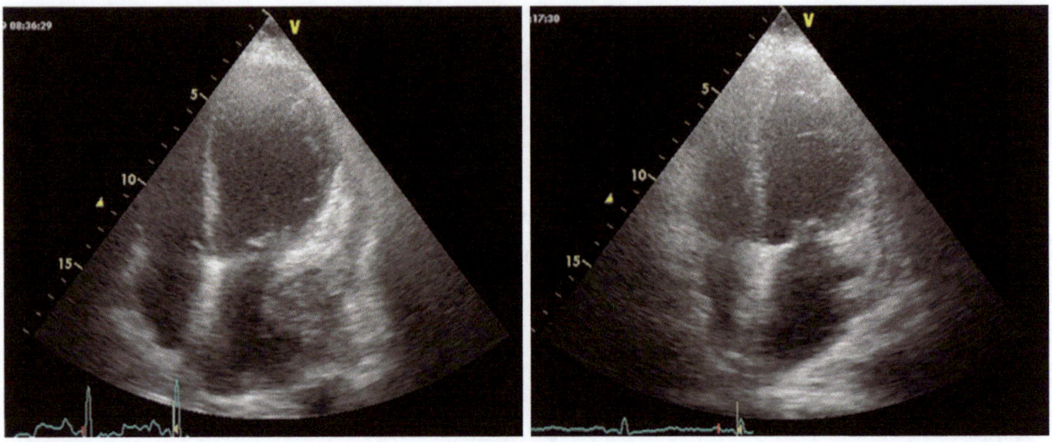

Fig. 12.1 Two-dimensional echocardiograms (apical four-chamber view) in a primary Non-Hodgkin lymphoma of the left atrium. (**a**) At diagnosis; (**b**) after two courses of R-CHOP chemotherapy (see text for acronym)

resection with negative margins is achieved in 20–45% of cases only [5, 7, 8, 11, 12]. For all these reasons, cardiac sarcomas are at higher risk of local or distant recurrence and they have a worse prognosis compared to STS of other more frequent anatomical sites, including extremities, superficial trunk, retroperitoneum, and head and neck [9].

The standard treatment for localized STS consists of adequate surgery with "wide" resection (i.e., with at least 1 cm of normal tissue around the tumor) followed by postoperative radiation therapy (RT) in most cases. Preoperative RT may be an option for large tumors or more critical tumor sites when adequate surgery with negative margins cannot be achieved [13, 14]. The role of adjuvant CT has not been yet defined so far, but clinical practice guidelines encompass it as an option in high-risk patients [14, 15].

The particular location of cardiac sarcomas makes both surgery with curative intent and the use of RT particularly challenging. While CT is mandatory in metastatic and/or locally advanced, unresectable disease, its use has been proposed for some critical locations, such as right heart/pulmonary artery sarcomas, in an attempt to increase the number of resections with negative margins [11, 16]. Therefore, a multimodality approach, including CT and/or RT before or after surgery, has been used by several authors even for localized, non-metastatic tumors, and it seems to be effective in prolonging both time to relapse and survival in some selected studies (Table 12.1). The outcome data reported in different papers are conflicting mainly for three reasons. There is a wide variety of tumor presentations (metastatic vs. non-metastatic, high-grade vs. low or intermediate grade, right vs. left heart, surgery limited to the heart or including the lung), there is no standardized surgical approach, and finally, in most studies, the multimodality therapy is limited to patients with incomplete resection or metastatic disease [11, 17–29]. Overall, when comparing studies with a multimodality approach, regardless of the surgical outcome, and historical studies with CT used in some subgroups of patients only, there seems to be a favorable trend for the multimodality approach (Fig. 12.3) [25, 29].

Systemic Therapy: Chemotherapy and Target Therapy (Table 12.2)

The "classic" and most commonly used CT regimens for soft tissue sarcomas are based on a combination of anthracyclines (ANTHRA) and ifosfamide (IFO). However, more than 50 distinct histological subtypes of sarcoma have been identified to date. Data are now available on the activity of some specific chemotherapeutic agents for some selected histological subtypes.

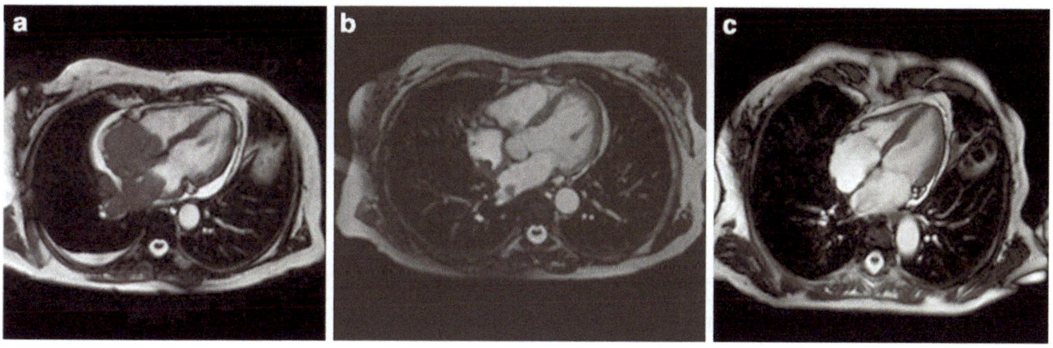

Fig. 12.2 Magnetic resonance imaging in a case of Non-Hodgkin lymphoma. (**a**) At diagnosis the mass occupies both atria, extending to pulmonary veins. (**b**) After three courses of R-CHOP chemotherapy there is a small residual mass within the left atrium. (**c**) At last follow-up after 2 years there is complete remission (see text for acronym). Courtesy of Dr. Sara Calamelli, General Hospital of Mirano (VE), Italy

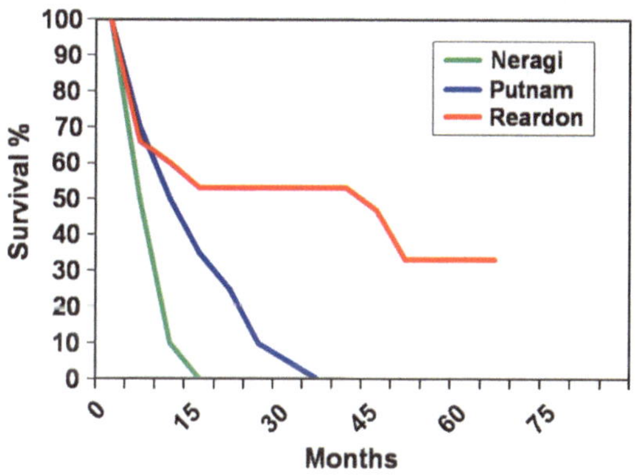

Fig. 12.3 Overall survival of patients treated with different approaches: literature cases of non-resected cases (Neragi), resected cases with or without chemotherapy (Putnam), multimodality treatment of left heart tumors with cardiac autotransplantation, and adjuvant chemotherapy (Reardon). Courtesy of Prof. Michael J. Reardon, Methodist DeBakey Heart and Vascular Center, Houston, TX, USA

This should allow, in the near future, a histology-driven CT approach for a better tailored treatment, including also cardiac sarcomas [30–33]. In addition, in the past 10 years, the increased understanding of surface receptors expression and activity as well as of the molecular pathogenesis of various tumors has led to the development of the so-called target therapy. Target therapy has significantly changed the treatment of some of these tumors such as gastrointestinal stromal tumors (GIST), dermatofibrosarcoma protuberans, and aggressive fibromatosis.

Angiogenesis, i.e., the formation of new blood vessels, is integral to the growth and metastasis of many malignancies, including STS, and it has been suggested that the balance between factors promoting the endothelial proliferation and vasal formation and factors inhibiting these processes are responsible for tumor progression [34]. Thus, a therapy affecting the creation, growth, and survival of new vessels (anti-angiogenic and/or angiotoxic) has the rationale to be effective in some tumors. The anti-angiogenic drugs showed different mechanisms of action; some may inhibit selectively a single angiogenic protein, whereas others may inhibit two, three, or a wide range of angiogenic proteins involved in endothelial proliferation and in microvascular sprouts. The drugs currently used or under evaluation in clinical trials for STS (and considered as possible options for cardiac sarcomas) are Bevacizumab, Sunitinib, Sorafenib, Dasatinib, Pazopanib, Thalidomide, and Paclitaxel [34, 35]. The successful administration of anti-angiogenic factors observed in small trials enrolling a variety of sarcomas may indicate a potential role in the treatment of highly vascular-nature cancers as heart angiosarcoma, which is the most frequent cardiac sarcoma. Anti-angiogenic therapy has some peculiar aspects compared to "classic" therapies. First, cytotoxic CT is often administered at the maximum tolerated dose with a long off-therapy interval; anti-angiogenic therapy requires endothelial cell exposure to steady blood levels of the inhibitor and anti-angiogenic

Table 12.1 Mean and median survival of patients with primary malignant tumors of the heart; literature data

Author (reference)	Years of recruitment	Year of publication	Institution	No. of patients	Treatment	Median survival (months)	Mean survival (months)	Notes
Putnam [17]	1964–1989	1991	MD Anderson	21	All treatments	11	15	
				5	Surgery	12	17	One alive
				6	Surgery + CT	17	18	One alive
				8	CT only +/– debulking	10		
Burke [18]	ND	1992	Armed Force Institute of Pathology	40	All treatments	6	11	30 complete, 10 incomplete resection; 7 perioperative deaths
				12	Surgery	3	7	
				21	Surgery + CT/RT	12	19	
Llombart-Cussac [3]	1978–1995	1998	Gustave Roussy	19	All treatments	11		
				6	Complete resection + CT	23		
				9	Incomplete resection + CT	7		
				4	CT only	5		
Centofanti [20]	1980–1997	1999	University of Turin	5	Wide resection	9	13	
Donsbeck [19]	1968–1996	1999	Multicenter	24	All treatments		16	
				8	Complete resection + CT/RT		NS	
				15	Incomplete resection/ biopsy + CT/RT	NS		
				1	No therapy			
Huo [22]	1990–2004	2006		12	All treatments	19		All pulmonary artery
				4	Surgery	9		2 alive, 1 lost to follow-up
				8	Surgery + CT/RT	21		4 alive, 2 lost to follow-up
Mayer [8]	1993–2006	2007	South West German Cancer Center	14	All treatments	15		
				6	Complete resection ± CT	15		
				4	Palliative resection + CT	15		
				4	CT only	15		
Thomas-de-Montpreville [24]	1986–2005	2007	Marie Lannelongue, Paris	8	All treatments	26	17	
				2	Complete resection	34	34	Both intermediate grade
				4	Resection + CT	18	17	All high grade
				2	Biopsy only	ND		

(continued)

Table 12.1 (continued)

Author (reference)	Years of recruitment	Year of publication	Institution	No. of patients	Treatment	Median survival (months)	Mean survival (months)	Notes
Simpson [5]	1975–2007	2008	Mayo Clinic	34	All treatments	12		
				15	Complete resection±CT/RT	15		
				8	Incomplete resection + CT	6		
				11	CT only or nothing	5		
Kim CH [6]	1994–2006	2008	Cornell University	24	All treatments	18		
				5	Complete resection	10		1 alive
				19	Incomplete resection + CT	25		4 alive
Kim HK [25]	1999–2007	2008	Samsung Medical Center	9	All treatments	19	19	All pulmonary artery, pneumonec-tomy
				4	Radical surgery	13	13	2 alive
				5	Radical sur-gery + CT/RT	22	25	1 alive
Zhang [10]	1975–2006	2008	Multicenter	27				4 postoperative deaths, 10 lost to follow-up
				3	Surgery	54	54	2 alive, NED
				3	Heart transplantation	27	39	All alive, NED
				7	Surgery + CT/RT	29	39	5 alive, 3 NED
Blackmon [29]	1998–2008	2008	Methodist DeBakey Heart Center	18	All treatments	29	28	All left heart; autotransplan-tation
				2	Surgery	3	3	
				16	Surgery + CT/RT	29	28	
Blackmon [26]	1999–2006	2009	Methodist DeBakey Heart Center	8	Complete resection + CT/RT	24		All pulmonary artery; 5 alive
Truong [7]	1990–2006	2009	British Columbia Cancer Agency	16	All treatments	8	14	
				10	Complete resection ± CT/RT		25	
				6	Incomplete resection/distant disease + CT/RT		6	
Hamidi [9]	1998–2005	2010	Multicenter	210	All treatments	6		Missing subgroup data
				125	With surgery	12		
				81	Without surgery	1		
				50	RT	11		
				159	No RT	4		

CT chemotherapy, *RT* radiotherapy, *ND* not determined, *NED* no evidence of disease

Table 12.2 Systemic schedules most frequently administered in cardiac sarcomas

	Epirubicin	*Ifosfamide*	
Dosage	60 mg/m²/die	1,8 g/m²/die	
Frequency	Days 1–2	Days 1–5	q3 weeks
Dosage	60 mg/m²/die	3 g/m²/die	
Frequency	Days 1–2	Days 1–3	q3 weeks
	Doxorubicin	*Ifosfamide*	
Dosage	50 mg/m²	5 g/m²	
Frequency	Day 1	Day 1	q3 weeks
Dosage	25 mg/m²/die continuous infusion	2 g/m²/die	
Frequency	Days 1–3	Days 1–5	q3 weeks
Dosage	30 mg/m²	3 g/m²	
Frequency	Day 1	Days 1–3	q3 weeks
	Dose intensive chemotherapy		
Dosage	75 mg/m² 72 h infusion	2 g/m²/day	
Frequency	Days 1–3	Day 1–5	q3 weeks
Dosage	90 mg/m² 72 h infusion	2.5 g/m²/day	
Frequency	Days 1–3	Days 1–4	q3 weeks
	Pegylated liposomal doxorubicin		
Dosage	20 mg/m²		
Frequency	Days 1, 15		q4 weeks
Dosage	30 mg/m²		
Frequency	Day 1		q3 weeks
	Paclitaxel		
Dosage	80 mg/m²		
Frequency	Days 1, 8, 15		q4 weeks
	Gemcitabine		
Dosage	1,000 mg/m²/die		
Frequency	Days 1, 8, 15		q4 weeks
	Gemcitabine	*Docetaxel*	
Dosage	900 mg/m²	100 mg/m²	
Frequency	Days 1, 8	Day 8	q3 weeks
Dosage	675 mg/m²	75 mg/m²	
Frequency	Days 1, 8	Day 8	q3 weeks
	Experimental drugs		
	Sorafenib		
Dosage	400 mg oral twice per day		
Frequency	Continuously		
	Imatinib		
Dosage	600 mg/die per os		
Frequency	Continuously		
	Bevacizumab		
Dosage	15 mg/kg		
Frequency	Day 1		q3 weeks

agents with a short half-life might need to be dosed daily and without any breaks [35]. Secondly, anti-angiogenic agents tend to have a biphasic, U-shaped dose–efficacy curve where blood levels that are too low or too high may be ineffective in the inhibition of angiogenesis; therefore, more is not necessarily better when it comes to anti-angiogenesis [33].

Anthracyclines and Ifosfamide

With the commonly employed first-line CT of STS, an objective response rate of 45%, including 10% of complete response and a median survival of 15 months, has been obtained [36, 37]. Accordingly, the standard systemic approach to patients with advanced/unresectable sarcomas of the heart and great vessels or to those who have progressed from earlier stages remains to be the chemotherapeutic ANTHRA-based regimen [33, 38].

Doxorubicin (DOX)-based CTs (DOX 50 mg/m^2/die on day 1 and IFO g/m^2/die on day 1 or DOX 25 mg/m^2/die on days 1, 2, and 3 and IFO 2 g/m^2/die per day on days 1–5) or epidoxorubicin (epiDOX)-based regimens (epiDOX 60 mg/m^2/die on days 1 and 2 and IFO 3 g/m^2/die on days 1–3) are now the conventional first-line treatments [39–41]. A Cochrane review showed that combination regimens, compared with single-agent DOX, achieved only marginal increases in response rates at the expense of increased toxic effects and with no improvements in overall survival [42]. Moreover, it should be emphasized that most of the CT agents used in cancer management have demonstrated a dose–response relationship. For DOX, in a randomized dose–response study the response rate was twice as high at the dose of 75 mg/m^2 as compared with 45 mg/m^2 [43]. Since response rate increases at higher doses, the increase of dose intensity may be an important strategy to favor the response rate and reduce the relapse rate. For IFO, the data are weaker, even if an higher response rate at higher doses has been reported [44]. In young patients with optimal performance status may be more useful to administer high doses of DOX (90 mg/m^2) and IFO (10 g/m^2) preceded by granulocytic growth factors and cardioprotective agents [45]. The pegylated liposomal form of DOX accumulates preferentially in tissues with increased microvascular permeability, such as the case of most tumors with active neoangiogenesis [46]. The first clinical studies with pegylated liposomal DOX in the treatment of extracardiac sarcomas have shown variable results in response rates with improved toxicity profile and at least equivalent activity in comparison to DOX [47–49]. Furthermore, pegylated liposomal ANTHRA have also produced satisfactory results in the treatment of angiosarcoma and lymphangiosarcoma [50, 51].

Taxanes

Paclitaxel and Docetaxel are natural alkaloids active for several tumor types from ovarian to breast and lung cancers. They act as cytotoxic drugs by inhibiting microtubular assembly. Paclitaxel has also anti-angiogenesis effects by inhibiting endothelial motility and proliferation as well as invasiveness [34, 52]. Many different anticancer drug combinations, including gemcitabine and docetaxel, have been demonstrated to have greater activity than gemcitabine alone [30, 53, 54]. Gemcitabine is given on days 1 and 8 at 900 mg/m^2 over 90 min and docetaxel at 100 mg/m^2 over 60 min. Typically the most sensitive histological type to the combination of gemcitabine and docetaxel in the salvage setting is fibrohistiocytic sarcoma (or malignant fibrous histiocytoma) [33]. Weekly paclitaxel has been shown to carry out an important role in the treatment of patients with heart angiosarcoma [55]. In a retrospective study enrolling 32 patients with pretreated angiosarcomas, 3 out of 5 patients with heart angiosarcoma showed stable disease or response to paclitaxel [56]. Not surprisingly, the weekly paclitaxel schedule (80 mg/m^2/die) is linked to diverse activities, from anti-angiogenesis to pro-apoptotic effects. In a series of in vitro and in vivo experiments it has been observed that low-dose schedules of paclitaxel were significantly capable of causing an inhibition in endothelial cell proliferation, motility, and invasiveness [52, 57, 58]. There is abundant evidence, therefore, that the weekly paclitaxel possesses different mechanisms of action compared with triweekly paclitaxel. However, the activity of taxanes is higher in scalp angiosarcoma than in primary angiosarcomas of other sites and ineffective for other histological subtypes of STS [59].

Target Therapy (Bevacizumab, Tyrosine Kinase Inhibitors)

Bevacizumab (Avastin®) is a humanized monoclonal antibody which neutralizes all isoforms of vascular endothelial growth factor (VEGF) and it is approved for the treatment of metastatic colorectal cancer, metastatic non-squamous non-small-cell lung cancer, metastatic breast cancer, recurrent glioblastoma multiforme, and metastatic renal cell carcinoma. Though the inhibition of tumor angiogenesis was originally thought to simply aggravate hypoxia, VEGF inhibition has also been shown to induce so-called *vascular normalization*, a restoration of normal structure, function, and flow to the disorganized vessels characteristic of malignant tumors, allowing an improvement of the delivery of oxygen, nutrients, and cytotoxic CT to the tumor. Bevacizumab has been shown to have a limited antitumoral activity as monotherapy; therefore it has been combined with cytotoxic or cytokine therapy. Data about the use of bevacizumab combined with DOX in STS are limited, and this approach deserves further investigation [34]. Some patients with cancer are or become refractory to VEGF-inhibitor treatment; a mechanism of acquired resistance is the increased reliance on alternative pro-angiogenetic factors that do not use the VEGF pathway. VEGF blockade inhibits sprouting angiogenesis, but may not be as efficient in suppressing other modes of tumor vascularization. Therefore, inhibitors of several pathways implicated in tumor growth angiogenesis and metastasis may offer advantages over inhibition of a single pathway. Sunitinib inhibits the tyrosine kinase receptors (RTKs) VEGFR1-3, platelet-derived growth factor receptor alpha (PDGFR-α), platelet-derived growth factor receptor beta (PDGFR-β), FMS-like tyrosine kinase 3 (FLT-3), c-KIT receptor, RET, and colony-stimulating factor receptor type 1, some of which have been implicated in tumor growth angiogenesis and metastasis. There is no clear evidence on utility and efficacy of this agent in the treatment of heart sarcomas since the available data come from anecdotal case reports and no prospective randomized trials have been conducted. On the other hand, it is also possible that sunitinib efficacy may be underestimated when local evaluation of anatomic response is performed using changes in tumor size according to RECIST criteria [60]. Sorafenib inhibits the RTKs VEGFR1-3, FLT-3, c-KIT, PDGFR-β, and p38 tyrosine kinases, which block the VEGF- and PDGF-dependent angiogenesis. In a phase II trial that evaluated the activity of sorafenib in patients with metastatic sarcoma, five of 37 patients with angiosarcoma had a partial response (response rate 14%); in this subgroup median progression-free survival was 3.8 months whereas median overall survival was 14.9 months. Therefore this study provides important information on the relative activity and safety profile of this drug used in this setting of patients [61], demonstrating that sorafenib has activity against angiosarcoma and minimal activity against other sarcomas. In a nother study imatinib (600 mg/die) used in patients with advanced or metastatic angiosarcoma attained a response rate about 12% whereas the non-progression rate was only 20% at 3 months [62]. Other angiogenic regulators as endostatin and caplostatin could carry out, in the future, an important role in the treatment of heart sarcomas [33, 63]. In conclusion, at the present, the recommended first-line regimen in cardiac sarcomas remains to be the ANTHRA/IFO; taxanes and/or gemcitabine have demonstrated a good activity, are used in the metastatic setting, and may be considered as first line for angiosarcomas (Figs. 12.4 and 12.5). New targeted drugs are under evaluation and may be used in relapsing or refractory tumors. An interesting new field of research in target therapy is focused on cancer stem cell characterization and on the proteomics approach, but it is still far from clinical application [64].

Radiation Therapy

Historically, RT has played a minor role in the management of patients with cardiac sarcomas primarily because of the low tolerance of the whole heart to RT and the challenge associated

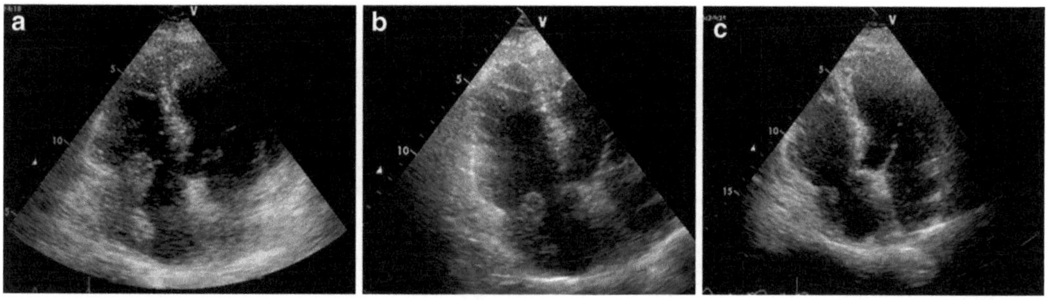

Fig. 12.4 Transthoracic two-dimensional echocardiogram (apical four-chamber view) in a case of angiosarcoma. (**a**) At diagnosis a large mass infiltrates the right atrial and right ventricular walls and prolapses through the tricuspid orifice. (**b**) After three courses of Taxol chemotherapy the mass is reduced in size. (**c**) After IMRT-Tomotherapy the mass is further reduced in size. At this time the patient underwent complete resection (see text for acronym)

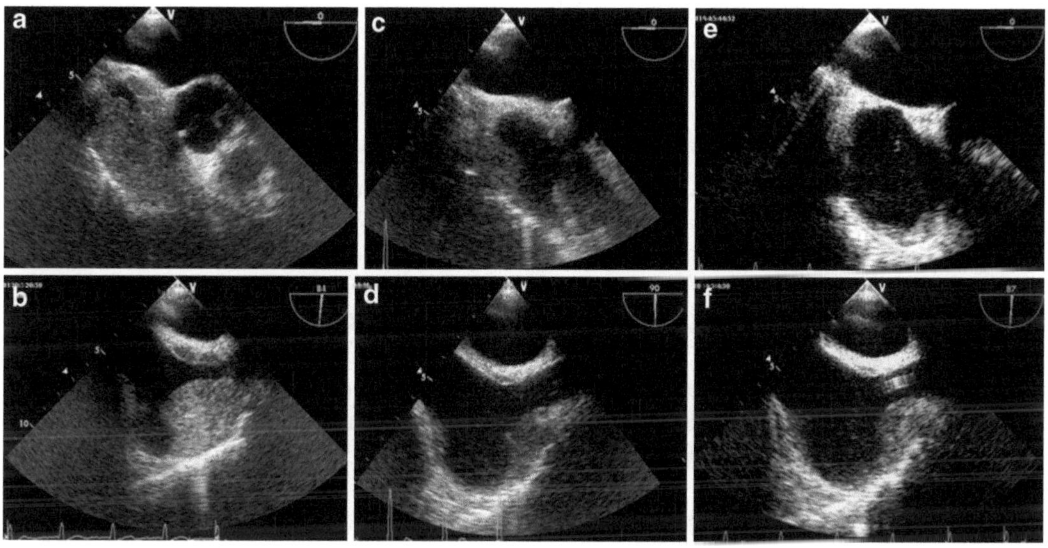

Fig. 12.5 Transesophageal echocardiogram in a case of right atrium angiosarcoma. Top horizontal plane, bottom sagittal plane. (**a**) At diagnosis a mass infiltrates extensively the right atrial walls, roof, and interatrial septum and is judged unresectable. (**b**) After chemotherapy with IFO plus liposomal DOX the mass is markedly reduced in size. (**c**) After tomotherapy the mass is further reduced in size; the interatrial septum is no more infiltrated. The patient underwent then successful removal of the whole residual mass (see text for acronyms)

with delivering highly conformal RT to the cardiac tumor, or tumor bed after resection, while sparing the non-tumor-bearing surrounding heart tissue. Although a clear correlation of dose-volume predictors for acute and late radiation-induced heart disease (RIHD) has not yet been defined, a risk >5% of RIHD after whole-heart RT of 30–35 Gy given over 4 weeks is reported [65]. Such dose of 30–35 Gy is lower than the dose required to eradicate the tumor.

Advancements that allow the safe delivery of higher dose RT to cardiac tumors include advanced imaging to improve tumor definition, 3-dimensional radiation (3D-CRT) planning techniques to deliver high dose which conform tightly to the tumor, image-guided RT (IGRT) to localize the tumor at the time of treatment, organ motion evaluation for appropriated planned target-volume definition, and improved knowledge of the partial volume tolerance of the heart

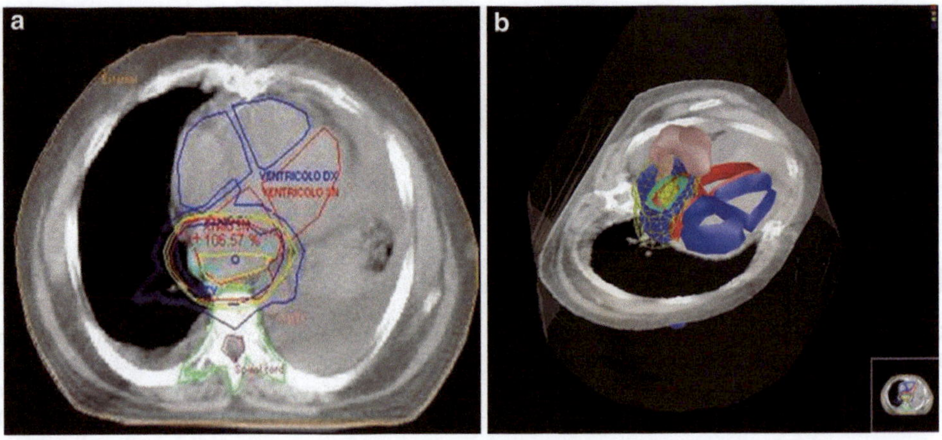

Fig. 12.6 Radiotherapy plan of 3D conformal radiotherapy for a left atrial sarcoma infiltrating the interatrial septum, atrial roof, lateral and posterior free wall, and posterior mitral annulus. (**a**) 2D plan, aiming to give 45 Gy in 25 fractions to include all the left atrium and the involved structures with organ motion margins (sparing uninvolved heart), and higher dose up to 59.4 Gy limited to the residual tumor mass. (**b**) 3D reconstruction

to radiation [66–69]. With such technological advances, it has been possible to deliver a higher dose to cardiac tumors than was previously possible with a low risk of complications. An example of a 3D-CRT plan for a patient with left atrial sarcoma is reported in Fig. 12.6.

Intensity-modulated RT (IMRT) is another technological advancement that facilitates the delivery of highly conformal RT. With IMRT, radiation is delivered with multiple small fields ("segments") within each beam, producing a modulated fluence pattern for each beam angle. Computer-aided, automated optimization of segments weights (or "inverse planning") is conducted to obtain to the best target coverage and sparing of dose to normal tissues. Clinical experience with IMRT for the treatment of cardiac sarcomas is limited. However, planning study comparison between IMRT and 3D-CRT suggests that IMRT may have a potential benefit for some patients with cardiac sarcomas [70]. The Tomotherapy system, a technological facility, is a dedicated IMRT linear accelerator that integrates IMRT by means of dynamic rotational therapy (helical tomotherapy) and IGRT by means of megavolt computerized tomography (MVCT) allowing an optimal, evaluated, and optimized target-volume dose distribution, and a daily accurate patient positioning [69]. An example of a IMRT-IGRT tomotherapy plan for a patient with right atrial sarcoma is reported in Fig. 12.7. With 3D-CRT or, more recently, by IMRT-IGRT Tomotherapy, it is possible to give RT dose as high as 45–59.4 Gy/25–33 fractions, over 5–6 weeks in patients with unresectable or partially resected cardiac sarcomas, as recently reported by our group [70]. Echocardiography examination was used in the treatment planning for organ motion evaluation and margin target-volume definition. Individualized dose constraints to left and right ventricle were included (Fig. 12.7). Two patients with unresectable tumor at presentation had major response to CT-RT and underwent a successful complete surgical resection. At a median follow-up of 22 months (range 3–84 months), nine patients were alive and six of them free of disease. In our experience, RT for cardiac sarcomas demonstrated a feasible approach, also when combined with CT and surgery. These results confirm previous published experiences in selected series of patients (Table 12.1). Technological advances in RT planning and delivery and further insight into RT cardiac tolerance appeared crucial in minimizing the risk of RIHD. Further experience is needed to confirm these encouraging results and to attempt a multidisciplinary approach with curative intent also in these unfavorable sarcomas.

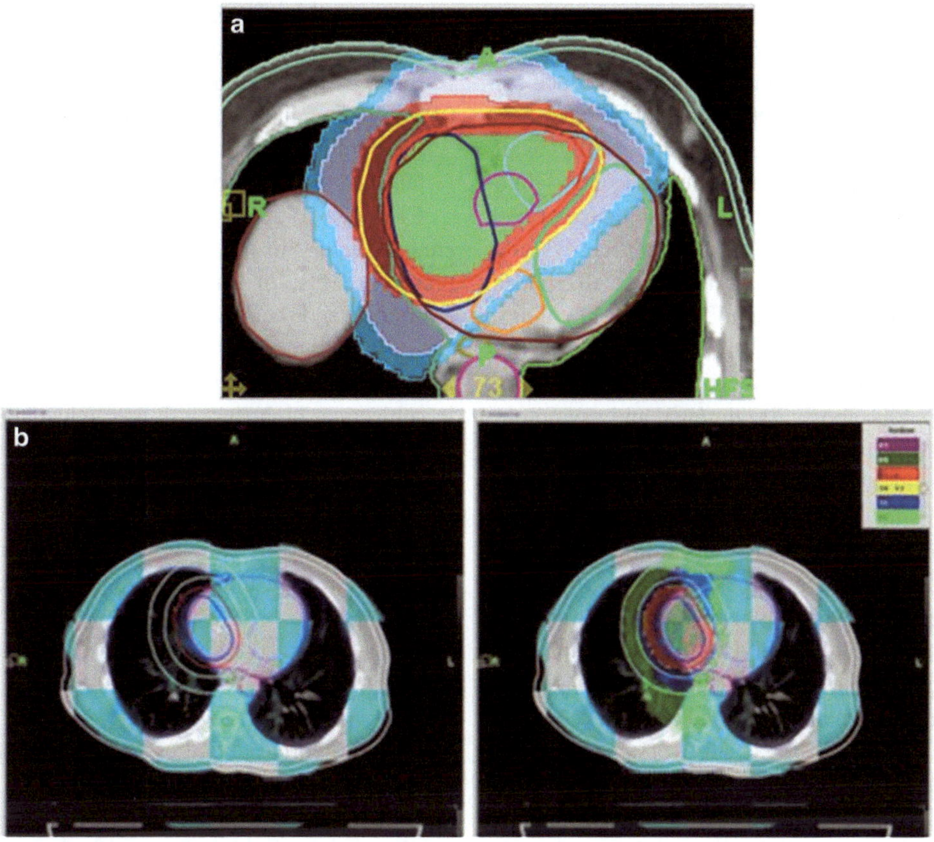

Fig. 12.7 Radiotherapy plan of preoperative IMRT-IGRT tomotherapy for a tumor involving the right atrium (roof, lateral free wall, tricuspid annulus). This patient had unresectable angiosarcoma and was treated with 45 Gy with a highly conformal plan with IMRT to include all the atrium with organ motion margins and a simultaneous dose escalation up to 54 Gy in 25 fractions limited to the tumor (equivalent to 60 Gy in 2 Gy fraction). Uninvolved heart was optimally spared (see text for acronyms). (**a**) Radiation planning before treatment. (**b**) Planning and treatment computed tomography fusion before each radiation fraction

Cardiotoxicity

Anthracyclines

Cardiotoxicity has been known as one of the most important and limiting side effects of DOX and other ANTHRA for decades. The exact pathophysiology has been debated for a long time, and is probably due to a complex interaction of several factors: iron-mediated formation of Reactive Oxygen Species (ROS), membrane lipid peroxidation, inhibition of nucleic acids and protein synthesis, altered calcium homeostasis, mitochondrial disruption, apoptotic response, formation of toxic alcoholic metabolites (DOXOL), and alterations of the cardiac-specific gene expression. The final myocyte damage is then both iron-dependent and iron-independent [71–73]. Ultrastructural early alteration in damaged myocytes consists of distension of sarcoplasmic reticulum to form sarcoplasmic vacuoles, followed by myofibrillar lysis and focal proliferation of sarcoplasmic reticulum, disruption of myofibrils, atrophy, and necrosis; interstitial edema and eventually fibrosis are observed in more severe forms; myocardial damage has been reported to be most severe in the left ventricle (LV) and in the ventricular septum, intermediate in the right ventricle and the left atrium, and least in the right atrium [74]. Each single dose of DOX causes an irreversible cardiac damage; for this reason the cardiotoxicity is cumulative, even for CT given many years apart. The final effect is diastolic and systolic left ventricular dysfunction and, in the most advanced stages, congestive heart failure (CHF). In an attempt to reduce cardiotoxicity, several DOX analogues have been developed: EpiDOX, Idarubicin (orally available), Mitoxantrone, and—more recently—liposomal DOX formulations. The incidence of both asymptomatic and symptomatic cardiac dysfunction depends mostly on the cumulative dose: CHF is rather low (around 5%) up to a total dose of 400 mg/sm of DOX and then increases exponentially (raising to 26% at a dose of 550 mg/m^2 and to 40% above 700 mg/m^2), and asymptomatic LV dysfunction is observed in 9% at a cumulative dosage of 250 mg/sm, and 65% above 550 mg/m^2 [75]. Several risk factors have been indentified for ANTHRA cardiotoxicity: age <18 and >60 years, preexisting cardiac disease (ischemic, hypertensive) and/or LV dysfunction, concomitant RT involving the heart, and high concentration of the single dose [75, 76]. Of particular concern is the delayed onset of cardiotoxicity in long-term cancer survivors; recent studies have demonstrated that the alcoholic metabolites (like DOXOL and EpiDOXOL) are retained within the myocardial cell much longer than the parent drug, and may represent a lifelong toxic reservoir inducing a heart frailty when exposed to other stressors and that these toxic metabolites increase when DOX is administered together with taxanes [71, 77]. A number of strategies have been explored to prevent or reduce ANTHRA cardiotoxicity: changes in infusion schedules; association of antioxidants (vitamin E, selenium, and so on), calcium-channel blockers, iron-chelators (as Dexrazoxane), angiotensin-converting enzyme (ACE) inhibitors, and beta-blockers; and cardiac monitoring with serial LV function assessment or with biomarkers as troponins. The most effective ways to prevent cardiotoxicity are [73, 78–81]:

(a) The concomitant use of dexrazoxane, an iron-chelating agent, that has been proven to significantly reduce cardiac dysfunction without affecting the antineoplastic effect of DOX.
(b) The use of prolonged infusions (>6 h; preferably 48–72 h continuous infusions) rather than bolus administration.
(c) The use of EpiDOX that is roughly 30% less cardiotoxic compared to DOX, and less potentiated by the concomitant use of taxanes.
(d) The use of liposomal formulations that limit the cardiac uptake of the drug leaving unaltered the tumor delivery.

CHF due to ANTHRA toxicity was considered refractory to medical therapy for years; at present, the use of conventional drugs as ACE-inhibitors and beta-blockers has been proven effective both in treating overt cardiotoxicity and in preventing the progression of LV dysfunction in subjects at high risk with preclinical signs of cardiac damage [82–85]. So, besides the above-mentioned strategies to prevent cardiotoxicity, a strict monitoring during the treatment is recommended; at the first signs of LV dysfunction therapy with ACE-inhibitors should be started.

Ifosfamide

The main reported toxicities of IFO are nephrotoxicity and neurotoxicity. From the cardiac point of view it has been usually considered safe, but cardiac toxicity in high-dose (>10 g/m^2) treated patients has been reported, and is significant (>10%) when using >15 g/m^2 [83, 86–88]. Possibly, there is a link between nephrotoxicity and cardiotoxicity: the LV dysfunction follows usually an increase in blood creatinine, and—according to a recent experimental study—IFO-induced Fanconi syndrome may cause a carnitine deficiency dangerous for the heart [87, 89]. Since IFO is usually given together with ANTHRA, a strict follow-up using echocardiography and myocardial damage biomarkers (in order to early diagnosing and treating LV dysfunction) is recommended [83].

Taxanes

Taxane cardiotoxicity is mainly evident as self-limiting supraventricular arrhythmias (atrial fibrillation, sinus bradycardia), but they may also increase DOX (much less EpiDOX) toxicity, as above mentioned, altering ANHTRA pharmacokinetics and possibly promoting the formation of toxic metabolites [71, 72, 87]. To prevent this problem, the two drugs should be administered apart, and DOX before taxanes. Cases of allergic myocarditis have also been reported, mostly with paclitaxel; some authors argued that they could be due not to the drug itself but to its solvent, the Cremophor EL [72, 87]. Moreover, anaphylactic reactions (ARs) have been frequently described with taxanes, with a mortality reported more often with docetaxel than paclitaxel; prophylactic pre-medications did not significantly impact mortality from ARs with docetaxel, but was associated with significantly lower mortality from ARs with paclitaxel [90].

Vascular Endothelial Growth Factor Blocking Agents and Tyrosine Kinase Inhibitors

Two types of side effects have to be considered: on-target (due to the same mechanisms acting as antitumoral; these effects may be also a biological marker of antineoplastic efficacy) and off-target. The VEGF block (by the monoclonal antibody Bevacizumab and the tyrosine kinase inhibitors (TKI) Sunitinib and Sorafenib) causes hypertension (mainly by reducing the nitric oxide release by the endothelial cells, by interfering with renal physiology, and by increasing the vascular resistance), thromboembolism, and hemorrhages [90–92]. Moreover, the activation of VEGF is crucial in wound repair, in maintaining capillary density in the hypertrophied heart, and for the neoangiogenesis in ischemic and diabetic heart disease; its block may then have deleterious effects in patients with preexisting cardiac diseases or undergoing cardiotoxic CT. There are some differences among the pharmacokinetics of these three drugs: Sunitinib and Sorafenib have an half-life of hours, while Bevacizumab half-life varies from 10 to 50 days (mean 20) in different patients: during prolonged treatments, then, Bevacizumab may cause a progressively worsening hypertension. After introducing in the market Sunitinib and Sorafenib, an unexpectedly high rate of cardiovascular side effects, including a direct myocardial damage, has been noticed. Besides the effects due to the VEGF block, in fact, there are a number of off-target effects common to the whole class of TKI: most important are myocardial damage and prolongation of QT interval at ECG (with the risk of life-threatening ventricular arrhythmias). Different molecules have different cardiotoxicity, and besides the dozens of TKI already in use, there are hundreds still under evaluation: the topic of TKI cardiotoxicity is an everyday changing field, and the mechanisms are still to be defined [92, 94]. In fact, the role in cardiac physiopathology of the 90 human tyrosine kinases (and, then, the effect of their block) is largely unknown; some of them protect the myocardial cell from ischemic or oxidative stress, are involved in the reparative process after myocardial ischemia, or have generally an antiapoptotic action. According to the most recent studies, TKI-induced LV dysfunction is due to a direct cytotoxic effect, with mechanisms different from ANTHRA cardiotoxicity, cannot be prevented by dexrazoxane, and is not always reversible upon withdrawal of the drug or even with commonly used cardiac therapy with ACE-inhibitors and beta-blockers; the risk is inversely proportional to the selectivity of TKI [94–96]. Since LV dysfunction seems to be more frequent in patients with uncontrolled hypertension, and according to the experimental data, probably the cardiotoxic effect of anti-VEGF drugs may be due to a combination of hypertensive stimulus and of inhibition of the homeostatic mechanisms protecting the myocardium from the pressure overload stress (on-target effect); as regards Sunitinib and other multitarget TKI, there might be additionally a direct cytotoxic effect (off-target effect). For these reasons, the only strategies to prevent LV dysfunction are presently an accurate management of hypertension and a regular echocardiographic follow-up.

Radiotherapy

Data about radiation heart disease are derived by studies in two kinds of human populations (the atomic bomb survivors and the long-term survivors of tumors—mostly Hodgkin's disease and left

Table 12.3 Echocardiographic ejection fraction (EF) before chemotherapy (CT), after CT and before radiotherapy (RT), and at last follow-up after RT

Sex, age (type of RT)	CT/RT INTENT (surgical status)	Site	EF before CT (%)	EF before RT (%)	EF after RT (%)	Follow-up (months)	State at follow-up
m 57 (3D-CRT)	Curative (unresectable)	LA	58	65	58	101	Alive NED
m 61 (IMRT)*	Adjuvant (R2 resection)	PA		64	68	20	Dead of 2nd neoplasm
m 25 (3D-CRT)	Curative (unresectable)	RA, SVC	60	62	49	36	Dead of local progression
f 58 (IMRT)	Adjuvant (R1 resection)	LA, LV	64	62	58	36	Alive with metastases
m 44 (3D-RT)	Curative (unresectable)	RA, RV	69	65	66	12	Dead of metastases
f 69 (IMRT)	Curative (incomplete resection	LA	72	72	70	15	Dead of metastases
m 39 (Tomo)	Adjuvant (R2 resection)	RA, IAS	68	58	63	20	Dead of metastases
m 72 (Tomo)§	Neoadjuvant #	RA, RV	70	69	59	16	Dead of local relapse
f 57 (Tomo)	Adjuvant (R2 resection)	RA, LA	72	72	68	21	Alive with local disease
m 39 (Tomo)	Palliative after local relapse	Pericardium	70	53	63	13 after relapse, 34 overall	Dead of local progression
m 44 (Tomo)	Neoadjuvant #	RA, IAS	62	64	65	16	Dead of metastases

Patient signed with: asterisk symbol did not receive any CT, signed with section symbol taxanes only, and signed with hash symbol had radical surgery after neoadjuvant CT/RT

3D-CRT 3-dimensional conformational RT, *IMRT* intensity-modulated RT, *Tomo* tomotherapy, *f* female, *m* male, *nd* not determined, *IAS* interatrial septum, *LA* left atrium, *LV* left ventricle, *PA* pulmonary artery, *RA* right atrium, *RV* right ventricle, *NED* no evidence of disease

breast cancer—undergone therapeutic irradiation), and by animal experiments. Ionizing radiation may cause acute symptomatic effects, and chronic or delayed effects. Coronary artery disease, valvular heart disease, and constrictive pericarditis are the typical chronic side effects affecting long-term survivors: they become clinically evident usually 10 years after treatment, with increasing incidence at longer follow-up [67]. Since the 5-years survival of patients with malignant cardiac tumors is still low, the main problem, in these particular patients, is the acute or medium-term cardiac toxicity. The first acute effect of irradiation is a pro-inflammatory effect, with endothelial damage of medium-large vessels and microvessels, pericarditis, and myocarditis; mast cells seem to have a protective effect [66–68]. Pericardium is the most frequently affected site: acute pericarditis is associated with edematous swelling of the pericardial layers: it may present in a painless effusive form with spontaneous recovery, or as an acute fibrinous pericarditis (with classical signs and symptoms of pericardial rubs and pain) that can be cured with Nonsteroidal Anti-inflammatory Drugs. In both cases, pericardial effusion is usually mild to moderate, and in 80% of cases there are no reliquates, while in 20% the disease evolves toward a constrictive pericarditis [97]. The microvessel damage is followed by a persistent decrease in capillary density and eventually leads to chronic myocardial ischemia and degeneration; an impairment in myocardial perfusion may be observed in the first months after RT, even if the increased risk of clinically evident RT-linked ischemic heart disease becomes statistically significant only after 10 years [68, 97–100]. In our experience, using modern radiation techniques, we did not observe any clinically relevant myocardial dysfunction on the short-medium term of observation in 11 patients with cardiac tumors treated with RT with or without previous CT, including three long-term >30 months survivors [70] (Table 12.3).

Conclusions

Malignant heart tumors are usually aggressive and have a dismal prognosis. The mainstay of therapy for sarcomas is radical surgery. Multimodality treatment including systemic therapy and/or RT seems to prolong the time to relapse and overall survival. Most of the treatments have a considerable risk of cardiac toxicity, but this risk should be balanced against the risk of tumor progression. Since the survival is usually limited to few years, the main concern is to prevent short- and medium-term toxicity. CT adverse effects may be prevented with careful dosage of drugs, cardioprotective agents, and strict monitoring of cardiac function. Short- and medium-term cardiac toxicity of RT may be limited using modern radiation techniques. A number of new targeted therapies are under evaluation and will hopefully improve the outcome of this severe pathology.

References

1. Flowers CR, Sinha R, Vose JM. Improving outcomes for patients with diffuse large B-cell lymphoma. CA Cancer J Clin. 2010;60:393–408.
2. Tilly H, Dreyling M, ESMO Guidelines Working Group. Diffuse large B-cell non-Hodgkin's lymphoma: ESMO clinical practice guidelines for diagnosis, treatment and follow-up. Ann Oncol. 2010;21 Suppl 5:v172–4.
3. Llombart-Cussac A, Pivot X, Contesso G, Rhor-Alvarado A, Delord JP, Spielmann M, Tűrsz T, Le Cesne A. Adjuvant chemotherapy for primary cardiac sarcomas: the IGR experience. Br J Cancer. 1998;78:1624–8.
4. Debourdeau P, Gligorov J, Teixeira L, Aletti M, Zammit C. Tumeurs cardiaques malignes. Bull Cancer. 2004;91:S136–46.
5. Simpson L, Kumar SK, Okuno SH, Schaff HV, Porrata LF, Buckner JC, Moynihan TJ. Malignant primary cardiac tumors. Review of a single institution experience. Cancer. 2008;112:2440–6.
6. Kim CH, Dancer JY, Coffey D, Zhai QJ, Reardon M, Ayala AG, Ro JY. Clinicopathologic study of 24 patients with primary cardiac sarcomas: a 10-year single institution experience. Hum Pathol. 2008;39:933–8.
7. Truong PT, Jones SO, Martens B, Alexander C, Paquette M, Joe H, Hart J, Allan SJ. Treatment and outcomes in adult patients with primary cardiac sarcoma: the British Columbia Cancer Agency experience. Ann Surg Oncol. 2009;16:3358–65.
8. Mayer F, Aebert H, Rudert M, Königsrainer A, Horger M, Kanz L, Bamberg M, Ziemer G, Hartmann JT. Primary malignant sarcomas of the heart and great vessels in adult patients. A single-center experience. Oncologist. 2007;12:1134–42.
9. Hamidi M, Moody JS, Weigel TL, Kozak KR. Primary cardiac sarcoma. Ann Thorac Surg. 2010;90:176–81.
10. Zhang PJ, Brooks JS, Goldblum JR, Yoder B, Seethala R, Pawel B, Gorman JH, Gorman RC, Huang JH, Acker M, Narula N. Primary cardiac sarcomas: a clinicopathologic analysis of a series with follow-up information in 17 patients and emphasis on long-term survival. Hum Pathol. 2008;39:1385–95.
11. Vaporciyan A, Reardon MJ. Right heart sarcomas. Methodist Debakey Cardiovasc J. 2010;6:44–8.
12. Reardon MJ. Malignant tumor overview. Methodist Debakey Cardiovasc J. 2010;6:35–7.
13. NCCN Practice Guidelines in Oncology (NCCN GuidelinesTM). Soft tissue sarcomas. Version 1. 2011. http://www.NCCN.org.
14. Casali PG, Blay JY, ESMO/CONTICANET/EUROBONET Consensus Panel of Experts. Soft tissue sarcomas: ESMO Clinical Practice Guidelines for diagnosis, treatment and follow-up. Ann Oncol. 2010;21 Suppl 5:v198–203 (Erratum in: Ann Oncol. 2010;21:1736).
15. Pervaiz N, Colterjohn N, Farrokhyar F, Tozer R, Figueredo A, Ghert M. A systematic meta-analysis of randomized controlled trials for adjuvant chemotherapy for localized soft tissue sarcoma. Cancer. 2008;113:573–81.
16. Blackmon SH, Reardon MJ. Pulmonary artery sarcoma. Methodist Debakey Cardiovasc J. 2010;6:38–43.
17. Putnam JB, Sweeney MS, Colon R, Lanza LA, Frazier OH, Cooley DA. Primary cardiac sarcomas. Ann Thorac Surg. 1991;51:906–10.
18. Burke AP, Cowan D, Virmani R. Primary sarcomas of the heart. Cancer. 1992;69:387–95.
19. Donsbeck A-V, Ranchere D, Coindre J-M, Le Gall F, Cordier J-F, Loire R. Primary cardiac sarcomas: an immunohistochemical and grading study with long-term follow-up of 24 cases. Histopathology. 1999;34:295–304.
20. Centofanti P, Di Rosa E, Deorsola L, Dato GM, Patanè F, La Torre M, Barbato L, Verzini A, Fortunato G, di Summa M. Primary cardiac tumors: early and late results of surgical treatment in 91 patients. Ann Thorac Surg. 1999;68:1236–41.
21. Bakaeen FG, Reardon MJ, Coselli JS, Miller CC, Howell JF, Lawrie GM, Espada R, Ramchandani MK, Noon GP, Weilbaecher DG, DeBakey ME. Surgical outcome in 85 patients with primary cardiac tumors. Am J Surg. 2003;186:641–7.
22. Huo L, Moran CA, Fuller GN, Gladish G, Suster S. Pulmonary artery sarcoma. Am J Clin Pathol. 2006;125:419–24.
23. Neragi-Miandoab S, Kim J, Vlahakes GJ. Malignant tumors of the heart: a review of tumor type, diagnosis and therapy. Clin Oncol. 2007;19:748–56.
24. Thomas-de-Montpréville V, Nottin R, Dulmet E, Serraf A. Heart tumors in children and adults:

clinicopathological study of 59 patients from a surgical center. Cardiovasc Pathol. 2007;16:22–8.
25. Kim HK, Choi YS, Kim K, Shim YM, Sung K, Lee YT, Park PW, Kim J. Surgical treatment for pulmonary artery sarcoma. Eur J Cardio-Thoracic Surg. 2008;33:712–6.
26. Blackmon SH, Rice DC, Correa AM, Mehran R, Putnam JB, Smythe WR, Walkes JC, Walsh GL, Moran C, Singh H, Vaporciyan AA, Reardon M. Management of primary pulmonary artery sarcomas. Ann Thorac Surg. 2009;87:977–84.
27. Bakaeen FG, Jaroszewski DE, Rice DC, Walsh GL, Vaporciyan AA, Swisher SS, Benjamin R, Blackmon S, Reardon MJ. Outcomes after surgical resection of cardiac sarcoma in the multimodality treatment era. J Thorac Cardiovasc Surg. 2009;137:1454–60.
28. Orlandi A, Ferlosio A, Roselli M, Chiariello L, Spagnoli LG. Cardiac sarcomas. An update. J Thorac Oncol. 2010;5:1483–9.
29. Blackmon SH, Patel AR, Bruckner BA, Beyer EA, Rice DC, Vaporciyan AA, Wojciechowski Z, Correa AM, Reardon MJ. Cardiac autotransplantation for malignant or complex primary left-heart tumors. Tex Heart Inst J. 2008;35:296–300.
30. Kopp HG, Patel S, Brücher B, Hartmann JT. Potential combination chemotherapy approaches for advanced adult-type soft-tissue sarcoma. Am J Clin Dermatol. 2008;9:207–17.
31. Chao J, Chow WA, Somlo G. Novel targeted therapies in the treatment of soft-tissue sarcomas. Expert Rev Anticancer Ther. 2010;10:1303–11.
32. Homsi J, Daud AI. Spectrum of activity and mechanism of action of VEGF/PDGF inhibitors. Cancer Control. 2007;14:285–94.
33. Ravi V, Benjamin RS. Systemic therapy for cardiac sarcomas. Methodist Debakey Cardiovasc J. 2010;6:57–60.
34. Ganjoo K, Jacobs C. Antiangiogenesis agents in the treatment of soft tissue sarcomas. Cancer. 2010;116:1177–83.
35. Kisker O, Becker CM, Prox D, Fannon M, D'Amato R, Flynn E, Fogler WE, Sim BK, Allred EN, Pirie-Shepherd SR, Folkman J. Continuous administration of endostatin by intraperitoneally implanted osmotic pump improves the efficacy and potency of therapy in a mouse xenograft tumor model. Cancer Res. 2001;15:7669–74.
36. Le Cesne A, Judson I, Crowther D, Rodenhuis S, Keizer HJ, Van Hoesel Q. Randomized phase III study comparing conventional-dose doxorubicin plus ifosfamide *versus* high-dose doxorubicin plus ifosfamide plus recombinant human granulocyte macrophage colony-stimulating factor in advanced soft-tissue sarcomas: a trial of the EORTC-STBSG. J Clin Oncol. 2000;18:2676–84.
37. Schütte J, Mouridsen HT, Stewart W, Santoro A, van Oosterom AT, Somers R, Blackledge G, Verweij J, Dombernowsky P, Thomas D. Ifosfamide plus doxorubicin in previously untreated patients with advanced soft tissue sarcoma. The EORTC Soft Tissue and Bone Sarcoma Group. Eur J Cancer. 1990;26:558–61.
38. Grimer R, Judson I, Peake D, Seddon B. Guidelines for the management of soft tissue sarcomas. Sarcoma. 2010;2010:506182.
39. Casali P, Pastorino U, Azzarelli A, Bertulli R, Zucchinelli P, Devizzi L, Santoro A. Perspectives on anthracyclines plus ifosfamide in advanced soft tissue sarcoma. Cancer Chemother Pharmacol. 1993;31 Suppl 2:S228–32.
40. Sarcoma Meta-analysis Collaboration. Adjuvant chemotherapy for localised resectable soft-tissue sarcoma of adults: metaanalysis of individual data. Lancet. 1997;350:1647–54.
41. Frustaci S, Gherlinzoni F, De Paoli A, Bonetti M, Azzarelli A, Comandone A, Olmi P, Buonadonna A, Pignatti G, Barbieri E, Apice G, Zmerly H, Serraino D, Picci P. Adjuvant chemotherapy for adult soft tissue sarcomas of the extremities and girdles: results of the Italian randomized cooperative trial. J Clin Oncol. 2001;19:1238–47.
42. Bramwell VH, Anderson D, Charette ML. Doxorubicin-based chemotherapy for the palliative treatment of adult patients with locally advanced or metastatic soft tissue sarcoma. Cochrane Database Syst Rev. 2003;CD003293
43. O'Bryan RM, Baker LH, Gottlieb JE, Rivkin SE, Balcerzak SP, Grumet GN, Salmon SE, Moon TE, Hoogstraten B. Dose response evaluation of Adriamycin in human neoplasia. Cancer. 1977;39:1940–8.
44. Patel SR, Vadhan-Raj S, Papadopolous N, Plager C, Burgess MA, Hays C, Benjamin RS. High-dose ifosfamide in bone and soft-tissue sarcomas: results of phase II and pilot studies-dose response and schedule dependence. J Clin Oncol. 1997;15:2378–84.
45. Patel SR, Vadhan-Raj S, Burgess MA, Plager C, Papadopolous N, Jenkins J, Benjamin RS. Results of 2 consecutive trials of dose-intensive chemotherapy with doxorubicin and ifosfamide in patients with sarcomas. Am J Clin Oncol. 1998;21:317–21.
46. Wu NZ, Da D, Rudoll TL, Needham D, Whorton AR, Dewhirst MW. Increased microvascular permeability contributes to preferential accumulation of Stealth liposomes in tumor tissue. Cancer Res. 1993;53:3765–70.
47. Garcia AA, Kempf RA, Rogers M, Muggia FM. A phase II study of Doxil (liposomal doxorubicin): lack of activity in poor prognosis soft tissue sarcomas. Ann Oncol. 1998;9:1131–3.
48. Skubitz KM. Phase II trial of pegylated-liposomal doxorubicin (Doxil™) in sarcoma. Cancer Invest. 2003;21:167–76.
49. Skubitz M, Haddad PA. Paclitaxel and pegylated-liposomal doxorubicin are both active in angiosarcoma. Cancer. 2005;15:361–6.
50. Eiling S, Lischner S, Busch J-O, Rothaupt D, Christophers E, Hauschild A. Complete remission of a radio-resistant cutaneous angiosarcoma of the scalp by systemic treatment with liposomal doxorubicin. Brit J Derm. 2002;147:150–3.
51. Verdier E, Carvalo P, Young P, Musette P, Courville P, Joly P. Lymphangiosarcoma treated with liposomal

doxorubicin. Ann Dermatol Venerol. 2007; 134:760–3.
52. Belotti D, Vergani V, Drudis T, Borsotti P, Pitelli MR, Viale G, Giavazzi R, Taraboletti G. The microtubule-affecting drug paclitaxel has anti-angiogenic activity. Clin Cancer Res. 1996;2:1843–9.
53. Patel SR, Gandhi V, Jenkins J, Papadopolous N, Burgess MA, Plager C, Plunkett W, Benjamin RS. Phase II clinical investigation of gemcitabine in advanced soft-tissue sarcomas and window evaluation of dose-rate on gemcitabine triphosphate accumulation. J Clin Oncol. 2001;19:3483–9.
54. Hensley ML, Maki R, Venkatraman E, Geller G, Lovegren M, Aghajanian C, Sabbatini P, Tong W, Barakat R, Spriggs DR. Gemcitabine and docetaxel in patients with unresectable leiomyosarcoma: results of a phase II trial. J Clin Oncol. 2002;20:2824–31.
55. Penel N, Bui BN, Bay JO, Cupissol D, Ray-Coquard I, Piperno-Neumann S, KerbratP, Fournier C, Taieb S, Jimenez M, Isambert N, Peyrade F, Chevreau C, Bompas E, Brain EG, Blay JY. Phase II trial of weekly paclitaxel for unresectable angiosarcoma: the AngioTax study. J Clin Oncol. 2008;26:5269–74.
56. Schlemmer M, Reichardt P, Verweij J, Hartmann JT, Judson I, Thyss A, Hogendoorn PCW, Marreaud S, Van Glabbeke M, Blay JY. Paclitaxel in patients with advanced angiosarcomas of soft tissue: a retrospective study of the EORTC soft tissue and bone sarcoma group. Eur Jof Cancer. 2008;44:2433–6.
57. Bocci G, Nicolaou KC, Kerbel RS. Protracted low-dose effects on human endothelial cell proliferation and survival *in vitro* reveal a selective anti-angiogenic window for various chemotherapeutic drugs. Cancer Res. 2002;62:6938–43.
58. Browder T, Butterfield CE, Kräling BM, Shi B, Marshall B, O'Reilly MS. Anti-angiogenic scheduling of chemotherapy improves efficacy against experimental drug-resistant cancer. Cancer Res. 2000;60:1878–86.
59. Verweij J, Lee SM, Ruka W, Buesa J, Coleman R, van Hoessel R, Seynaeve C, di Paola ED, van Glabbeke M, Tonelli D, Judson IR. Randomized phase II study of docetaxel versus doxorubicin in first-line and second-line chemotherapy for locally advanced or metastatic soft tissue sarcomas in adults: a study of the European Organization for Research and Treatment of Cancer Soft Tissue and Bone Sarcoma Group. J Clin Oncol. 2000;18:2081–6.
60. George S, Merriam P, Maki RG, Van den Abbeele AD, Yap JT, Akhurst T, Harmon DC, Bhuchar G, O'Mara MM, D'Adamo DR, Morgan J, Schwartz GK, Wagner AJ, Butrynski JE, Demetri GD, Keohan ML. Multicenter phase II trial of sunitinib in the treatment of nongastrointestinal stromal tumor sarcomas. J Clin Oncol. 2009;27:3154–60.
61. Maki RG, D'Adamo DR, Keohan ML, Saulle M, Schuetze SM, Undevia SD, Livingston MB, Cooney MM, Hensley ML, Mita MM, Takimoto CH, Kraft AS, Elias AD, Brockstein B, Blachère NE, Edgar MA, Schwartz LH, Qin LX, Antonescu CR, Schwartz GK. Phase II study of sorafenib in patients with metastatic or recurrent sarcomas. J Clin Oncol. 2009;27:3133–40.
62. Chugh R, Wathen JK, Maki RG, Benjamin RS, Patel SR, Meyers PA, Priebat DA, Reinke DK, Thomas DG, Keohan ML, Samuels BL, Baker LH. Phase II multicenter trial of imatinib in 10 histologic subtypes of sarcoma using a Bayesian hierarchical statistical model. J Clin Oncol. 2009;27:3148–53.
63. Penel N, Marreaud S, Robin YM, Hohenberger P. Angiosarcoma: state of the art and prospectives. Crit Rev Oncol/Hematol 2011;80:257–63.
64. Ordonez JL, Martins AS, Osuna D, Madoz-Gùrpide J, de Alava E. Targeting sarcomas: therapeutic targets and their rational. Sem Diagn Pathol. 2008;25: 304–16.
65. Gagliardi G, Constine LS, Moiseenko V, Correa C, Pierce LJ, Allen AM, Marks L. Radiation dose-volume effects in the heart. Int J Radiat Oncol Biol Phis. 2010;76(3 Suppl):S77–85.
66. Basavaraju SR, Easterly CE. Pathophysiological effects of radiation on atherosclerosis development and progression, and the incidence of cardiovascular complications. Med Phys. 2002;29:2391–403.
67. Boerma M, Wang J, Wondergem J, Joseph J, Qui X, Kennedy RH, Hauer-Jensen M. Influence of mast cells on structural and functional manifestations of radiation-induced heart disease. Cancer Res. 2005;65: 3100–7.
68. Schultz-Hector S, Trott KR. Radiation-induced cardiovascular diseases: is the epidemiologic evidence compatible with the radiobiologic data? Int J Radiat Oncol Biol Phys. 2007;67:10–8.
69. Goitein M. Organ and tumor motion: an overview. Semin Radiat Oncol. 2004;14:2–9.
70. De Paoli A, Lestuzzi C, Santini F, Boz G, Innocente R, Buonadonna A, Canzonieri V, Frustaci S. Primary cardiac sarcomas: experience with an evolving multidisciplinary approach with focus on the radiation therapy component. In: Proceedings of the 16th connective tumors oncology society annual meeting, 2010; #60. p. 118.
71. Minotti G, Menna P, Salvatorelli E, Cairo G, Gianni L. Anthracyclines: molecular advances and pharmacologic developments in antitumor activity and cardiotoxicity. Pharmacol Rev. 2004;56:185–229.
72. Simůnek T, Stérba M, Popelová O, Adamcová M, Hrdina R, Gersl V. Anthracycline-induced cardiotoxicity: overview of studies examining the roles of oxidative stress and free cellular iron. Pharmacol Rep. 2009;61:154–71.
73. Senkus E, Jassem J. Cardiovascular effects of systemic cancer treatment. Cancer Treat Rev. 2011;37: 300–11.
74. Bristow MR, Mason JW, Billingham ME, Daniels JR. Dose-effect and structure-function relationships in doxorubicin cardiomyopathy. Am Heart J. 1981;102:709–18.
75. Swain SM, Whaley FS, Ewer MS. Congestive heart failure in patients treated with doxorubicin:

a retrospective analysis of three trials. Cancer. 2003;97:2869–79.
76. Singal PK, Iliskovic N. Doxorubicin-induced cardiomyopathy. N Engl J Med. 1998;339:900–5.
77. Menna P, Salvatorelli E, Minotti G. Cardiotoxicity of antitumor drugs. Chem Res Toxicol. 2008;21: 978–89.
78. van Dalen EC, Caron HN, Dickinson HO, Kremer LC. Cardioprotective interventions for cancer patients receiving anthracyclines. Cochrane Database Syst Rev. 2008;16:CD003917.
79. Grenader T, Goldberg A, Hadas-Halperin I, Gabizon A. Long-term response to pegylated liposomal doxorubicin in patients with metastatic soft tissue sarcomas. Anticancer Drugs. 2009;20:15–20.
80. Lipshultz SE, Scully RE, Lipsitz SR, Sallan SE, Silverman LB, Miller TL, Barry EV, Asselin BL, Athale U, Clavell LA, Larsen E, Moghrabi A, Samson Y, Michon B, Schorin MA, Cohen HJ, Neuberg DS, Orav EJ, Colan SD. Assessment of dexrazoxane as a cardioprotectant in doxorubicin-treated children with high-risk acute lymphoblastic leukaemia: long-term follow-up of a prospective, randomised, multicentre trial. Lancet Oncol. 2010;11:950–61.
81. Smith LA, Cornelius VR, Plummer CJ, Levitt G, Verrill M, Canney P, Jones A. Cardiotoxicity of anthracycline agents for the treatment of cancer: systematic review and meta-analysis of randomised controlled trials. BMC Cancer. 2010;10:337.
82. Tallaj JA, Franco V, Rayburn BK, Pinderski L, Benza RL, Pamboukian S, Foley B, Bourge RC. Response of doxorubicin-induced cardiomyopathy to the current management strategy of heart failure. J Heart Lung Transplant. 2005;24:2196–201.
83. Cardinale D, Colombo A, Sandri MT, Lamantia G, Colombo N, Civelli M, Martinelli G, Veglia F, Fiorentini C, Cipolla CM. Prevention of high-dose chemotherapy-induced cardiotoxicity in high-risk patients by angiotensin-converting enzyme inhibition. Circulation. 2006;114:2474–81.
84. Cardinale D, Colombo A, Lamantia G, Colombo N, Civelli M, De Giacomi G, Rubino M, Veglia F, Fiorentini C, Cipolla CM. Anthracycline-induced cardiomyopathy: clinical relevance and response to pharmacologic therapy. J Am Coll Cardiol. 2010;55:213–20.
85. Wells QS, Lenihan DJ. Reversibility of left ventricular dysfunction resulting from chemotherapy: can this be expected? Prog Cradiovasc Dis. 2010;53:140–8.
86. Quezado ZMN, Wilson WH, Cunnion RE, Parker MP, Reda D, Bryant G, Ognibene FP. High-dose ifosfamide is associated with severe, reversible cardiac dysfunction. Ann Int Med. 1993;118:31–6.
87. Saintigny P, Chouhania K, Charniot J-C, Breau JL. Cardiovascular toxicity of some cancer agents (others than anthracyclines, fluoropyrimidines and trastuzumab). Bull Cancer. 2004;91:S174–84.
88. Tascilar M, Loos WJ, Seynaeve C, Verweij J, Sleijfer S. The pharmacologic basis of ifosfamide use in adult patients with advanced soft tissue sarcomas. Oncologist. 2007;12:1351–60.
89. Sayed-Ahmed MM, Darweesh AQ, Fatani AJ. Carnitine deficiency and oxidative stress provoke cardiotoxicity in an ifosfamide-induced Fanconi syndrome rat model. Oxid Med Cell Longev. 2010;3:266–74.
90. Raisch DW, Campbell W, Garg P, Qureshi ZP, Bookstaver PB, Norris LAB, Bennet CL. Description of anaphylactic reactions to paclitaxel and docetaxel reported to the FDA, with a focus on the role of premedication. Expert Opin Drug Saf. 2011;10:521–8.
91. Mourad JJ, des Guetz G, Debbabi H, Levy BI. Blood pressure rise following angiogenesis inhibition by bevacizumab. A crucial role for microcirculation. Ann Oncol. 2008;19:927–34.
92. Vaklavas C, Lenihan D, Kurzrock R, Tsimberidou AM. Anti-vascular endothelial growth factor therapies and cardiovascular toxicity: what are the important clinical markers to target? Oncologist. 2010;15: 130–41.
93. Syrigos KN, Karapanagiotou E, Boura P, Manegold C, Harrington K. Bevacizumab-induced hypertension: pathogenesis and management. BioDrugs. 2011;25:159–69.
94. Force T, Kolaja KL. Cardiotoxicity of kinase inhibitors: the prediction and translation of preclinical models to clinical outcomes. Nat Rev Drug Discov. 2011;10:111–26.
95. Hasinoff BB, Patel D. Mechanisms of myocyte cytotoxicity induced by the multikinase inhibitor sorafenib. Cardiovasc Toxicol. 2010;10:1–8.
96. Hasinoff BB, Patel D. The lack of target specificity of small molecule anticancer kinase inhibitors is correlated with their ability to damage myocytes in vitro. Toxicol Appl Pharmacol. 2010;249:132–9.
97. Berry GJ, Jorden M. Pathology of radiation and anthracycline cardiotoxicity. Pediatr Blood Cancer. 2005;44:630–7.
98. Fajardo LF, Stewart JR. Capillary injury preceding radiation-induced myocardial fibrosis. Radiology. 1971;101:429–33.
99. Marks LB, Yu X, Prosnitz RG, Zhou SM, Hardenbergh PH, Blazing M, Hollis D, Lind P, Tisch A, Wong TZ, Borges-Neto S. The incidence and functional consequences of RT-associated cardiac perfusion defects. Int J Radiat Oncol Biol Phys. 2005;63:214–23.
100. Veinot JP, Edwards WD. Pathology of radiation-induced heart disease: a surgical and autopsy study of 27 cases. Hum Pathol. 1996;27:766–75.

Novelties in Immunohistochemical and Molecular Study of Cardiac Tumors

13

Augusto Orlandi and Luigi Giusto Spagnoli

Introduction

Cardiac tumors are rare entities [1, 2]. Because of the rarity, it is difficult to investigate systematically large series of cardiac tumors using ancillary or biomolecular and experimental methods of investigation. As a consequence, scarce innovative information is available concerning the histogenesis of the majority of cardiac tumors. Myxomas are the most frequent neoplasms, accounting for 50% of all tumors [1, 2], and the most investigated primary cardiac tumor. Nevertheless, the origin of myxoma remains uncertain. In this chapter, we summarize the most recent novelties in the biomolecular, immunohistochemical and genetic investigation of primary cardiac tumors.

Cardiac Myxoma

Novelties in Immunohistochemical Findings

Myxoma is the most frequent primary tumor of the heart [1]. Its name derives from myxoid appearance of a mucopolysaccharide-rich extracellular matrix [2]. Myxoma usually arises from the inter-atrial septum, more frequently on the left side [1, 2]. The histogenesis of cardiac myxoma was for a long time considered uncertain, because of the nature of the morphological and immunohistochemical findings obtained after the characterization of this tumor. In fact, a variable expression of proteins typical of different adult cell phenotypes has been reported, even in the same tumor, suggesting an epithelial, endothelial, myogenic, myofibroblastic, or neural origin, respectively [3–10]. In adult myocardium, two sarcomeric actins, α-cardiac and α-skeletal actin, are co-expressed and represent the predominant isoforms [11]; in addition, α-smooth muscle actin (α-actin) is transiently observed in cardiomyocytes during the early stage of fetal cardiac development [12]. In Table 13.1 are reported the comparisons between microscopic and immunohistochemical findings (as percentages of positive cardiac myxoma cells) in a series of thirty tumors [13]. Although cardiac myxomas variably expressed vimentin, Notch1, CALB2, and smooth muscle antigens such as α-actin and caldesmon were the most frequently observed with a diffuse cytoplasmic immunoreactivity, followed by CD34. It is worth noting that α-cardiac actin was observed in a few cases and α-skeletal actin was always absent. Single or multinucleated cells were CD34 positive mainly in the superficial areas of tumors, whereas interstitial or perivascular cells were more α-smooth muscle actin positive. The immunophenotype of vascular structures of cardiac myxoma has been also investigated [13]. As concerning the complex vascular

A. Orlandi, M.D. (✉) • L.G. Spagnoli, M.D.
Department of Biomedicine and Prevention,
Institute of Anatomic Pathology,
Tor Vergata University of Rome,
Via Montpellier, Rome 00133, Italy
e-mail: orlandi@uniroma2.it

C. Basso et al. (eds.), *Cardiac Tumor Pathology*, Current Clinical Pathology,
DOI 10.1007/978-1-62703-143-1_13, © Springer Science+Business Media New York 2013

Table 13.1 Comparison of microscopic and immunohistochemical features in a series of 30 cardiac myxomas

Microscopic findings	(% of positive cases)
Smooth	63.3
Irregular surface	36.7
Superficial collagenization	43.3
Myxomatous areas (>50%)	56.6
Ki-67 positive cells (>5%)	6.7
Calcification	6.7
Small superficial thrombi	40
Extramedullary hematopoiesis	6.7
Ring structures	80
Vascular-like lacunae	16.7
Arterial-like vessels	60
Glandular structures	0.6
Immunohistochemical findings	
Cytokeratins	6.7
Vimentin	90
α-Smooth muscle actin	83.3
α-Cardiac actin	10
α-Skeletal actin	0
Notch1	86.7
Calretinin	86.7
CD34	66.7
Factor VIII	36.7
Caldesmon	86.7
Tenascin C	80
MMP-1	36.7
MMP-2	36.7
TIMP-1	36.7
S-100	13.3
Flt-1	26.7
c-kit	0

[a]Modified from Orlandi et al. [13].

structures, enlarged ring structures are in the majority of cases CD34 positive and only focally α-actin positive. Lacunae, other complex vascular-like structures of cardiac myxoma, are characterized by wide vascular-like spaces covered by single or multilayered CD34 positive and α-actin negative cells, whereas parietal cells are positive for the myocytic marker α-actin, suggesting an endothelial and pericyte-like differentiation, respectively (Fig. 13.1). Rarely, parietal cells of ring structures were also focally α-cardiac actin positive. Thick arterial-like structures of cardiac myxoma were of two different types: the first, larger and with a thick wall, covered by CD34 positive endothelial-like cells with α-actin positive parietal cells, were observed throughout the entire myxoma tissue; the second type, smaller and mainly at the parietal edge, resembled morphologically and immunohistochemically the normal atrial vasculature. Finally, confocal microscopy well documents the presence of CD34 and α-actin positive myxoma cells; rare myxoma cells, including multinucleated cells, focally co-expressed both proteins (Fig. 13.2), suggesting a precursor or an intermediate cell phenotype [13].

Biomolecular Analysis of Cardiac Myxomas

The availability of methods of investigation of gene expression, in particular reverse transcriptase-polymerase chain reaction (RT-PCR) and Real Time-PCR, may help to better characterize phenotypic features of cardiac tumor cells. Unfortunately, the optimal results are obtained after mRNA extraction from fresh tissue and, for their intrinsic rarity, a systematized tissue banking of cardiac tumor tissues is quite difficult. When possible, gene transcripts recapitulating specific phenotypes can be also useful to trace differentiation of tumor cells. In cardiac myxoma, PCR analysis performed on RNA extracted from frozen tissue from eight consecutive cases of cardiac myxoma [13] revealed CALB2 (calretinin) and Sox9 transcripts in all cases, Notch1 and NFATcI transcripts in 87.5 and 37.5% of cases, respectively, whereas all cases were negative for ErbB3 and Wilms' tumor transcription factor (Fig. 13.3).

Myxoma Cell Phenotype and Clinical Behavior of Cardiac Myxomas

Cardiac myxomas are benign tumors which are unable to infiltrate the myocardium or give rise to metastases [1, 2]. Nevertheless, they are considered "clinically malignant" tumors because of their susceptibility to embolize to distant

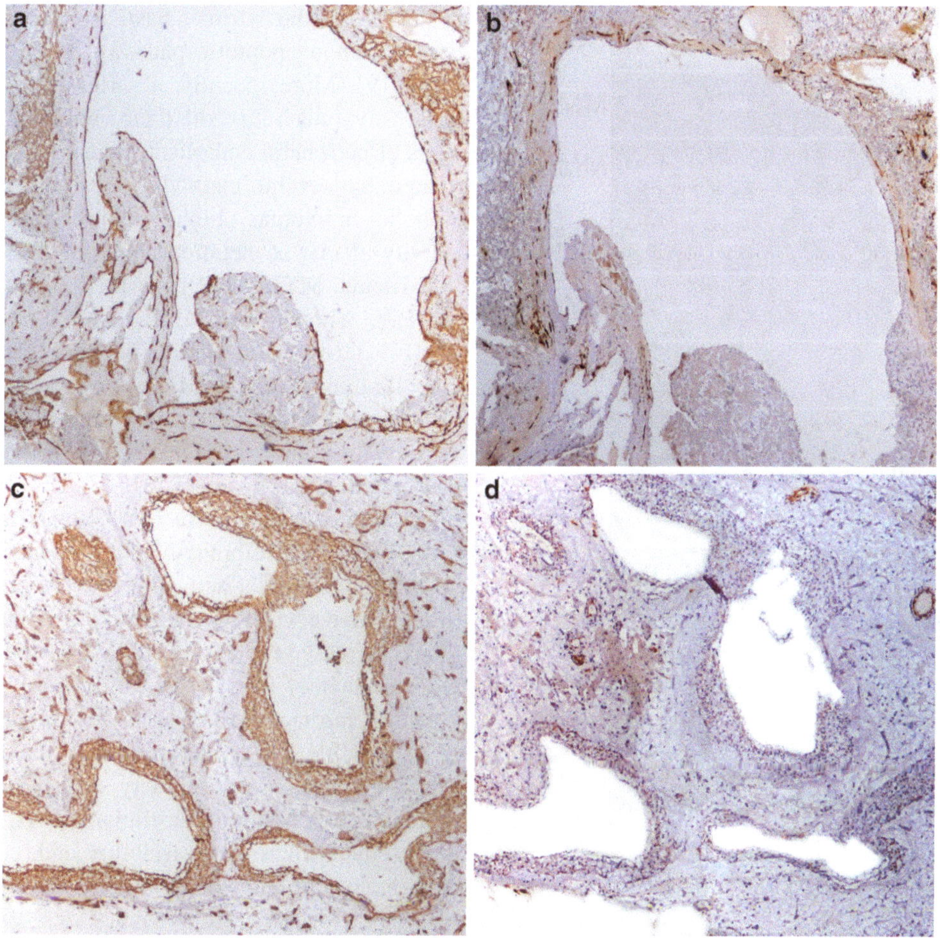

Fig. 13.1 Immunohistochemical characterization of vascular complex structures of cardiac myxoma. (**a**, **b**) Complex structures from wide vascular-like spaces with a thin wall constituted by one or more layers of flattened (**a**) CD34 positive and (**b**) focally α-smooth muscle actin positive cells. (**c**, **d**) Elongated multilayered structures, with (**c**) abundant CD34 positive and (**d**) rare parietal α-smooth muscle actin positive cells. Diaminobenzidine as chromogen; original magnification, ×125

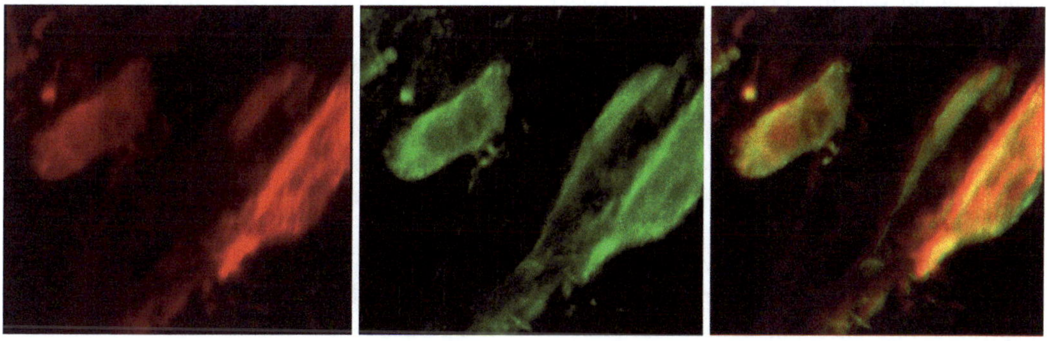

Fig. 13.2 Co-expression of endothelial and myogenic markers in cardiac myxoma. Immunofluorescent staining of α-smooth muscle actin (*left*, *red*) and CD34 (*middle*, *green*) of cardiac myxoma cell, sometimes multinucleated; merged image (*right*) shows co-expression of both endothelial and myocytic antigens. Original magnification, ×400

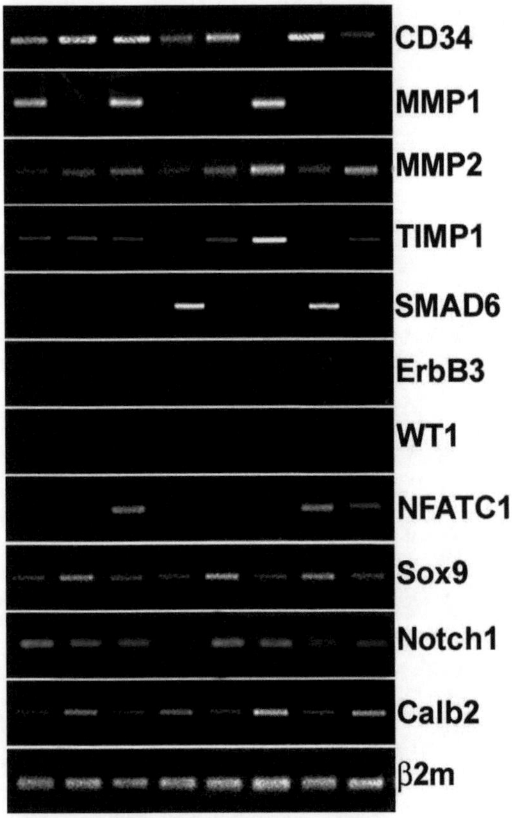

Fig. 13.3 Primitive mesenchymal markers gene expression in cardiac myxoma. Agarose gel after ethidium bromide staining documents RT-PCR analysis of transcripts from eight consecutive cardiac myxomas mRNA showing variable CD34, MMP-2, TIMP-1, Sox9, CALB2, and Notch1 transcripts, while ErbB3 and WT1 transcripts are absent; β2microglobulin is used as housekeeping gene. Modified from Orlandi et al. [13]

organs [1, 2, 14]. As a matter of fact, clinical signs of tumor embolism represent the primary manifestation in 30–50% of cases. Since most myxomas are left atrium-located, emboli prevalently involve peripheral districts, in particular cerebral arteries, including retinal artery [1, 2, 14]. Echocardiographic polypoid and irregular macroscopic aspects, changes in the composition of the myxomatous matrix, as well as the autocrine production of IL-6 have been considered [14–17]. Another hypothesis considers apoptosis as relevant for myxoma tissue remodeling and, consequently, for the clinical behavior of these cardiac tumors [18]. Successively, other researchers identified at both mRNA and protein levels the extrinsic Fas/FasL-dependent final common apoptotic pathway of myxoma cells [19]. More recently, a series of 27 left atrial myxomas, 10 of them with clinical signs of peripheral embolism, have been investigated by several methods, documenting in embolic myxomas higher expression and activity of matrix metalloproteinases (MMPs), in particular MT1-MMP, pro-MMP-2, and pro-MMP-9, whereas pro-MMP-1, MMP-3, and TIMP-1 levels were similar to those of non-embolic tumors [20]. MMPs are a large family of zinc-dependent proteolytic enzymes that degrade the extracellular matrix in both normal and pathological processes [21–23]. MMPs are released into the extracellular milieu in a proenzyme state or membrane-bound enzymes that undergo intracellular activation and are proteolitically active when inserted into the cell membrane. Increased expression of MMPs associated more frequently with the irregular or polypoid aspect of cardiac myxomas [20]. Consequently, it is possible to hypothesize that increased MMP expression and activity can induce a remodeling of tumor extracellular matrix, with a consequent increase of friability and, consequently, of the risk of embolism of cardiac myxoma. Nevertheless, in some cases of non-embolic irregular myxomas, MMP expression did not significantly differ from non-embolic smooth tumors, suggesting that embolism is not the natural consequence of the irregular macroscopic appearance. Moreover, these studies in vivo do not clarify if increased MMP activity is an intrinsic feature of myxoma cells or, alternatively, it is related to an increased susceptibility to locally delivered cytokines [17]. Nevertheless, embolic myxoma cells retain higher MT1-MMP and pro-MMP-2 levels in basal condition and after stimulation with IL-1β and IL-6 in vitro [20].

The Origin of Cardiac Myxoma: An Update

The heterogeneous phenotype of myxoma cells gave origin to several interpretations concerning the histogenesis of cardiac myxoma. The presence of endothelial marker and cytoplasmic neuropeptides such as protein gene product 9.5, S100 protein and neuron-specific enolase in more than half of a series of cardiac myxomas supports the hypothesis that myxoma cells originate from pluripotent mesenchymal cells capable of neural and endothelial differentiation [9]. Another explanation for heterogeneous differentiation in cardiac myxoma is its origin from a pluripotential cell or from a subendothelial vasiform reserve cell, on the basis of the expression of transcripts characteristic of cardiac cushion development and/or primitive cardiac mesenchymal differentiation [3, 4, 24]. Some morphologic homologies between cardiac myxoma cells and those of embryonic cardiac cushion cells support this hypothesis. A cardiomyogenic derivation of cardiac myxomas was based on the finding of transcripts for Nkx2.5/Csx, typical of the cardiac homeobox gene, recapitulating a primitive cardiomyocytic phenotype and supporting an embryonic cardiomyocytic progenitor cell as precursor [25]. Although Nkx2.5/Csx encodes for a gene required for specification of cardiac precursor cells, its expression is maintained throughout development [25]. Moreover, Nkx2.5/Csx is documented during development of other tissues, including skeletal myoblasts and promotes neuronal differentiation in vitro [26, 27]. This explains the previously reported expression of neural markers [9] as a demonstration of a possible neurogenic origin of cardiac myxoma cells. Investigation of actin isoform expression can be useful to trace the origin of cardiac myxoma cells. In particular, the diffuse presence of α-smooth muscle actin, the paucity of α-cardiac actin, and the absence of α-skeletal actin isoform expression have been described in cardiac myxomas [20]; α-smooth muscle actin is reported to be transiently expressed in human cardiomyocytes during early stages of fetal development [28]. This finding supports that myxoma cells are phenotypically reconducible to a more primitive cardiac progenitor or primordial cardiac stem cell. In fact, in the 20-week-old fetal heart, a time when septation is complete and the heart exhibits all the morphological characteristics of the adult heart, α-cardiac actin is the major isoform and uniformly expressed [12]. The mesenchymal origin and the subsequent endothelial differentiation are further supported from ultrastructural study of cardiac myxomas [20, 29, 30]. The presence of a limited number of myxoma cells co-expressing the primitive endothelial and myocytic markers CD34 and α-actin supports the hypothesis that myxoma cells can derive from a common cardiac early precursor cell [25]. The origin of cardiac myxoma in atrial cavity in association with fibrous septa or fossa ovalis suggests a relationship with fibrous cardiac structures and their development [1, 2]. Endocardial cushions are the precursors of mature heart valves and cardiac septa [31–34]. Embryonic endocardial cells of the outflow tract and atrioventricular canal change their phenotype from endothelial to mesenchymal cells during the so-called endothelial–mesenchymal transformation, leading to cardiac septation and mature valve formation. During this phase, embryonic endocardial cells progressively express α smooth muscle actin and lose endothelial antigens [33]. Cardiac jelly, an acellular matrix rich in fibronectin and proteoglycans, separates the primitive endocardium from myocardium and favors the initiation of the endothelial–mesenchymal transformation [31–34]. Cardiac jelly appears very similar to extracellular matrix of cardiac myxoma. Transient ectopic activation of Notch1 in zebrafish embryos leads to hypercellular cardiac valves, whereas its inhibition prevents valve development [35]. Notch activation in endothelial cells determines downregulation of endothelial markers and upregulation of mesenchymal ones, including α-smooth muscle actin and fibronectin [35]. Moreover, RT-PCR shows in cardiac myxomas the presence of Sox9 and NFATcI transcripts [20]. Sox9 has been indicated to play an essential role in early phases of endocardial cushion differentiation, when endocardial endothelial cells migrate into the cardiac jelly [36]. NFATcI expression is critical during signal-transduction processes required for cardiac valve formation and is normally abolished after endocardial cushion cell migration [37]. The presence of phenotypic markers of endothelial–mesenchymal transformation may be related to the persistence of developmental remnants or stem cells in adult heart or, alternatively, to de novo re-expression of a developmental phenotype in adult cardiac cells.

Carney's Complex

Carney's complex is a neuroendocrine-cardiac syndrome characterized by (a) familial recurrent myxomas; (b) pigmented skin lesions, schwannomas, and recurrent mucocutaneous myxomas; and (c) endocrine abnormalities, including Cushing syndrome and acromegaly, and malignancies [38]. One-third of the patients with Carney's syndrome display at presentation mucocutaneous myxomas of the eyelid, external ear canal, breast, and oropharynx. About two-thirds of these patients have cardiac tumors, and 75% various skin pigmented lesions, including blue nevi and café au lait spots [39]. Carney's complex is characterized by an autosomal dominant transmission with incomplete penetrance. Linkage studies have revealed genetic foci at 2p16 and 17q22–24 [40, 41]. Among the families mapping to 17q, mutations in the gene encoding the protein kinase A type I-α regulatory subunit have been identified [42]. In patients with Carney's complex, cardiac tumors recur in more than 20% of cases, and account for more than 50% of causes of death [39]. Consequently, patients with established Carney's complex require vigorous screening for cardiac tumors, in particular to exclude multiple locations. Routinary echocardiographic screening of the first-degree relatives seems appropriate for familial myxomas [43].

Genetic Features of Cardiac Non-myxomatous Tumors

Non-myxomatous cardiac benign tumors are rare and sometimes arising in the setting of genetic syndromes (Table 13.2). Molecular genetic investigation of cardiac primary non-myxomatous tumors has provided relevant information to elucidate many mechanisms of cardiac cell developmental growth. Cytogenetic studies have targeted candidate chromosomal loci that may be perturbed during the pathogenesis of cardiac lipoma. Common cutaneous lipomas have been associated with rearrangements of chromosome band 12q15. Cytogenetic analysis of an unusual giant cardiac lipoma in a patient with a history of multiple lipomatosis demonstrated no abnormalities of chromosome 12, but a translocation (2, 19) (p13; p13.2) [48]. Rhabdomyoma, the most common pediatric cardiac neoplasm, is frequently associated with tuberous sclerosis by mutations in the tuberous sclerosis complex-1 and - 2 that codify two proteins, hamartin and tuberin. Tuberous sclerosis complex is a genetic disorder characterized by the formation of hamartomas in multiple organs, including rhabdomyomas in the heart [49]. Hamartin and tuberin antagonize the mammalian target of rapamycin signaling pathway, thus regulating cell growth and proliferation. Nonsense mutations in the hamartin and tuberin genes have been identified as causative of cardiac rhabdomyomas [49]. Many complications have been reported in association with nevoid basal cell carcinoma syndrome, also known as Gorlin–Goltz or Gorlin syndrome [50, 51]. The hallmark of this syndrome is the

Table 13.2 Cardiac tumors and related genetic syndromes

	Genetic syndrome(s)	Gene(s) mutation	Chromosome	Refs.
Rhabdomyoma	Tuberous sclerosis	TSC1/TSC2	9q34/16p13	[44]
Myxoma	Carney complex	PRKAR1A	2p16, 7q22, q17	[20, 40, 41, 45]
Fibroma	Gorlin–Goltz syndrome	PTCH1	9q22.3	[46]
Paraganglioma	Neurofibromatosis type 1, Von Hippel–Lindau syndrome, 2B Familial pheochromocytoma–paraganglioma syndrome	VHL NF1 RET SDHB SDHC SDHD	3p25, 17q11, 1p36, 10q11, q21, 11q23	[47]

Table 13.3 Main immunohistochemical findings in cardiac sarcomas[1]

	CD34	FVIII	CD31	S100	α-Smooth muscle actin	Desmin	CK	Vimentin	Myogenin
Angiosarcoma	+	+	+	–	–	–	R*	+	–
Undifferentiated pleomorphic sarcoma	–	–	–	–	R	–	R	+	–
Rhabdomyosarcoma	–	–	–	–	+	+	–	+	+
Fibrosarcoma	–	–	–	–	R	–	–	+	–
Leiomyosarcoma	–	–	–	–	+	+	R	–	+
Synovial sarcoma	–	–	–	–	R	–	+	+	–
Liposarcoma	–	–	–	+	–	–	–	+	–

FVIII factor VIII, *CK* cytokeratins, *R* rare and focal, + positive, – negative, *asterisk* diffusely positive in epithelioid variant

[8]Modified from Orlandi et al. [52]

presence of multiple basal cell carcinomas, which may appear early in infancy. Other associated features may include craniofacial, central nervous system, musculoskeletal, and genitourinary anomalies. Approximately 3% of cases are associated with cardiac fibromas, which may present later during adulthood rather than the typical infancy or childhood period [51]. Consequently, cardiac fibromas are generally not considered part of the syndrome and judged as minor diagnostic criteria [50]. Nevertheless, the investigation of Gorlin syndrome has shed light on the etiology of cardiac fibromas. It is caused by mutations in the *PTCH1* gene, which acts as a cell cycle regulator and regulates cell growth, commitment, and differentiation [51].

Cardiac Sarcomas

Introduction

Primary cardiac sarcomas are by definition malignant neoplasms deriving from mesenchymal cells and confined to the heart at the time of diagnosis. Most cardiac sarcomas have the same histological appearance as their soft tissue counterpart. Primary heart sarcomas are exceptionally rare and represent approximately 10% of total primary cardiac tumors [2, 52]; cardiac metastases at autopsy are 20–40 times more frequent than primary tumors [53]. For many years, no universally accepted classification of primary cardiac sarcomas existed. The difficulty derived from the rarity and lack of systematic studies, with only a few series of cardiac sarcomas in the literature. Virtually, all soft tissue sarcoma types have also been found to arise in the heart. The recent WHO classification system of cardiac tumors proposed in 2004 [54] is largely based on the soft tissue classification counterpart and only the most frequent malignant entities are listed, since the majority of cardiac sarcomas have limited areas with morphologically recognizable differentiation. Moreover, despite a careful immunohistochemical investigation, they frequently lack tissue-specific antigens.

Immunohistochemical Features of Cardiac Sarcomas

Despite a careful immunohistochemical investigation, cardiac sarcomas generally lack tissue-specific antigens. Main immunohistochemical findings are schematically reported in Table 13.3 and can be useful in supporting morphological criteria of diagnosis in some specific cases. Angiosarcoma is microscopically characterized by vascular differentiation with channels covered by endothelial cells exhibiting marked atypia. Factor VIII or CD34 positive immunodetection of malignant cells represents useful markers of endothelial differentiation; moreover, cytokeratins can be diffusely positive in epithelioid areas of angiosarcoma [2]. Undifferentiated sarcoma is defined as a cardiac sarcoma with no specific histological pattern or undifferentiated [53]. Nowadays, undifferentiated sarcoma is considered synonymous with pleomorphic malignant fibrous histiocytoma [54]. Undifferentiated sarcoma must be distinguished from embryonal rhabdomyosarcoma and metastatic small cell cancer. Immunostaining is crucial, epithelial, neural, or endothelial markers being usually negative and vimentin typically positive; high grade undifferentiated sarcomas can exhibit focal α-actin positive areas, but the latter are generally limited in their extension [54]. Leiomyosarcoma is a malignant tumor showing phenotypic and ultrastructural smooth muscle differentiation. Immunostaining for desmin and α-actin is usually diffusely positive, whereas epithelial, vascular, and neural markers are negative [55, 56]. Rhabdomyosarcoma is considered as a malignant tumor showing striated muscle differentiation [2, 54]. Rhabdomyosarcoma usually arises in the ventricular wall and is microscopically composed of small cells with the presence of recognizable rhabdomyoblasts with the characteristic cross striations by Masson's trichrome and a diffuse desmin positive immunostaining [2, 57]. Rhabdomyosarcoma can express other muscle markers, including myogenin, myoD1, sarcomeric actin, muscle-specific actin, and myoglobin. Among these, myogenin and myoD1 seem to be more specific [58]. Synovial sarcoma is a biphasic malignant tumor usually located in the atria or pericardial surface. The latter localization should be considered for distinction from malignant mesothelioma. In the heart, the monophasic variant of synovial sarcoma is more common. A differential diagnosis between malignant mesothelioma and synovial sarcoma may be challenging on the basis of morphological aspect and immunophenotype, both being positive for cytokeratins, calretinin, and vimentin [54].

Genetic Features of Cardiac Sarcomas

At present, the molecular histogenesis of cardiac sarcomas is poorly known and there are no specific genetic mutations reported. This is likely due to the rarity and consequent absence of a systematically characterized large series of cardiac sarcomas. Moreover, as concerning genetic characterization of cardiac sarcomas, K-ras mutation and the absence of p53 mutations have been observed in three cases of angiosarcomas and two of rhabdomyosarcomas [59]. p53 mutations in two primary cardiac angiosarcomas have been reported [60]. Cytogenetic features can represent a useful diagnostic tool and can be detected by using reverse transcriptase-polymerase chain reaction or fluorescence in situ hybridization techniques. Accordingly, synovial sarcomas typically harbor t(X; 18)(p21.2; q11.2) resulting in SS18-SSX1 fusion transcripts, including the reported unique case with a cardiac localization in the examined series [61]. The same SYT-SSX1 fusion transcript identified by molecular genetic studies has been also reported in two cases of primary cardiac synovial sarcoma arising in left atrium and ventricle and on the anterior mitral leaflet [62, 63]. Cytogenetic analysis has been reported to help to distinguish low-grade fibromyxoid sarcoma from either more benign or more malignant tumor types [64]. Cytogenetic investigation also identified a recurrent balanced translocation t(7; 16)(q32–34; p11), later shown by molecular genetic approaches to result in a FUS/CREB3L2 fusion gene. Reverse transcriptase-polymerase chain reaction analysis disclosed a FUS/CREB3L2 fusion transcript in 96% of cases classified as low-grade fibromyxoid sarcoma after the histological reevaluation and from which RNA of sufficient quality could be extracted, whereas a FUS/CREB3L2 fusion transcript was absent in other tumor types [65]. The proteins encoded by a CREB3L1 and CREB3L2 genes belong to the basic leucine-zipper family of transcription factors. A similar t(7;16)(q32–34; p11) translocation by FISH analysis was documented in a primary intracardiac large low-grade fibromyxoid sarcoma of the right atrium [65]. Cytogenetic and molecular genetic studies performed in one case [66] of pleomorphic malignant fibrous histiocytoma removed from the left atrium of a 15-year-old girl [65] revealed several alterations previously associated with adult malignant fibrous histiocytoma, including abnormalities of 11p11 and 19p13 chromosomal bands. Moreover, pleomorphic malignant fibrous histiocytoma demonstrated homogeneously staining regions and double minute chromosomes, in particular the co-amplification of the 12q13–14 chromosome; the latter amplicon was not previously detected in pediatric malignant fibrous histiocytoma. This cytogenetic and molecular genetic evidence suggests that pediatric and adult malignant fibrous histiocytoma, although histogenetically related, are distinct malignancies [66].

References

1. Reynen K. Cardiac myxomas. N Engl J Med. 1995;333:1610–7.
2. Burke AP, Virmani R. Tumors of the heart and great vessels. In: Burke AP, Virmani R, editors. Atlas of tumor pathology. 3rd ed. Washington DC: Armed Forced Institute of Pathology; 1996. p. 121–46.
3. Lie JT. The identity and histogenesis of cardiac myxomas. A controversy put to rest. Arch Pathol Lab Med. 1989;113:724–6.
4. Tazelaar HD, Locke TJ, McGregor CG. Pathology of surgically excised primary cardiac tumors. Mayo Clin Proc. 1992;67:957–65.
5. Boxer ME. Cardiac myxoma: an immunoperoxidase study of histogenesis. Histopathology. 1984;8:861–72.
6. Goldman BI, Frydman C, Harpaz N, Ryan SF, Loiterman D. Glandular cardiac myxomas. Histologic, immunohistochemical, and ultrastructural evidence of epithelial differentiation. Cancer. 1987;59:1767–75.
7. Govoni E, Severi B, Cenacchi G, Laschi R, Pileri S, Rivano MT, Alampi G, Branzi A. Ultrastructural and immunohistochemical contribution to the histogenesis of human cardiac myxoma. Ultrastruct Pathol. 1988; 12:221–33.
8. Landon G, Ordonez NG, Guarda LA. Cardiac myxomas. An immunohistochemical study using endothelial, histiocytic, and smooth-muscle cell markers. Arch Pathol Lab Med. 1986;110:116–20.
9. Pucci A, Gagliardotto P, Zanini C, Pansini S, di Summa M, Mollo F. Histopathologic and clinical characterization of cardiac myxoma: review of 53 cases from a single institution. Am Heart J. 2000;140:134–8.
10. McComb RD. Heterogeneous expression of factor VIII/von Willebrand factor by cardiac myxoma cells. Am J Surg Pathol. 1984;8:539–44.
11. Vandekerckhove J, Bugaisky G, Buckingham M. Simultaneous expression of skeletal muscle and heart actin proteins in various striated muscle tissues and cells. A quantitative determination of the two actin isoforms. J Biol Chem. 1986;261:1838–43.
12. Suurmeijer AJ, Clement S, Francesconi A, Bocchi L, Angelini A, Van Veldhuisen DJ, Spagnoli LG, Gabbiani G, Orlandi A. Alpha-actin isoform distribution in normal and failing human heart: a morphological, morphometric, and biochemical study. J Pathol. 2003;199:387–97.
13. Orlandi A, Ciucci A, Ferlosio A, Genta R, Spagnoli LG, Gabbiani G. Cardiac myxoma cells exhibit embryonic endocardial stem cell features. J Pathol. 2006;209:231–9.
14. Ha JW, Kang WC, Chung N, Chang BC, Rim SJ, Kwon JW, Jang Y, Shim WH, Cho SY, Kim SS, Cho SH. Echocardiographic and morphologic characteristics of left atrial myxoma and their relation to systemic embolism. Am J Cardiol. 1999;83:1579–82.
15. Kairemo KJ, Blomqvist CP, Miettinen M. Cardiac myxomas. N Engl J Med. 1996;334:1407–8.
16. Negishi M, Sakamoto H, Sakamaki T, Ishikawa O, Kanda T, Tamura J, Kurabayashi M, Nagai R. Disaccharide analysis of glycosaminoglycans synthesized by cardiac myxoma cells in tumor tissues and in cell culture. Life Sci. 2003;73:849–56.
17. Parissis JT, Mentzikof D, Georgopoulou M, Gikopoulos M, Kanapitsas A, Merkouris K, Kefalas C. Correlation of interleukin-6 gene expression to immunologic features in patients with cardiac myxomas. J Interferon Cytokine Res. 1996;16:589–93.
18. Suzuki M, Hamada M, Hiwada K. Apoptosis in cardiac myxoma. Ann Intern Med. 2000;132:681.
19. Liu CC, Jung SM, Orlandi A, Yeh TS, Lin YS, Shiu TF, Wu HH, Chu JJ, Lin PJ, Chu PH. The Fas-mediated apoptotic pathway in cardiac myxoma. Int J Surg Pathol. 2010;18:493–8.
20. Orlandi A, Ciucci A, Ferlosio A, Pellegrino A, Chiariello L, Spagnoli LG. Increased expression and activity of matrix metalloproteinases characterize embolic cardiac myxomas. Am J Pathol. 2005;166:1619–28.
21. Oh J, Takahashi R, Kondo S, Mizoguchi A, Adachi E, Sasahara RM, Nishimura S, Imamura Y, Kitayama H, Alexander DB, Ide C, Horan TP, Arakawa T, Yoshida H, Nishikawa S, Itoh Y, Seiki M, Itohara S, Takahashi C, Noda M. The membrane-anchored MMP inhibitor RECK is a key regulator of extracellular matrix integrity and angiogenesis. Cell. 2001;107:789–800.
22. Dollery CM, McEwan JR, Henney AM. Matrix metalloproteinases and cardiovascular disease. Circ Res. 1995;77:863–8.
23. Singer CF, Kronsteiner N, Marton E, Kubista M, Cullen KJ, Hirtenlehner K, Seifert M, Kubista E. MMP-2 and MMP-9 expression in breast cancer-derived human fibroblasts is differentially regulated by stromal–epithelial interactions. Breast Cancer Res Treat. 2002;72:69–77.
24. Markwald RR, Fitzharris TP, Manasek FJ. Structural development of endocardial cushions. Am J Anat 1977;148:85–119.

25. Kodama H, Hirotani T, Suzuki Y, Ogawa S, Yamazaki K. Cardiomyogenic differentiation in cardiac myxoma expressing lineage-specific transcription factors. Am J Pathol. 2002;161:381–9.
26. Schwartz RJ, Olson EN. Building the heart piece by piece: modularity of cis-elements regulating Nkx2.5 transcription. Development. 1999;126:4187–92.
27. Riazi AM, Lee H, Hsu C, Van Arsdell G. CSX/Nkx2.5 modulates differentiation of skeletal myoblasts and promotes differentiation into neuronal cells in vitro. J Biol Chem. 2005;280:10716–20.
28. Sugi Y, Lough J. Onset of expression and regional deposition of alpha-smooth and sarcomeric actin during avian heart development. Dev Dyn. 1992;193:116–24.
29. Valente M. Structural profile of cardiac myxoma. Appl Pathol. 1983;1:251–63.
30. Zhang PF, Jones JW, Anderson WR. Cardiac myxomas correlative study by light, transmission, and scanning electron microscopy. Am J Cardiovasc Pathol. 1989;2:295–300.
31. Sugi Y, Markwald RR. Formation and early morphogenesis of endocardial endothelial precursor cells and the role of endoderm. Dev Biol. 1996;175:66–83.
32. Gitler AD, Lu MM, Jiang YQ, Epstein JA, Gruber PJ. Molecular markers of cardiac endocardial cushion development. Dev Dyn. 2003;228:643–50.
33. Nakajima Y, Mironov V, Yamagishi T, Nakamura H, Markwald RR. Expression of smooth muscle alpha-actin in mesenchymal cells during formation of avian endocardial cushion tissue: a role for transforming growth factor beta3. Dev Dyn. 1997;209:296–309.
34. Moorman A, Webb S, Brown NA, Lamers W, Anderson RH. Development of the heart: (1) formation of the cardiac chambers and arterial trunks. Heart. 2003;89:806–14.
35. Noseda M, McLean G, Niessen K, Chang L, Pollet I, Montpetit R, Shahidi R, Dorovini-Zis K, Li L, Beckstead B, Durand RE, Hoodless PA, Karsan A. Notch activation results in phenotypic and functional changes consistent with endothelial-to-mesenchymal transformation. Circ Res. 2004;94:910–7.
36. Akiyama H, Chaboissier MC, Behringer RR, Rowitch DH, Schedl A, Epstein JA, de Crombrugghe B. Essential role of Sox9 in the pathway that controls formation of cardiac valves and septa. Proc Natl Acad Sci USA. 2004;101:6502–7.
37. Ranger AM, Grusby MJ, Hodge MR, Gravallese EM, de la Brousse FC, Hoey T, Mickanin C, Baldwin HS, Glimcher LH. The transcription factor NF-ATc is essential for cardiac valve formation. Nature. 1998;392:186–90.
38. Carney JA, Gordon H, Carpenter PC, Shenoy BV, Go VL. The complex of myxomas, spotty pigmentation, and endocrine overactivity. Medicine (Baltimore). 1985;64:270–83.
39. Pinede L, Duhaut P, Loire R. Clinical presentation of left atrial cardiac myxoma: a series of 112 consecutive cases. Medicine (Baltimore). 2001;80:159–72.
40. Stratakis CA, Carney JA, Lin JP, Papanicolaou DA, Karl M, Kastner DL, Pras E, Chrousos GP. Carney complex, a familial multiple neoplasia and lentiginosis syndrome: analysis of 11 kindreds and linkage to the short arm of chromosome 2. J Clin Invest. 1996;97:699–705.
41. Dijkuizen T, van den Berg E, Molenaar WM, Meuzelaar JJ, de Jong B. Rearrangements involving 12p12 in two cases of cardiac myxoma. Cancer Genet Cytogenet. 1995;82:161–2.
42. Kirscher LS, Carney JA, Pack SD, Taymans SE, Giatzakis C, Cho YS, Cho-Chung YS, Stratakis CA. Mutations of the gene encoding the protein kinase A type I-alpha regulatory subunit in patients with the Carney complex. Nat Genet. 2000;26:89–92.
43. Grebenc ML, Rosado-de-Christenson ML, Green CE, Burke AP, Galvin JR. Cardiac myxoma: imaging features in 83 patients. Radiographics. 2002;22:673–89.
44. Curatolo P, Bombardieri R, Jozwiak S. Tuberous sclerosis. Lancet. 2008;372:57–668.
45. Wilkes D, Charitakis K, Basson CT. Inherited disposition to cardiac myxoma development. Nat Rev Cancer. 2006;6:157–65.
46. Lo Muzio L. Nevoid basal cell carcinoma syndrome (Gorlin syndrome). Orphanet J Rare Dis. 2008;3:32.
47. Callender GG, Rich TA, Perrier ND. Multiple endocrine neoplasia syndromes. Surg Clin North Am. 2008;88:863–95.
48. Vaughan CJ, Weremowicz S, Goldstein MM, Casey M, Hart M, Hahn RT, Devereux RB, Girardi L, Schoen FJ, Fletcher JA, Morton CC, Basson CT. A t(2;19)(p13; p13.2) in a giant invasive cardiac lipoma from a patient with multiple lipomatosis. Genes Chromosomes Cancer. 2000;28:133–7.
49. Madueme P, Hinton R. Tuberous sclerosis and cardiac rhabdomyomas: a case report and review of the literature. Congenit Heart Dis. 2011;6:183–7.
50. Evans DG, Ladusans EJ, Rimmer S, Burnell LD, Thakker N, Farndon PA. Complications of the naevoid basal cell carcinoma syndrome: results of a population based study. J Med Genet. 1993;30:460–4.
51. Gorlin RJ. Nevoid basal cell carcinoma (Gorlin) syndrome. Genet Med. 2004;6:530–9.
52. Orlandi A, Ferlosio A, Roselli M, Chiariello L, Spagnoli LG. Cardiac sarcomas: an update. J Thorac Oncol. 2010;9:1483–9.
53. Lymbumer R. Tumours of the heart: histopathological and clinical study. Can Med Assoc J. 1934;30:368–73.
54. Burke A, Veinot J, Loire R. Tumours of the heart. In: Travis W, Brambilla E, Müller H, Harris C, editors. Tumours of the lung, pleura, thymus and heart. Lyon: IARC Press; 2004. p. 251–88.
55. Mazzola A, Spano JP, Valente M, Gregoriani R, Villani C, Di Eusanio M, Ciocca M, Minuti U, Giancola R, Basso C, Thiene G. Leiomyosarcoma of the left atrium mimicking a left atrial myxoma. J Thorac Cardiovasc Surg. 2006;131:224–6.
56. Basso C, Valente M, Poletti A, Casarotto D, Thiene G. Surgical pathology of primary cardiac and pericardial tumors. Eur J Cardiothorac Surg. 1997;12:730–7.

57. Castorino F, Masiello P, Quattrocchi E, Di Benedetto G. Primary cardiac rhabdomyosarcoma of the left atrium: an unusual presentation. Tex Heart Inst J. 2000;27:206–8.
58. Cessna MH, Zhou H, Perkins SL, Tripp SR, Layfield L, Daines C, Coffin CM. Are myogenin and myoD1 expression specific for rhabdomyosarcoma? A study of 150 cases, with emphasis on spindle cell mimics. Am J Surg Pathol. 2001;25:1150–7.
59. Garcia JM, Gonzalez R, Silva JM, Dominguez G, Vegazo IS, Gamallo C, Provencio M, España P, Bonilla F. Mutational status of K-ras and TP53 genes in primary sarcomas of the heart. Br J Cancer. 2000;82:1183–5.
60. Naka N, Tomita Y, Nakanishi H, Araki N, Hongyo T, Ochi T, Aozasa K. Mutations of p53 tumor-suppressor gene in angiosarcoma. Int J Cancer. 1997;71:952–5.
61. Amary MF, Berisha F, Bernardi Fdel C, Herbert A, James M, Reis-Filho JS, Fisher C, Nicholson AG, Tirabosco R, Diss TC, Flanagan AM. Detection of SS18-SSX fusion transcripts in formalin-fixed paraffin-embedded neoplasms: analysis of conventional RT-PCR, qRT-PCR and dual color FISH as diagnostic tools for synovial sarcoma. Mod Pathol. 2007;20:482–96.
62. Hazelbag HM, Szuhai K, Tanke HJ, Rosenberg C, Hogendoorn PC. Primary synovial sarcoma of the heart: a cytogenetic and molecular genetic analysis combining RT-PCR and COBRA-FISH of a case with a complex karyotype. Mod Pathol. 2004;17:1434–9.
63. Miller DV, Deb A, Edwards WD, Zehr KJ, Oliveira AM. Primary synovial sarcoma of the mitral valve. Cardiovasc Pathol. 2005;14:331–3.
64. Mertens F, Fletcher CD, Antonescu CR, Coindre JM, Colecchia M, Domanski HA, Downs-Kelly E, Fisher C, Goldblum JR, Guillou L, Reid R, Rosai J, Sciot R, Mandahl N, Panagopoulos I. Clinicopathologic and molecular genetic characterization of low-grade fibromyxoid sarcoma, and cloning of a novel *FUS/CREB3L1* fusion gene. Lab Invest. 2005;85:408–15.
65. Jakowski JD, Wakely Jr PE. Primary intrathoracic low-grade fibromyxoid sarcoma. Hum Pathol. 2008;39:623–8.
66. Palmer JL, Masui S, Pritchard S, Kalousek DK, Sorensen PH. Cytogenetic and molecular genetic analysis of a pediatric pleomorphic sarcoma reveals similarities to adult malignant fibrous histiocytoma. Cancer Genet Cytogenet. 1997;95:141–7.

Index

C. Basso et al. (eds.), *Cardiac Tumor Pathology*, Current Clinical Pathology,
DOI 10.1007/978-1-62703-143-1, © Springer Science+Business Media New York 2013

MIX
Papier aus verantwortungsvollen Quellen
Paper from responsible sources
FSC® C105338

If you have any concerns about our products,
you can contact us on
ProductSafety@springernature.com

In case Publisher is established outside the EU,
the EU authorized representative is:
Springer Nature Customer Service Center GmbH
Europaplatz 3, 69115 Heidelberg, Germany

Printed by Libri Plureos GmbH
in Hamburg, Germany